Cancer and Stress: Psychological, Biological and Coping Studies

Edited by

CARY L. COOPER

University of Manchester Institute of Science and Technology, UK

and

MAGGIE WATSON

The Institute of Cancer Research and The Royal Marsden Hospital, UK

JOHN WILEY & SONS

Chichester · New York · Brisbane · Toronto · Singapore

Other Wiley Editorial Offices

John Wiley & Sons, Inc., 605 Third Avenue,
New York, NY 10158-0012, USA

Jacaranda Wiley Ltd, G.P.O. Box 859, Brisbane,
Queensland 4001, Australia

John Wiley & Sons (Canada) Ltd, 5353 Dundas Road West, Fourth Floor
Etobicoke, Ontario M9B 6H8, Canada

John Wiley & Sons (SEA) Pte Ltd, 37 Jalan Pemimpin 05-04,
Block B, Union Industrial Building, Singapore 2057

Library of Congress Cataloging-in-Publication Data:

Cancer and stress: psychological, biological, and coping studies /
    edited by Cary L. Cooper and Maggie Watson
        p.   cm.
    Includes bibliographical references and index.
    ISBN 0 471 93061 X (cloth)   ISBN 0 471 93307 4 (paper)
    1. Cancer—Psychological aspects. 2. Psychoneuroimmunology.
    3. Adjustment (Psychology) I. Cooper, Cary L. II. Watson, M.
    [DNLM: 1. Adaptation, Psychological. 2. Neoplasms—etiology.
    3. Neoplasms—psychology. 4. Stress, Psychological. QZ 200
    C21507]
    RC262.C269   1991
    616.99′4′0019—dc20
    DNLM/DLC   91-16867
    for Library of Congress   CIP

British Library Cataloguing in Publication Data:

A catalogue record for this book is
available from the British Library

ISBN 0 471 93061 X (cloth)
ISBN 0 471 93307 4 (paper)

Typeset by MCS Typesetters Ltd, Salisbury, Wiltshire, England
Printed and bound in Great Britain by
Biddles Ltd, Guildford and King's Lynn

Contents

SECTION III – COPING AND PSYCHOSOCIAL INTERVENTIONS

Contributors

CARY L. COOPER
Editor

Manchester School of Management, University of Manchester Institute of Science and Technology, UK

MAGGIE WATSON
Editor

Cancer Research Campaign, Psychological Medicine Group, The Institute of Cancer Research and The Royal Marsden Hospital, London, UK

JOAN R. BLOOM

School of Public Health, University of California, Berkeley, California, USA

HANS J. EYSENCK

Institute of Psychiatry, University of London, UK

TIMOTHY L. GORDON

Department of Psychology, Kent State University, Kent, Ohio, USA

JOHN GREEN

Psychology Department, St. Mary's Hospital, London, UK

GUO YAN-RONG

Beijing Institute for Cancer Research, Beijing, China

BARBARA HEDGE

Psychology Department, St. Mary's Hospital, London, UK

EDGAR HEIM

Department of Psychiatry, University of Bern, Bern, Switzerland

JIMMIE C. HOLLAND

Psychiatry Service, Memorial Sloan-Kettering Cancer Center, New York, USA

PAUL B. JACOBSEN

Psychiatry Service, Memorial Sloan-Kettering Cancer Center, New York, USA

SOO H. KANG

School of Public Health, University of California, Berkeley, California, USA

CYNTHIA M. MATHIESON   *Department of Psychology, University of Calgary, Alberta, Canada*

SUSANNE M. MEEHAN   *Department of Psychology, Kent State University, Kent, Ohio, USA*

BENJAMIN H. NEWBERRY   *Department of Psychology, Kent State University, Kent, Ohio, USA*

AMANDA RAMIREZ   *Imperial Cancer Research Fund, Clinical Oncology Unit and Division of Psychiatry, Guy's Hospital, London, UK*

PATRICK ROMANO   *School of Public Health, University of California, Berkeley, California, USA*

MARZIO E. E. SABBIONI   *Department of Neurology Psychiatry Service, Memorial Sloan-Kettering Cancer Center, New York, USA*

HENDERIKUS J. STAM   *Department of Psychology, University of Calgary, Alberta, Canada*

ZHANG ZONG-WEI   *Beijing Institute for Cancer Research, Beijing, China*

Foreword

Theoretically cancer and stress can be reciprocally related through both biological and psychological interactions: stress might affect cancer incidence or physical progress, or it might affect incidence or change in psychological events; and conversely, cancer might affect the incidence of stress or its changes, as well as any physical or psychological events that may accompany it. For our present purposes it is important to note that almost all of the psychological factors examined in both case-control and cohort studies have stress as an important component of their effect, and thus examination of these factors falls well within the scope of this book. To help maintain a realistic view of matters it is also valuable to remember that most of the psychological factors examined have produced few replicated relationships, even though the reverse might seem true because the various authors cite and emphasize only the one or two for which they have found a relationship.

The literature has discussed a number of elements in these relationships, and focussed on a few. Early in the era of interest in these matters many personality characteristics were examined, and a considerable number were reported to be related to cancer incidence or progress. Very few writers have suggested that what a cancer patient reported or how he or she reacted could be influenced by the physiological consequences of disease (hormonal changes, immune changes, neurotropic effects) and might therefore not reflect premorbid or pretesting status. Nor did many mention the possible effect that knowledge of or even *belief* in having cancer might have on measured personality states or reported feelings, past events, or impact of such events on the subject. This failure to consider these possible effects applied, up to very recent times, even to prebiopsy studies where, presumably, diseased and non-diseased were equally uncertain of their status. Nor did they, for the most part, consider the paraneoplastic physical effects mentioned above. Only recently have we come to realize that a large number of factors can affect the creation of a malignant tumour and its development once it has appeared. This understanding was well described in certain chapters of the editor's previous book, *Stress and Breast Cancer*.

As we do more research we become more aware of what is needed to produce stable scientific positions that have gone beyond hypothesis and theory to accepted fact, like the germ theory of disease, the existence of unconscious psychological processes, or, to cite the most recent, that the nervous system influences the immune system. That awareness, in turn, allows progress toward such a stable position regarding the relationship of stress to cancer initiation and growth, and treatment of its stressful psychological sequelae. Thus, for retrospective and prebiopsy studies, a view of the most recent developments, as is afforded by this book, is very important.

One would think that prospective studies would produce a more secure scientific position than retrospective ones, and they do, for well-known reasons. But we also observe that they can produce contradictory findings in apparently similar studies, just as do retrospective ones. It may be fruitful to examine what seems like a reasonable scenario to help explain, in some degree, such contradictory findings. This scenario is grounded on a basic fact that has been all but ignored as a possibility in both types of studies. That fact is that the larger the number of uncontrolled variables that can affect an outcome the greater the probability that one or some may by chance happen to exert an unusual or extreme effect in any given study. In the general dose–response situation, the stronger the factor the greater the effect and the weaker the factor the weaker the effect; they tend to cancel each other out. Similarly, if there are many uncontrolled variables the positive and negative extreme deviations tend to cancel each other out.

In this case, however, I hypothesize that a special circumstance leads to the biased appearance of too many positive effects, apparently due to the experimental variable but actually due to such chance deviations, more often than would appear in orthodox dose–response studies that do not relate to cancer. In those we find, most often, a symmetric situation with as much reduced effect as there is enhanced effect, and the influences of different variables tend to cancel each other out. Thus extreme upward chance deviations of confounders (above a critical threshold) increase the probability of cancer and hence the apparent effect of stress. However, in the case examining cancer incidence, extreme downward chance deviations do not decrease the *observed* probability of cancer, since they yield the same result as the average or non-extreme value of the confounder – namely, no cancer – and they do not discriminate the non-appearance of cancer based on average confounder values from those based on extremely low values of the confounder. Overall, this picture yields more apparent effects showing stress to be associated with cancer than not. The same rationale applies, in somewhat altered form, to progress of cancer.

If the underlying effect of stress on cancer is small, such a scenario will yield just the contradictory mix of results in both retrospective and prospective studies. In large cohorts where the researcher has tried to achieve random selection, the odds of a randomly discrepant sample are smaller, and one can have more confidence that the results reflect the true state of affairs.

In view of the above, what should we do? At first view one might suggest either several large cohort studies as was done in the case of non-clinical depression, or a considerable number of smaller studies where one does not expect any one or two to define correctly the "true" state of affairs, but where the overall mass of data suggests the "true" state of affairs. A good meta-analysis would be valuable at that point. Right now we do not have enough similar studies on one variable to carry out a proper meta-analysis, since its requirements are rarely met. But such difficulties can be overcome in the long run with proper planning.

It thus becomes important to add to our store of studies since, in the long run, the more variables we control the less the chance of bias appearing. While, overall, studies in this field are moving towards better controls, there is a long way to go. Reporting on new results, as does this book, can produce a better fix on the actual state of affairs in regard to stress and the aetiology and progress of cancer.

Because of the unsettled state of this field and in view of the above discussion, it is important to measure as many suspected confounders as possible. A researcher should also have at hand the values of all the measured variables in a study, for analysis by others. In such an unsettled state it is further important to weigh carefully the reported results of studies, their controlled (and uncontrolled) variables, and the assumptions underlying the conduct of the study.

I subscribe wholeheartedly to the objectives of the editors of this book, as well as to their cautions and their clear position that we can gain understanding in this field only by rigorous, careful and cross-validated investigations.

Bernard H. Fox
March 6, 1991

Introduction

THE PSYCHOBIOLOGICAL MODEL

The idea that stress or psychological factors play a role in the onset or progress of cancer continues to excite considerable interest and heated debate. It is, also, a rapidly moving area of study, thus making it important to update reviews in order to keep abreast of findings and evaluate current models. Opinions on the possible role of stress in cancer are widely divergent. At one extreme is the view espoused in Angell's (1985) editorial that "our belief in disease as a direct reflection of mental state is largely folklore." At the other extreme is the notion, reported by some of the gurus, that it is possible to think, or love, away your tumour. Of course, it is no more possible to think away a tumour than the nose upon your face. Neither of these views is absolutely correct and the reality lies somewhere in between.

The idea that disease is multifactorial in origin and a result of interrelationships between genetic, endocrine, nervous and immune systems is by no means new. Sir William Osler, often considered the father of modern medicine, was said to have observed that in order to predict the outcome of pulmonary tuberculosis, it was as important to know what was going on in a man's head as what was going on in his chest.

Any psychobiological model of cancer must satisfy certain basic criteria before it could be considered scientifically acceptable. First, it would be necessary to identify particular psychological responses and confirm their more frequent occurrences in either those who develop cancer or those with shorter than average survival time. Second, it would be necessary to know something of the physical implications of the psychological responses identified. Third, it would be important to know whether the identified physical responses contribute in any way to cancer aetiology and/or progression.

The psychobiological model of cancer has, indeed, a long history, with Galen's view on melancholic women being often quoted. However, more recent progress in the development of a psychoneuroimmunology model has brought this topic out from the speculative and into the scientific domain.

An examination of available studies indicates that the first issue; namely, evidence of specific psychological responses, is the most frequently addressed. The incidence of stressful life events, particular personality variables, coping styles and the social characteristics of cancer patients are among the topics covered in the chapters to follow. The concept of the cancer-prone personality has received substantial attention with some authors reporting quite spectacular results (Grossarth-Maticek *et al.*, 1988). However, as already pointed out elsewhere (Johnston, 1991), these claims require careful independent replication before they should be accepted. The second area, relating to associated biological response, has been addressed only more recently. Of course, the literature on biological concomitants of stress is somewhat older and owes much to the seminal work of Selye (1976). Some of this work has helped to lay the ground for more recent research on stress and cancer. The currently fashionable model involves the idea that psychological factors can affect the release of stress hormones which in term act upon immune responses, thus weakening the body's defence system. Also, there is no doubt that Ader's (1981) work on the conditionability of the immune system has contributed to the popularity of the psychoimmunology model of cancer progression. Interestingly, Ader, although providing an important body of evidence on the conditionability of immune responses, has never argued that these changes contribute to ill-health or, for that matter, cancer (Ader, 1990). Indeed, an increasing number of studies have appeared over the last decade which have shown immune responses, in animals and humans, to be conditionable. The statistical differences found in comparisons for human immune responses are interesting but, on the whole, are of little clinical significance. Indeed, in a relatively young science like immunology, researchers still have difficulty in defining what constitutes a "pathological" immune response in the sense of the one that is damaging to the system. It is likely that the current focus on immune response as the underlying mechanism is both unwarranted and premature. It is too early to close the area to other biological factors. This is especially so in cancer because different cancers have different aetiologies and different prognoses.

Taking the issue one step further, and asking whether the biological responses observed in this currently fashionable model contribute to cancer, raises further difficulties. The literature regarding the role of the immune system in carcinogenesis is controversial, as Kripke's (1988) excellent review points out. The original model, as developed by Burnet (1970), involved the idea that the immune system served as a means of controlling carcinogenesis. Damage to the immune system in the form of immunode-pression would increase the likelihood of precancerous cells escaping the surveillance system and developing into full-blown cancers. This model can be tested by examining those individuals immunosuppressed by specific immune deficiencies or by organ transplant procedures, and lately by the AIDS virus. A number of studies (Fraumeni and Hoover, 1977; Purtillo, 1984; see also Kripke, 1988 for a further review) have shown that where cancers develop in these groups they are of a specific nature and do not include the most prevalent cancers such as lung, breast, stomach and colon. It has been concluded (Kripke, 1988) that overall "the general immunological reactivity of the host need not be impaired for most neopla-sias to occur and progress". Immunological research has thus shifted in focus from examining systemic changes to examining the effects on local tumour-specific function. In general, the concept of systemic immunore-gulation of cancer aetiology and/or progression is not strongly supported. However, local immune changes surrounding the tumour site may well play a role alongside other factors in tumour progression, and this merits further investigation.

THE CONCEPT OF CARE

When examining stress and cancer the remit does not have to be limited to psychosomatic or psychobiological models. Indeed, many would argue that the primary focus ought to be on how best to care for cancer patients, enhance their wellbeing and reduce stress. The importance of psychosocial and psychiatric services to cancer patients and their families has been increasingly promulgated in the more recent literature. The acknowledged high level of psychological morbidity and psychiatric sequelae have fuelled the argument that better support and rehabilitation services are needed. These issues are addressed in some of the chapters to follow.

ORGANISATION OF THE BOOK

This book is organised into three sections. The first two sections, com-prising two and four chapters respectively, explore the psychological mechanisms in the link between stress and cancer, and the psychosocial and personality factors. These two sections update the literature from the previous volume on psychosocial stress and cancer (Cooper, 1984). The next section, Coping and Psychosocial Interventions, comprises four chap-ters which explore issues on the way in which people cope with the diag-nosis and treatment of cancer, interventions to help people cope, their adaptation to the disease and the role of counselling. This latter section adds a new dimension to the relationship of stress to cancer, which has not been fully explored in previous volumes in the field.

In the first section, Psychobiological Mechanisms, Chapter 1 (Sabbioni) explores psychobiological processes by reviewing psychoneuroimmunology, and in doing so provides the reader with a good basis from which to approach this very complex area. The author expresses a view, increasingly voiced, that close collaboration between different disciplines is essential. Clearly, interdisciplinary training needs to progress further if we are to see penetrating research across these areas in the future. Chapter 2 (Newbury, Gordon and Meehan) on the other hand, reviews the animal literature, and outlines the insights which might be gained from this work, and the contribution of stress to animal models of carcinogenesis.

In the second section of the book, Psychosocial and Personality Factors, we explore the psychological factors in cancer prognosis, the link between cancer and personality, and the impact of social support on the stress–cancer relationship. In addition, we invited a distinguished Chinese oncologist to describe the work being undertaken in China assessing the psychosocial and personality factors. Although the work may not in some regards be as advanced as in the West, the differences in the nature and approach of their work proves novel and enlightening. In this section, Chapters 3 (Watson and Ramirez) and 4 (Eysenck) deal with the possible link between personality/behaviour/life events and cancer. Some of the views expressed await independent replication and until such replication studies are completed, it is wise to view findings with some caution. Studies of cancer progression are notoriously difficult to mount; requiring large numbers of patients, control for initial disease stage and incorporation of subsequent medical treatments into the analysis. Only careful, rigorous research, taking account of all such factors, will provide any satisfactory results on the role of psychological factors in either carcinogenesis or disease progression. Nevertheless, some of the latest research in the field is explored in these two chapters. Chapter 5 (Bloom, Kang and Romano) provides a far-reaching review of the possible role of social support in cancer prognosis. This is an area of great importance, where much further research is likely to take place, and further information on social factors is likely to enhance our understanding of the psychobiological model in cancer. Chapter 6 (Zhang and Guo) describes a study underway in China which aims to examine the psychobiological model of stress and cancer. It also requires, in the description of traditional Chinese medicine, that we make a conceptual leap to another domain of thinking. Some elements of Chinese medicine (e.g. acupuncture) have been accepted into the Western medical approach, and we must remain open to many different perspectives. Zhang and Guo's chapter is fascinating in providing an understanding of Chinese research in this field, and their methods of prevention and treatment.

The last section of the book, Coping and Psychosocial Interventions, deals with the issues of coping, adaptation and intervening to deal with the stress of cancer. Chapter 7 (Jacobsen and Holland) reviews the now extensive literature on psychological and psychiatric sequelae following cancer diagnosis and treatment. These authors point to important goals and directions for future research. Chapter 8 (Mathieson and Stam) attempts to provide a balance to the view that psychological factors play a role in carcinogenesis and disease progression. The authors reflect, to a certain extent, the increasing concern that the idea of "heroic self-healing" (Gray and Doan, 1990) causes psychological damage to some patients. They draw attention to the issues which arise as part of "the patient's larger social world". As such they represent a counterbalance to those who advocate that personality is of primary importance. The reader will find here also a useful review of the methods of psychological support for cancer patients. Chapter 9 (Heim) looks at coping adaptation, providing a considerable review of the complexities in this area, and the trends to date. Finally, Chapter 10 (Green and Hedge) takes us into the domain of patients with AIDS-related tumours, describing possible psychobiological models and an excellent model of patient care. Although the orientation is counselling with AIDS patients, its relevance and importance to cancer care is obvious.

It is hoped that this volume will help readers to achieve several objectives. First, to update researchers on the most recent material on the link between stress and cancer, and the stress of cancer. Second, to highlight the various current research methodologies in the field so that they may be improved upon. Third, to attempt to encourage more work on the coping and intervention aspects of the stress of cancer and in cancer prevention. And finally, to continue the momentum in the academic community to be open to all possible precursors and interventions that may in the long run bring cancer under control. This book does not provide any definitive answers or solutions, but is, we hope, another incremental step up the research ladder in trying to understand the nature and process of the relationship between life stress, personality, social support and cancer.

Cary L. Cooper
Maggie Watson

REFERENCES

Ader, R. (1981) *Psychoneuroimmunology*. Academic Press, New York.

Ader, R. (1990) *Conditional Immune Responses*. Paper presented at First International Congress of Behavioral Medicine, Uppsala, Sweden.

Angell, M. (1985) Editorial. *New Engl. J. Med.*, **312**, 1570–1572.

Burnet, F.M. (1970) The concept of immunological surveillance. *Prog. Exp. Tumor Res.*, **13**, 1–27.

Cooper, C.L. (1984) *Psychosocial Stress and Cancer*. John Wiley, Chichester.

Fraumeni, J.F. and Hoover, R. (1977) Immunosurveillance and cancer: epidemiologic observation. *Natl Cancer Inst. Monographs*, **47**, 121–126.

Gray, R.E. and Doan, B.D. (1990) Heroic self-healing and cancer: clinical issues for the health professions. *J. Palliative Care*, **6**, 32–41.

Grossarth-Maticek, R., Eysenk, H.J., Vetter, H. and Schmidt, P. (1988) Psychosocial types and chronic disease: results of the Heidelberg prospective psychosomatic intervention study. In Maes, S., Speilberger, C.D., Defares, P.B. and Sarason, I.G. (eds) *Topics in Health Psychology*. John Wiley, Chichester, pp. 57–75.

Johnston, D.W. (1991) Behavioural Medicine: the application of behaviour therapy to physical health. *Behav. Psychother.*, **19**, 100–108.

Kripke, M.L. (1988) Immunoregulation of carcinogenesis: past, present and future. *J. Natl Cancer Inst.*, **80**, 722–727.

Purtillo, D.T. (1984) Biology of disease. Defective immune surveillance in viral carcinogenesis. *Lab Invest.*, **51**, 373–385.

Selye, H. (1976) *Stress in Health and Disease*. Butterworths, Reading, Mass.

Section I
PSYCHOBIOLOGICAL MECHANISMS

1

Cancer and Stress: A Possible Role for Psychoneuroimmunology in Cancer Research?

MARZIO E. E. SABBIONI

Department of Neurology Psychiatry Service, Memorial Sloan-Kettering Cancer Center, New York, USA

Psychoneuroimmunology, an emerging interdisciplinary field of research studying the interactions between the central nervous system and the immune system, may elucidate some of the questions regarding the possible influence of psychosocial factors on cancer. Cancer affects not only the physical but also the psychological and social wellbeing of patients (Holland and Rowland, 1989; Redd and Jacobsen, 1988). The patient has to adjust to different medical factors including diagnosis, prognosis, treatment and the clinical course. The growing knowledge about stage-, treatment- and site-specific psychological issues can be applied to help the patient as well as his or her family and underscores one possible direction of the relationship between psychosocial factors and cancer.

The inverse direction of the relationship is also of interest. Two separate areas of research on the influence of psychosocial factors in the development and progression of cancer can be distinguished.

First, specific behaviors can increase the risk for cancer, e.g. cigarette smoke, diet, exposure to sunlight, alcohol, sexual habits, environmental and occupational exposure to carcinogens and delay in seeking treatment (Razavi and Holland, 1990). The mediating mechanisms between these behaviors and cancer are biologically evident. The effect can even be

Cancer and Stress: Psychological, Biological and Coping Studies
Edited by C. L. Cooper and M. Watson. © 1991 John Wiley & Sons Ltd

quantified for some of these behavioral factors, e.g. 30% of deaths from cancer are due to cigarette smoke (Holland, 1989).

Secondly, it is of interest to know whether psychosocial factors may influence cancer risk or survival by as yet unknown changes of the "internal milieu" (Holland, 1989). Socioeconomic status, social ties, personality, coping style, emotional states and stress have been linked to cancer risk and survival (Holland, 1989). The mediating factors are still hypothetical and controversial. Since human neoplasm shows considerable biological heterogeneity and the development of clinically detectable disease requires a multitude of steps over a long period, very different mechanisms may be involved (Pettingale, 1985). Tumor cells may be hormone sensitive, therefore different levels of hormones and different quantities or sensitivities of hormone receptors may link psychosocial factors and the risk or prognosis of cancer (Razavi *et al.*, 1990). Distress can affect DNA repair, indicating another possible pathway (Kiecolt-Glaser *et al.*, 1985).

The purpose of this chapter is to discuss the possibility that the immune system is involved in linking psychosocial factors with cancer risk or outcome. I will focus on studies carried out in humans.

PATHWAYS OF INTERACTION OF THE NERVOUS, ENDOCRINE AND IMMUNE SYSTEM

Research in psychoneuroimmunology has been greatly encouraged by the growing evidence of an integration of the nervous, immune and endocrine systems in a common network. Several examples will be discussed in this section, highlighting the fact that information is carried back and forth from the central nervous system (CNS) to the periphery by means of all three systems.

Lesions or stimulation of various CNS areas, particularly within the hypothalamus, result in altered immune responses, such as reduction of mitogen (Cross *et al.*, 1980), antigen driven lymphocyte proliferation (Roszman *et al.*, 1985; Stein, *et al.*, 1981) or reduced or abolished natural killer (NK) cell activity (Forni *et al.*, 1983). Information is sent from the CNS to the immune system via the autonomic nervous system. Lymphoid organs (thymus, bone marrow, spleen and lymph nodes) are richly innervated with sympathetic nerves which regulate not only blood flow but also their immune function (Felten *et al.*, 1987; Giron *et al.*, 1980; Williams and Felten, 1981; Williams *et al.*, 1981; Bulloch and Moore, 1981).

Neuroendocrine pathways of information delivery have also been described: besides the well-known hypothalamo-hypophyseal-adrenal axis and the sympatho-adrenomedullary axis, the involvement of opioid peptides and of neuropeptides such as substance P, somatostatin and vasoactive intestinal peptide have also been demonstrated. These pathways are highly interconnected and build a network of regulatory and counter-regulatory loops (Khansari *et al.*, 1990; Dantzer and Kelley, 1989; Grossman, 1989). Receptors for hormones, neurotransmitters and neuropeptides have been detected on leukocytes (Bost, 1988; Calabrese *et al.*, 1987; Plaut, 1987). Immune response modulation by hormones, neurotransmitters and neuropeptides has been demonstrated (Blalock, 1989). Among many other substances, catecholamines (Besedovsky *et al.*, 1985; Irwin *et al.*, 1988), the hormones of the hypothalamo-pituitary-adrenal axis (Berczi, 1986), and the opioid peptides have been studied as possible immunomodulators (Lewis *et al.*, 1985; Morley *et al.*, 1985; Plotnikoff, 1985): the effect on immunocompetent cells is cell specific and may be dose dependent.

These findings support the theory that stress can have an impact on immune response by alterations of the endocrine system: research has shown an activation of the hypothalamo-hypophyseal-adrenal axis, the sympatho-adrenomedullary axis, increased endogenous opioid release, and increased secretion of growth hormone and prolactin among other effects related to the experience of stress (Dantzer and Kelly, 1989; Grossman, 1989; Khansari *et al.*, 1990). However, the variance of physiological responses to stressors, such as the often-found dissociation of the activation of the hypothalamo-hypophyseal-adrenal and sympatho-adrenomedullary axis, has yet to be fully understood.

The immune system receives information from, and delivers it to the CNS; it could also be envisaged as a sensory organ detecting stimuli such as viruses, bacteria or tumors (Blalock, 1984). Increased rates of firing of hypothalamic neurons have been associated with the induction of an immune response (Besedovsky *et al.*, 1977). Two pathways of communication between the immune system and the central nervous system have been identified: (1) biologically active neuroendocrine peptide hormones such as adrenocorticotropic hormone (ACTH) can be synthesized by leukocytes; (2) neuroendocrine tissues can be influenced by cytokines, peptides produced by immunocompetent cells (Blalock, 1988; Smith, 1988) and by thymosins, peptides produced by the epithelial cells of the thymus (Hall *et al.*, 1985). For example, the activation of T-cells requires two signals: an antigen presented by an antigen-presenting cell and interleukin-1 (IL-1), a cytokine produced by the antigen-presenting cell. Interleukin-1 also induces ACTH production (Woloski *et al.*, 1985), increases corticosteroid synthesis (Besedovsky *et al.*, 1986a) and is an endogenous pyrogen, increasing the set point for body temperature. Fever in turn can augment a number of protective immune mechanisms (Dinarello, 1984). Other effects of IL-1 reported in animals are promotion of slow-wave sleep and loss of appetite (Farrar *et al.*, 1987).

The immune system has an extensive capacity for self-regulation, mechanisms including cell-to-cell contact and secretion of regulatory factors such as cytokines (Roitt, 1988). There is a multitude of possible mechanisms by which neural signals (via autonomic nervous system or neuroendocrine system) may interact with an immune reaction but whether neural signals have only a generic influence on the immune system (such as a nonspecific suppression or enhancement of immune responses), or whether a more specific modulation of definite responses is possible, is still unclear. Neural signals could directly influence effector cells of the immune system. The interaction could also occur via modulation of the complex regulatory mechanisms within the immune system. Present knowledge is still fragmentary, but the functional significance of these pathways is indicated by the evidence for feedback (Besedovsky *et al.*, 1986b) and feedforward regulation (Bovbjerg and Ader, 1986) of the immune system by the CNS. The influence – through admittedly unknown neural processes – of psychosocial factors on immune responses in humans is therefore not contrary to the knowledge gathered, rather it is a further example for the existence of a (psycho-)neuroendocrine–immune network (Bovbjerg, 1989).

THE ROLE OF THE IMMUNE SYSTEM IN THE HOST RESPONSE TO NEOPLASMS

The discussion which follows focuses on immune responses which may be influenced by psychosocial factors and may play a role in the host response to tumors. Spontaneous regressions document the existence of a host response to tumors (Everson and Cole, 1966). Immunologic responses considered critical in cancer involve both specific and nonspecific cellular immune responses (Rosenberg *et al.*, 1989). The relevance, for psychoneuroimmunological research in cancer patients, of the limited efficacy of the immune response to cancer, the implications of the present knowledge for the immunosurveillance concept, and insights derived from adoptive immunotherapy to overcome tumor-induced suppression of immune responses will be discussed further. However, a review of the role of the immune system in cancer risk and survival is not within the scope of this chapter, and the reader is referred to appropriate reviews and textbooks (Rosenberg *et al.*, 1989; Reif and Mitchel, 1985).

The demonstration of tumor-specific antigens, a precondition for a specific immune response, has proven difficult (Lennox, 1985; Hellström and Hellström, 1989). Tumor-associated differentiation antigens have been described in human tumors, but are also found on embryonic cells and the difference between normal and tumor cells is quantitative, not qualitative (Hellström and Hellström, 1989). Intratumoral antigenic heterogeneity has been described in several types of human cancer (Prehn and Prehn, 1989), as have antigenic differences between the primary tumor and metastases (Heppner and Miller, 1989).

The concept of immunosurveillance relies on the assumption that a great number of tumor cells arise daily, that these tumor cells are antigenic, and that they are recognized and killed by a specific cell-mediated immune response. However, neoplastic cells seem not to arise frequently, and only some are antigenic enough to be detected and eliminated by the immune system (Den Otter, 1986). The evidence available from animal experiments does not support the concept of immunosurveillance in the host defense against neoplasm (Stutman, 1985). Effector cells (NK cells) able to lyse target cells without the need to recognize a specific antigen have been discovered (Herberman, 1985). This property would make NK cells the ideal effector cells for the hypothesized immunosurveillance; unfortunately they seem to lyse only a restricted number of *fresh* tumor cells (Rosenberg *et al.*, 1989).

If the immune system plays a role in the development of tumors, immunocompromised patients should show a higher risk of cancer. Transplant patients receiving immunosuppressive therapy over a period of years, showed an increase over that seen in an age-matched population in non-Hodgkin's lymphoma, Kaposi's sarcoma, skin and lip cancers, and *in situ* carcinoma of the uterine cervix (Penn, 1986). This cannot be attributed solely to the immunosuppressed status of these patients. Other factors play a role: oncogenic viruses, the carcinogenic effect of the chemotherapeutic or immunosuppressive agents, chronic antigenic stimulation, disturbed immunoregulation, genetic and environmental factors (Penn, 1986).

Tumors show a varying degree of infiltration with cells of the immune system and immune reaction at the tumor site does not always lead to tumor rejection (Evans, 1986). Tumors seem to suppress cell-mediated immune responses, particularly in advanced stages (Pierce, 1978; North, 1985; Eura *et al.*, 1988). There may be an optimal level of immune reaction for tumor growth, and any change in level could inhibit tumor growth (Prehn and Prehn, 1989).

The importance of the suppressive effect of a tumor on the immune response has been highlighted by the recently developed possibilities of adoptive immunotherapy (Foon, 1989). Two cell types appear very promising: tumor infiltrating lymphocytes (TIL) and lymphokine activated killer cells (LAK). The former develop from T-cell precursors and seem to be specific for the tumor from which they are derived (Belldegrun *et al.*, 1989). Interleukin-2 (IL-2) enhances their cytotoxicity. TIL are ineffective until the host is immunosuppressed with cyclophosphamide or with total body irradiation, suggesting that some cell populations, possibly suppressor cells, must be eliminated before TIL can be effective. The tumor specificity of TIL can be lost in long term cultures (Klein and Leitman, 1989). The latter-type (LAK) originate from T-cells and are probably a heterogenous population. They are cytolytic for a broad range of fresh and cultured human and murine tumors, do not attack normal cells and are not MHC (major histocompatibility complex) restricted in their specificity. They are collected from peripheral blood, expanded in cultures with IL-2 and reinfused to the patient. LAK need exogenous IL-2 in order to be effective (Rayner *et al.*, 1985; Klein and Leitman, 1989). Preliminary results are encouraging despite significant toxicity (Glassman, 1989; Herberman, 1989).

Cell-mediated immune responses can be demonstrated in the host's response to several neoplasms which may or may not involve the detection of tumor antigens (Rosenberg *et al.*, 1989). However, the prognostic value of measures of cellular immunity is controversial (Nathanson, 1977; Pierce, 1978). *In vitro* immune responses to different autologous neoplasms have been associated with outcome (Cannon *et al.*, 1981; Vanky *et al.*, 1983a,b). *In vitro* lymphoproliferative responses to mitogens and antigens in breast cancer patients were less consistently related to outcome (positive association: Hacene *et al.*, 1986; Burford-Mason *et al.*, 1989; lack of association: Krown *et al.*, 1980). *In vitro* NK cell activity has had prognostic value in colorectal cancer patients (Tartter *et al.*, 1987). Delayed-type hypersensitivity to autologous breast cancer (Black *et al.*, 1989) and less consistently to recall antigens in patients with breast cancer and other neoplasms (Pierce, 1978; Nathanson, 1977) has been associated with outcome. However, these measures are not in current clinical use for evaluation of prognosis of cancer patients.

THE ROLE OF PSYCHOSOCIAL FACTORS ON CANCER RISK AND SURVIVAL

The influence of psychosocial factors on cancer risk and survival (without considering studies that have focused on behavioral factors such as cigarette smoking, alcohol intake, social status, etc.) by as yet unknown changes of the "internal milieu" is still controversial (for reviews, see Holland, 1989; Hürny, 1985; Fox, 1983). For in-depth discussion of the possible influence of psychosocial factors on cancer see elsewhere in this book (Section II).

It is possible to categorize the psychosocial factors examined in psycho-oncological research as follows: (1) A "cancer-prone personality" is hypothesized and characterized, for example by the inability to express emotions and to have satisfactory relationships. (2) The experience of depressive symptoms, feelings of hopelessness/helplessness, or of bereavement is believed to be associated with cancer risk or survival. (3) The experience of distress, or the chance to buffer stress by improving coping or by providing social support have been considered to influence cancer risk or survival.

Cancer-prone personality

The development or progression of cancer has been associated with a type C personality, characterized by suppression of emotional reactions, especially anger, and by conformity/compliance (Temoshok and Fox, 1984; Greer and Watson, 1985). Most available studies have focused on characteristics associated with type C personality, but the construct has not been prospectively investigated. For example, significant association was found between a cancer-prone personality comparable to the type C construct (Eysenck, 1988) and death from cancer in two large follow-up studies (Grossarth-Maticek *et al.*, 1985, 1988). In a semiprospective study patients with breast cancer were characterized as having poorly organized neurosis or psychosis (following the classification of Marty, 1983), excessive self-esteem, hysterical disposition and unresolved recent grief (Jasmin *et al.*, 1990). Some of these characteristics could be comparable with the concept of a type C personality (Hürny, 1990b).

The concept of a cancer-prone personality has still to be clarified in terms of psychological characterization and biological implications, and verified in large prospective studies. Of particular interest would be the demonstration that subjects with a premorbid cancer-prone personality show some kind of altered immune or endocrine responses or an impaired DNA repair process (at baseline, under stress or while recovering from stress), explaining higher cancer risk or lower cancer survival.

Depressive mood, hopelessness/helplessness, fighting spirit

Several studies have examined the possible influence of psychosocial factors on cancer relapse or survival. "Fighting spirit" and optimism after surgery for breast cancer were related to recurrence-free survival (Greer *et al.*, 1979, 1990; Hislop *et al.*, 1987). However, the lack of association between psychosocial factors and time of relapse in patients with stage I and II melanoma or stage II breast cancer has also been reported (Cassileth *et al.*, 1985; Holland *et al.*, 1986).

In several large prospective studies over 10–17 years depressive mood was found not to be associated with cancer risk or survival (Zonderman *et al.*, 1989; Kaplan and Reynolds, 1988; Hahn and Pettiti, 1988). Other authors reported an association between depressive symptoms with 20-year incidence and mortality from cancer (Persky *et al.*, 1987).

Bereavement has been associated with increased morbidity and mortality, but Ewertz (1986) found no association between marital status, length of widowhood and the development of breast cancer. Other studies on loss of spouse have not demonstrated a significant association between bereavement and cancer risk and survival (Hürny, 1990a; Chochinov and Holland, 1989).

The effect of depressive mood on cancer risk and survival seems to be small (Fox, 1989). However, findings related to the experience of hopelessness/helplessness and fighting spirit on cancer survival indicate a possible influence on cancer outcome.

Stress, coping modes and social support

A case-control study (Ramirez *et al.*, 1989) has found an increased relative risk of breast cancer recurrence associated with severe life events and difficulties during the postoperative disease-free interval. In patients with malignant melanoma, death or severe disease progression was associated with high levels of distress and dysphoric emotions on self-report scales (Temoshok, 1985). Patients with metastatic breast cancer randomly assigned to weekly supportive group therapy over a year, aimed at reducing distress through therapeutic social support and improvement of coping, had longer survival compared with patients in a control group (Spiegel *et al.*, 1989). The prognostic significance of the emotional network was supported by another study (Hislop *et al.*, 1987).

Intervention studies are a means of testing the relevance of psychosocial factors in humans. Interestingly, one of the most convincing studies demonstrating the importance of psychosocial factors in cancer survival is an intervention study influencing social support and coping with illness and illness- or treatment-related issues (Spiegel *et al.*, 1989).

Conclusions

In animal studies the existence of a direct influence of "psychosocial factors" – operationalized as stress and control over stress, and as stress buffering through such factors as different housing conditions – on cancer can be demonstrated, but the mechanisms are still unclear (Anisman and Sklar, 1985; Justice, 1985). There is consensus that stress-associated infectious or neoplastic pathologies will not be observed, despite the presence of stress, if no underlying disease is present (Riley, 1981). Knowledge gained from animal studies can be very stimulating for human research, but cannot be directly transferred to the human situation, particularly because of the tumor models used.

The possible direct influence of psychosocial factors on cancer risk and survival is still unresolved. The assumption that all tumors are equally affected by psychosocial factors must be dismissed because of the biological heterogeneity of different neoplasms. Furthermore, the influence of psychosocial factors on cancer morbidity and mortality may be very different. However, the assumption can be made that there is a small but significant contribution of psychosocial factors to cancer risk and survival, which might vary depending upon the specific neoplasm considered.

PSYCHOSOCIAL FACTORS AND THE IMMUNE SYSTEM

The focus of this section is to discuss cell-mediated immune responses that are affected by psychosocial factors and have been shown in some studies to be associated with cancer. Almost all studies considered here have been carried out in healthy subjects or in non-cancer patients. Since a review of psychoneuroimmunology is not intended the interested reader should refer to several books (Ader, 1981; Ader *et al.*, 1990; Berczi, 1986; Blalock and Bost, 1988; Jankovic *et al.*, 1987) and recent review articles (Biondi and Kotzalidis, 1990; Geiser, 1989; Gorman and Locke, 1989; Khansari *et al.*, 1990; Locke and Gorman, 1989) for an in-depth discussion.

Personality and immune responses

There are few studies evaluating differences in immune measures associated with a specific personality or personality traits. Comparison of studies is limited by the use of different concepts of personality. Pettingale *et al.* (1977) found an association between serum IgA levels and the tendency to suppress anger in a group of female patients with benign and malignant breast disease. Kropiunigg *et al.* (1989) reported that healthy students have higher lymphocyte and suppressor/cytotoxic T-cell counts, and higher lymphoproliferative responses to phytohaemagglutinin (PHA) and IL-2 during a stressful self-awareness seminar. Subjects with a higher need for succorance/nurturance had lower helper/inducer T-cells; more achievement- and order-oriented individuals showed higher suppressor/cytotoxic T-cell counts during the course. Jemmott *et al.* (1990) combined three studies to show low NK cell activity in subjects with stressed power motivation syndrome and a high NK cell activity in subjects with unstressed affiliation motivation syndrome.

Depressive symptoms, loss of significant others and immune responses

According to Schleifer *et al.* (1984) controls had higher lymphocyte stimulation to PHA, concanavalin A and pokeweed mitogen than hospitalized depressed patients. No difference existed between controls and depressed outpatients (Schleifer *et al.*, 1985). Significant age-related differences were found between controls and depressed patients in mitogen responses and in the number of T4 lymphocytes (Schleifer *et al.*, 1989). Immune changes were also associated with severity of depression and hospitalization status. The authors concluded that altered immunity is not a correlate of major depressive disorder but may occur only in subtypes of depressed patients. A 50% reduction of NK activity has been reported in a different study in hospitalized depressed patients in comparison to non-stressed and non-depressed controls (Irwin *et al.*, 1990). Non-depressed controls experiencing high levels of distressing life events and difficulties showed a similar reduction in NK cell activity.

Bereaved spouses have been reported to show decreased proliferative response to mitogens (Bartrop *et al.*, 1977; Linn *et al.*, 1984; Schleifer *et al.*, 1983) and lower NK cell activity (Irwin *et al.*, 1987) as early as one month after the death of the spouse. The changes in immune response were associated with the severity of depressive symptoms. Delayed-type hypersensitivity to recall antigens was unaffected by bereavement (Bartrop *et al.*, 1977; Linn *et al.*, 1984).

Stress, coping modes, social support and immune responses

A number of studies have indicated that cellular immune measures are affected by naturally occurring stressors. Two studies have compared assessments pre- and postexamination with partially contradictory results. Dorian and associates (1982) reported an increase of T and B lymphocyte counts and an impairment of plaque-forming cells and mitogen responsiveness two weeks before the examination in highly stressed psychiatry trainees, compared with controls. Halvorsen and Vassend (1987) found a decreased expression of IL-2 receptor before an examination, and decreased lymphoproliferative responses to mitogens, antigens and pooled allogenic cells two weeks after. The impact of distress of an academic examination on immunity was evaluated in other studies by comparing two assessments carried out (1) several weeks before and (2) during an examination period (Kiecolt-Glaser *et al.*, 1984b, 1986; Glaser *et al.*, 1985, 1986, 1987). Depressed interferon production by concanavalin A-stimulated leukocytes and decreased NK cell activity were found during the examination period (Glaser *et al.*, 1986). The decrease of interferon gamma production was replicated (Glaser *et al.*, 1987) in a later study. In addition, the authors reported an increase in antibody titers to Epstein–Barr virus (EBV) during the examination period, as well as a decline of T-cell killing by memory T lymphocytes of Epstein–Barr virus-transformed autologous B lymphocytes.

Changes in immune measures may be associated with stressful events other than an academic examination. Locke and associates (1984) found that the NK cell activity was higher in subjects with fewer psychologic symptoms and high life-change stresses in the past year than in subjects with higher levels of psychological symptoms and life-change stress. Negative results are reported when milder levels of stress are considered (Moss *et al.*, 1989).

Ironson and associates (1990) studied changes in psychological and immunological functioning preceding and following notification of serostatus in homosexual males taking the HIV-1 antibody test. Seronegative subjects showed a decrease in blastogenic responses to PHA and pokeweed mitogen before the notification compared with controls not undergoing testing. Proliferative responses to PHA were back in the normal range five weeks after notification. In seropositive subjects, blastogenic responses to mitogens remained unchanged. At the time of notification NK cell activity was negatively associated with anxiety levels of the preceding week in both groups (Ironson *et al.*, 1990).

The effects of an intervention aimed at reducing distress or improving coping on stress-induced decreased immune measures are controversial. Kiecolt-Glaser *et al.* (1986) found that NK cell activity and the percentage of helper T lymphocytes decreased at the time of exams compared with one month before. The percentage of helper T lymphocytes was higher in subjects participating in an intervention group practising relaxation. An intervention aimed at counteracting anticipated negative psychosocial effects of unemployment had no effect on measures of cell-mediated immunity, but proliferative responses to PHA decreased over time during unemployment (Arentz *et al.*, 1987). Healthy students have been reported to have higher lymphoproliferative response to mitogens after disclosure of past traumatic events (Pennebaker *et al.*, 1988), but this interpretation of the results has been challenged (Neale *et al.*, 1988).

Social support as a stress-buffering factor has been emphasized by stress research. Lower proliferative responses of lymphocytes to PHA and lower levels of NK cell activity have been reported in non-psychotic psychiatric inpatients with high scores on the UCLA loneliness scale (Kiecolt-Glaser *et al.*, 1984a). Students with high loneliness scores during an examination period had lower NK cell activity (Kiecolt-Glaser *et al.*, 1984b) and high antibody titers to EBV, reflecting an impaired cellular immunity to the virus (Glaser *et al.*, 1985).

Personal relationships may influence immune measures (Kennedy *et al.*, 1988). Lower lymphoproliferative responses to PHA and higher EBV anti-body titers were found in women with poorer marital quality. Women who had recently separated from their partners showed higher antibody titers to EBV, lower percentages of helper lymphocytes and NK cells and lower proliferative responses to PHA (Kiecolt-Glaser *et al.*, 1987a). Family carers of patients with Alzheimer's disease had significant lower percentages of total T lymphocytes and helper T lymphocytes, and lower helper/suppressor cell ratios (Kiecolt-Glaser *et al.*, 1987b).

Cell-mediated immune responses may be influenced by short-term changes in emotions or short-term distress. After a 40-min recall of stressful experiences lymphoproliferative response to PHA and concanavalin A decreased significantly (Knapp *et al.*, 1990). Futterman and colleagues (1990) found an increase in proliferative response to PHA during experimentally induced short-term positive mood states with high arousal and a decrease of response in negative mood states with high arousal. These findings underscore the sensitivity of some immune measures to psychosocial factors, and highlight the need to define clearly the circumstances of the assessments.

Conditioned immune responses

The possibility of modulating immune response through classic conditioning has been demonstrated in animal studies. These experiments are among the best evidence available of a functional relationship between the CNS and the immune system. Suppression, as well as enhancement, of measures of immune functions have been conditioned. These studies have been extensively reviewed elsewhere (Ader and Cohen, 1985, 1990). Successful conditioning of the effects of drugs such as cyclophosphamide, a chemotherapeutic agent with immunosuppressive properties, has been reported (Ader and Cohen, 1975); also stress-induced endocrine (Stanton and Levine, 1988) and immunologic changes (Lysle *et al.*, 1988). The conditioned immune responses were important enough to have an impact on the survival of mice (1) developing a systemic lupus erythematosus-like disease with a lethal glomerulonephritis (Ader and Cohen, 1982), or (2) being injected with a syngeneic plasmocytoma (Groczynski *et al.*, 1985). The graft-versus-host response was also reduced in conditioned mice (Bovbjerg *et al.*, 1982).

Conclusions

The influence of psychosocial factors on immune measures has been independently demonstrated by several authors, but the clinical importance of the effect in humans has yet to be determined. The use of terms such as "immunosuppression" to describe, for example, a decrease in proliferative responses to mitogen without demonstrating increased morbidity or mortality is therefore questionable. The specific mechanisms involved in the modulation of immune responses by psychosocial factors are still unclear. The mediating effect of cortisol (Landmann *et al.*, 1984; Bartrop *et al.*, 1977; Arentz *et al.*, 1987; Schleifer *et al.*, 1989; Kiecolt-Glaser *et al.*, 1984a), catecholamines (Landmann *et al.*, 1984), opioid peptides (Jamner *et al.*, 1988), intracellular cyclic adenosine monophosphate, interferon gamma, leukocyte migration inhibition factor (Glaser *et al.*, 1987), IL-2 receptor gene expression and IL-2 production (Glaser *et al.*, 1990) have been investigated in humans. However, the highly interesting results of these studies can only be considered preliminary and are not yet conclusive.

The measures of cellular immunity found to be influenced most often by psychosocial factors are subsets of lymphocytes, proliferative responses of peripheral blood mononuclear cells to mitogens or antigens and NK cell activity. The value of these *in vitro* measures of cellular immunity with regard to cancer risk or outcome is controversial, at present limiting the interpretation of findings. The activity of NK cells may be of prognostic value in specific neoplasms (Tartter *et al.*, 1987; Herberman, 1985).

PSYCHONEUROIMMUNOLOGICAL STUDIES IN CANCER PATIENTS

Three different approaches to the study of psychoneuroimmunological issues in cancer patients can be identified: (1) study of the association between psychosocial factors, cancer outcome and measures of immune function; (2) investigation of the psychological and immunological responses to stressful, cancer-related issues and of the impact of interventions aimed at reducing distress and improving coping and adjustment; (3) research on the possibility that patients could develop anticipatory immune changes associated with chemotherapy treatment, in analogy to the development of anticipatory nausea and vomiting.

An example of the first approach is reported by Levy and colleagues (1985, 1987). In 71 patients with breast cancer stage I or II NK cell activity after surgery was related to nodal status, known to be an important prognostic factor. Of the variance of NK cell activity 51% could be explained by patient "adjustment", lack of social support and fatigue/depression symptoms. At a second assessment three months later, 30% of the variance could be explained by baseline NK cell activity, lack of social support and fatigue/depression symptoms. In a later study 61 stage I and II breast cancer patients were evaluated after surgery (Levy *et al.*, 1990). NK cell activity was associated with perception of high quality emotional support from a spouse or intimate other, perceived social support from the patient's physician and utilization of social support as a coping strategy. However, NK cell activity was associated with estrogen/progesterone receptor negative tumor status, but not with number of positive lymph nodes. Mood and adjustment scores were only marginally associated with NK cell activity.

In a prospective study reported by Grossarth-Maticek and Eysenck (1989) 50 patients with breast cancer with visceral metastasis receiving chemotherapy and 50 patients refusing chemotherapy were randomly assigned to psychotherapy or non-psychotherapy. Survival time was significantly longer in patients receiving chemotherapy; psychotherapy alone also had a positive effect on survival. Patients receiving both chemotherapy and psychotherapy had longer survival times and higher percentages of lymphocytes before the beginning of the next chemotherapy treatment than did patients receiving chemotherapy alone.

The second approach is reported by Fawzy and colleagues (1990) who randomly assigned patients with malignant melanoma stage I and II to a six-week intervention group ($n = 35$) or a control group ($n = 28$). The group intervention included health education, enhancement of problem-solving skills, stress management (e.g. relaxation techniques) and psychological support. Patient distress in the intervention group was reduced at the end of the intervention and to a greater extent at six-month follow up. An increase in percentage of large granular lymphocytes and NK cells, an increase in interferon-alpha-augmented NK cell activity, and a decrease of helper/inducer T-cells were found at six-month follow up in the intervention group compared to the control group. The authors avoided any prognostic implication of these changes because of the controversial prognostic value of the immune measures.

The third approach – that anticipatory immune changes can be detected in analogy to anticipatory nausea and vomiting as a result of inadvertent classical conditioning in patients receiving chemotherapy – has been investigated by Bovbjerg and colleagues (1990). Proliferative responses to T-cell mitogens (PHA, concanavalin A) were lower in twenty patients assessed in their homes several days before chemotherapy than immediately before chemotherapy. Increased anxiety was not related to these differences. Patients with lower proliferative responses to PHA in the clinic showed higher levels of anticipatory nausea consistent with the assumption that both were conditioned responses to stimuli associated with the clinic after multiple pairings with chemotherapy.

The results of the reported studies are highly interesting, but need to be replicated and extended. These results must therefore be considered preliminary, but indicate that psychoneuroimmunological research can be carried out in cancer patients. Studies of the impact of psychosocial factors on cancer have become more complex with the inclusion of immune responses as possible mediating factors. Several methodological problems such as control for interfering factors (such as sleep, nutrition, etc.), necessity to assess simultaneously behavior, immunity and illness, restrictions imposed by discrete assessments of ongoing processes, etc., must be addressed (Kiecolt-Glaser and Glaser, 1988; Sabbioni and Hürny, 1990).

The prognostic value of available immune measures is controversial, and the choice of the measures will inevitably be arbitrary. Psychoneuroimmunological research strongly depends upon advances in tumor immunology. This limitation should be an incentive to focus on possible mechanisms involved in modulation of immune responses by psychosocial factors in patients with, or at risk for, specific neoplasms.

The findings in HIV seropositive subjects, where the infection itself seemed to override the effects of psychosocial factors on the immune system in asymptomatic subjects (Ironson *et al.*, 1990), urge careful appraisal of the effects of illness on immune responses in psychoneuroimmunological studies in cancer patients. However, it is possible that significant relationships between immune responses and neoplasm have been obscured by the lack of consideration of the potential impact of psychosocial variables on immune measures (Bovbjerg, 1990).

What is the potential of psychoneuroimmunology in cancer? The evidence presented in this review supports the assumptions that: (1) cell-mediated immunity particularly can play a role in the host's response and in the outcome of some neoplasms: (2) psychosocial factors such as emotions, stress, social support, coping modes and eventually specific personality traits can influence the outcome of some neoplasms; and (3) measures of cell mediated immunity such as lymphoproliferative responses to mitogens and antigens, and particularly NK cell activity, can be modulated by most of the aforementioned psychosocial factors. The results of these three independent research fields overlap enough to make an interdisciplinary research approach promising, and here lies the potential of psychoneuroimmunology in cancer. At present, there is not enough evidence from psychoneuroimmunological research to support clinical consequences for the treatment of cancer patients or the prevention of cancer. Nevertheless, the possibility that advances due to psychoneuroimmunological research in cancer patients may be of any benefit in future for some patients, or may at least elucidate some of the questions regarding the mind–body relationship, depends upon the close collaboration of all the research fields involved and can be considered optimistically.

ACKNOWLEDGEMENTS

The fellowship at Memorial Sloan-Kettering Cancer Center and the writing of this chapter was made possible by a research grant from the Bernese Cancer League, Switzerland. The author would like to thank William H. Redd PhD, Ann Futterman PhD, Paul B. Jacobsen PhD and Dana Bovbjerg PhD for their comments on the manuscript. A special thank you goes to Nancy R. Anton for her editorial assistance.

REFERENCES

Ader, R. (ed.) (1981) *Psychoneuroimmunology*. Academic Press, New York.

Ader, R. and Cohen, N. (1975) Behaviorally conditioned immunosuppression. *Psychosom. Med.*, **37**, 333–340.

Ader, R. and Cohen, N. (1982) Behaviorally conditioned immunosuppression and murine systemic lupus erythematosus. *Science*, **214**, 1534–1536.

Ader, R. and Cohen, N. (1985) CNS-immune system interactions: conditioning phenomena. *Behav. Brain Sci.*, **8**, 379–395.

Ader, R. and Cohen, N. (1991) The influence of conditioning on immune responses. In Ader, R., Felton, D. and Cohen, N. (eds) *Psychoneuroimmunology*, second edition. Academic Press, New York, pp. 611–646.

Ader, R., Felton, D.L. and Cohen, N. (eds) (1990) *Psychoneuroimmunology*, second edition. Academic Press, New York.

Anisman, H. and Sklar, L.S. (1985) Stress as a moderator variable in neoplasia. In White L., Tursky, B. and Schwartz, G.E. (eds) *Placebo, Theory, Research, and Mechanisms*. The Guilford Press, New York, pp. 351–394.

Arentz, B.B., Wasserman, J., Petrini, B., Brenner, S.O., Levi, L., Eneroth, P., Salovaara, H., Hjelm, R., Salovaara, L., Theorell, T. and Petterson, I.L. (1987) Immune function in unemployed women. *Psychosom. Med.*, **49**, 3–12.

Bartrop, R.W., Luckhurst, E., Lazarus, L., Kiloh, L.G. and Penny, R. (1977) Depressed lymphocyte function after bereavement. *Lancet*, **i**, 834–836.

Belldegrun, A., Kasid, A., Uppenkamp, M., Topalian, S.L. and Rosenberg, S.A. (1989) Human tumor infiltrating lymphocytes. *J. Immunol.*, **142**, 4520–4526.

Berczi, L. (ed.) (1986) *Pituitary Function and Immunity*. CRC Press, Boca Raton, Florida.

Besedovsky, H.O., Sorkin, E., Felix, D. and Hass, H. (1977) Hypothalamic changes during an immune response. *Eur. J. Immunol.*, **7**, 325–328.

Besedovsky, H., del Rey, A. and Sorkin, E. (1985) Immunological-neuroendocrine feedback circuits. In Guillemin, R., Cohn, M. and Melnechuk, T. (eds) *Neural Modulation of Immunity*. Raven Press, New York, pp. 165–177.

Besedovsky, H., del Rey, A., Sorkin, E. and Dinarello, C.A. (1986a) Immuno-regulatory feedback between Interleukin-1 and glucocorticoid hormones. *Science*, **233**, 652–654.

Besedovsky, H., del Rey, A. and Sorkin, E. (1986b) Regulatory immune-neuro-endocrine feedback signals. In Berzci, I. (ed.) *Pituitary Function and Immunity*. CRC Press, Boca Raton, Florida, pp. 241–249.

Biondi, M. and Kotzalidis, G.D. (1990) Human psychoneuroimmunology today. *J. Clin. Lab. Anal.*, **4**, 22–38.

Black, M.M., Zachrau, R.E., Ashikari, R.H. and Hankey, B.F. (1989) Prognostic significance of cellular immunity to autologous breast carcinoma and glyco-protein 55. *Arch. Surg.*, **124**, 202–206.

Blalock, J.E. (1984) The immune system as a sensory organ. *J. Immunol.*, **132**, 1067–1070.

Blalock, J.E. (1988) Production of neuroendocrine peptide hormones by the immune system. *Prog. Allergy*, **43**, 1–13.

Blalock, J.E. (1989) A molecular basis for bidirectional communication between the immune and neuroendocrine system. *Physiol. Rev.*, **69**, 1–32.

Blalock, J.E. and Bost, K.L. (eds) (1988) Neuro-immunoendocrinology. *Prog. Allergy*, **43**.

Bost, K.L. (1988) Hormone and neuropeptide receptors on mononuclear leukocytes. *Prog. Allergy*, **43**, 68–83.

Bovbjerg, D.H. (1990) Psychoneuroimmunology: Implications for oncology? *Cancer* (in press).

Bovbjerg, D. (1989) Psychoneuroimmunology and cancer. In Holland, J.C. and Rowland, J.H. (eds) *Handbook of Psychooncology. Psychological Care of the Patient with Cancer.* Oxford University Press, London, pp. 727–734.

Bovbjerg, D. and Ader, R. (1986) The central nervous system and learning: feedforward regulation of immune responses. In Berzci, I. (ed.) *Pituitary Function and Immunity.* CRC Press, Boca Raton, Florida, pp. 252–257.

Bovbjerg, D., Ader, R. and Cohen, N. (1982) Behaviorally conditioned suppression of a graft-vs-host response. *Proc. Natl. Acad. Sci. USA*, **79**, 583–585.

Bovbjerg, D.H., Redd, W.H., Maier, L.A., Holland, J.C., Lesko, L.M., Niedzwiecki, D., Rubin, S.C. and Hakes, T.B. (1990) Anticipatory immune suppression and nausea in women receiving cyclic chemotherapy for ovarian cancer. *J. Consult. Clin. Psychol.*, **58**, 153–157.

Bulloch, K. and Moore, R.Y. (1981) Innervation of the thymus gland by brain stem and spinal cord in mouse and rat. *Am. J. Anat.*, **162**, 157–166.

Burford-Mason, A., Gyte, G.M.L. and Watkins, S.M. (1989) Phytohaemagglutinin responsiveness of peripheral lymphocytes and survival in patients with primary breast cancer. *Breast Cancer Res. Treat.*, **13**, 243–250.

Calabrese, J.R., King, M.A. and Gold P.W. (1987) Alterations in immunocompetence during stress, bereavement and depression: Focus on neuroendocrine regulations. *Am. J. Psychiatry*, **144**, 1123–1134.

Cannon, G.B., Dean, J.H., Keels, M. and Alford, C. (1981) Lymphoproliferative responses to autologous tumour extracts as prognostic indicators in patients with resected breast cancer. *Int. J. Cancer*, **27**, 131–138.

Cassileth, B.R., Lusk, E.J., Miller, D.S., Brown, L.L. and Miller, C. (1985) Psychological correlates of survival in advanced malignant disease. *New Engl. J. Med.*, **312**, 1551–1555.

Chochinov, H. and Holland, J.C. (1989) Bereavement: A special issue in oncology. In Holland, J.C. and Rowland, J.H. (eds) *Handbook of Psychooncology. Psychological Care of the Patient with Cancer.* Oxford University Press, London, pp. 612–627.

Cross, R.J., Markesbery, W.R., Brooks, W.H. and Roszman, T.L. (1980) Hypothalamic–immune interactions. I. The acute effect of anterior hypothalamic lesions on the immune response. *Brain Res.*, **196**, 79–87.

Dantzer, R. and Kelley, K.W. (1989) Stress and immunity: An integrated view of relationships between the brain and the immune system. *Life Sci.*, **44**, 1995–2008.

Den Otter, W. (1986) Immune surveillance and natural resistance: An evaluation. *Cancer Immunol. Immunother.*, **21**, 85–92.

Dinarello, C. (1984) Interleukin-1. *Rev. Infect. Dis.*, **6**, 51–95.

Dorian, B., Garfinkel, P., Brown, G., Shore, A., Gladman, D. and Keystone, E. (1982) Aberration in lymphocyte subpopulations and function during psychological stress. *Clin. Exp. Immunol.*, **50**, 132–138.

Eura, M., Maehara, T., Ikawa, T. and Ishikawa, T. (1988) Suppressor cells in the effector phase of autologous cytotoxic reactions in cancer patients. *Cancer Immunol. Immunother.*, **27**, 147–153.

Evans, R. (1986) The immunological network at the site of tumor rejection. *Biochim. Biophys. Acta*, **865**, 1–11.

Everson, T.C. and Cole, W.H. (1966) *Spontaneous Regression of Cancer*. W.B. Saunders, Philadelphia.

Ewertz, M. (1986) Bereavement and breast cancer. *Br. J. Cancer*, **53**, 701–703.

Eysenck, H.J. (1988) Personality, stress and cancer: Prediction and prophylaxis. *Br. J. Med. Psychol.*, **61**, 57–75.

Farrar, W.L., Hill, J.M., Harel-Bellan, A. and Vinocur, M. (1987) The immune logical brain. *Immunol. Rev.*, **100**, 361–378.

Fawzy, F.I., Kemeny, M.E., Fawzy, N.W., Elashoff, R., Morton, D., Cousins, N. and Fahey, J.L. (1990) A structured psychiatric intervention for cancer patients. II. Changes over time in immunological measures. *Arch. Gen. Psychiatry*, **47**, 729–735.

Felten, D.L., Felten, S.Y., Bellinger, D.L., Carlson, S.L., Ackerman, K.D., Madden, K.S., Olschowki, J. and Livnat, S. (1987) Noradrenergic sympathetic neural interactions with the immune system: Structure and function. *Immunol. Rev.*, **100**, 225–260.

Foon, K.A. (1989) Biological response modifiers: The new immunotherapy. *Cancer Res.*, **49**, 1621–1639.

Forni, G., Bindoni, M., Santoni, A., Belluardo, N., Marchese, A.E. and Giovarelli, M. (1983) Radiofrequency destruction of the tuberoinfundibular region of hypothalamus permanently abrogates NK cell activity in mice. *Nature*, **306**, 181–184.

Fox, B. (1983) Current theory of psychogenic effects on cancer incidence and prognosis. *J. Psychosoc. Oncol.*, **1**, 17–31.

Fox, B.H. (1989) Depressive symptoms and risk of cancer. *JAMA*, **262**, 1231.

Futterman, A.D., Kemeny, M.E. and Fahey, J.L. (1990) Short term immune changes associated with experimentally-induced positive and negative mood states. *First International Congress of the International Society for Neuroimmunomodulation*, Florence, Italy, May 23–26 (Abstract).

Geiser, D.S. (1989) Psychosocial influences on human immunity. *Clin. Psychol. Rev.*, **9**, 689–715.

Giron, L.T., Crutcher, K.A. and Davis, J.N. (1980) Lymph nodes – a possible site for sympathetic neural regulation of immune responses. *Ann. Neurol.*, **8**, 520–525.

Glaser, R., Kiecolt-Glaser, J.K., Speicher, C.E. and Holliday, J.E. (1985) Stress, loneliness, and changes in Herpesvirus latency. *J. Behav. Med.*, **8**, 249–260.

Glaser, R., Rice, J., Speicher, C.E., Stout, J.C. and Kiecolt-Glaser, J.K. (1986) Stress depresses interferon production by leukocytes concomitant with a decrease in Natural Killer cell activity. *Behav. Neurosci.*, **100**, 675–678.

Glaser, R., Rice, J., Sheridan, J., Fertel, R., Stout, J., Speicher, C., Pinsky, D., Kotur, M., Post, A., Beck, M. and Kiecolt-Glaser, J.K. (1987) Stress-related immune suppression: Health implications. *Brain Behav. Immunol.*, **1**, 7–20.

Glaser, R., Kennedy, S., Lafuse, W.P., Bonneau, R.H., Speicher, C., Hillhouse, J. and Kiecolt-Glaser, J.K. (1990) Psychological stress-induced modulation of Interleukin-2 receptor gene expression and Interleukin-2 production in peripheral blood leukocytes. *Arch. Gen. Psychiatry*, **47**, 707–712.

Glassman, A.B. (1989) Interleukin-2 and Lymphokine Activated Killer cells: Promises and cautions. *Ann. Clin. Lab. Sci.*, **19**, 51–55.

Gorman, J.R. and Locke, S.E. (1989) Neural, endocrine and immune interactions. In Kaplan, H.I. and Sadock, B.J. (eds) *Comprehensive Textbook of Psychiatry*, 5th edition. Williams and Wilkins, Baltimore, pp. 111–125.

Greer, S. and Watson, M. (1985) Towards a biological model of cancer: Psychological considerations. *Soc. Sci.*, **20**, 773–777.

Greer, S., Morris, T. and Pettingale, K.W. (1979) Psychological response to breast cancer. Effect on outcome. *Lancet*, **ii**, 785–787.

Greer, S., Morris, T., Pettingale, K.W. and Haybittle, J.L. (1990) Psychological response to breast cancer and 15 year outcome. *Lancet*, **335**, 49–50.

Groczynski, R.M., Kennedy, M. and Ciampi, A. (1985) Cimetidine reverses tumor growth enhancement of plasmocytoma tumors in mice demonstrating conditioned immune suppression. *J. Immunol.*, **134**, 421–426.

Grossarth-Maticek, R., Bastiaans, J. and Kanazir, D.T. (1985) Psychosocial factors as strong predictors of mortality from cancer, ischemic heart disease and stroke: The Yugoslav prospective study. *J. Psychosom. Res.*, **29**, 167–176.

Grossarth-Maticek, R., Eysenck, H.J. and Vetter, H. (1988) Personality type, smoking habit and their interaction as predictors of cancer and coronary heart disease. *Person. Indiv. Diff.*, **9**, 479–495.

Grossarth-Maticek, R. and Eysenck, H.J. (1989) Length of survival and lymphocyte percentage in women with mammary cancer as a function of psychotherapy. *Psychol. Rep.*, **65**, 315–321.

Grossman, A.B. (1989) Stress and counter-stress: A critical role for opioid peptides. In Casanueva, F.F. and Dieguez, C. (eds) *Recent Advances in Basic and Clinical Neuroendocrinology*. Elsevier, Amsterdam, pp. 197–206.

Hacene, K., Desplaces, A., Brunet, M., Liderau, R., Bourguignat, A. and Oglobine, J. (1986) Competitive prognostic value of clinicopathologic and bio-immunologic factors in primary breast cancer. *Cancer*, **57**, 245–250.

Hahn, R.C. and Petitti, D.B. (1988) Minnesota Multiphasic Personality Inventory-rated depression and the incidence of breast cancer. *Cancer*, **61**, 845–848.

Hall, N.R., McGillis, J.P., Spangelo, B.L. and Goldstein, A.L. (1985) Evidence that thymosin and other biological response modifiers can function as neuroactive immunotransmitters. *J. Immunol.*, **135**, 806s–811s.

Halvorsen, R. and Vassend, O. (1987) Effects of examination stress on some cellular immunity functions. *J. Psychosom. Res.*, **31**, 693–701.

Hellström, K.E. and Hellström, I. (1989) Oncogene-associated tumor antigens as targets for immunotherapy. *FASEB J.*, **3**, 1715–1722.

Heppner, G.H. and Miller, B.E. (1989) Therapeutic implications of tumor heterogeneity. *Sem. Oncol.*, **16**, 91–105.

Herberman, R.B. (1985) Natural Killer (NK) cells: Characteristics and possible role in resistance against tumor growth. In Reif, A.E. and Mitchel, M.S. (eds) *Immunity to Cancer*. Academic Press, Orlando, pp. 217–227.

Herberman, R.B. (1989) Interleukin-2 therapy of human cancer: potential benefits versus toxicity. *J. Clin. Oncol.*, **7**, 1–4.

Hislop, T.G., Waxler, N.E., Coldman, A.J., Elwood, J.M. and Kan, L. (1987) The prognostic significance of psychosocial factors in women with breast cancer. *J. Chron. Dis.*, **40**, 729–735.

Holland, J.C. (1989) Behavioral and psychosocial risk factors in cancer: Human studies. In Holland, J.C. and Rowland, J.H. (eds) *Handbook of Psychooncology. Psychological Care of the Patient with Cancer*. Oxford University Press, London, pp. 705–726.

Holland, J.C., Korzun, A.H., Tross, S., Cella, D.F., Norton, L. and Wood, W. (1986) Psychosocial factors and disease-free survival in Stage II breast cancer. *Proc. Am. Soc. Clin. Oncol.*, **5**, 237 (Abstract).

Holland, J.C. and Rowland, J.H. (eds) (1989) *Handbook of Psychooncology. Psychological Care of the Patient with Cancer*. Oxford University Press, London.

Hürny, C. (1985) Psychoonkologische Forschung. In Meerwein, F. (ed.) *Einführung in die Psycho-Onkologie*. Hans Huber, Berne, pp. 13–57.

Hürny, C. (1990a) Psychosocial factors in cancer. In Holland, J.C. and Zittoun, R. (eds) *Psychosocial Aspects of Oncology*, Monographs/European School of Oncology. Springer, Berlin, pp. 75–82.

Hürny, C. (1990b) Psyche and cancer. *Ann. Oncol.*, **1**, 6–8.

Ironson, G., LaPierre, A., Antoni, M., O'Hearn, P., Schneiderman, N., Klimas, N. and Fletcher, M.A. (1990) Changes in immune and psychological measures as a function of anticipation and reaction to news of HIV-1 antibody status. *Psychosom. Med.*, **52**, 247–270.

Irwin, M., Daniels, M., Smith, T.L., Bloom, E. and Weiner, H. (1987) Impaired natural killer cell activity during bereavement. *Brain Behav. Immunity*, **1**, 98–104.

Irwin, M.R., Hauger, R.L., Brown, M. and Britton, K.T. (1988) CRF activates the autonomic nervous system and reduces Natural Killer cytotoxicity. *Am. J. Physiol.*, **255**, R744–R747.

Irwin, M., Patterson, T., Smith, T.L., Caldwell, C., Brown, S.A., Gillin, J.C. and Grant I. (1990) Reduction of immune function in life stress and depression. *Biol. Psychiatry*, **27**, 22–30.

Jamner, L.D., Schwartz, G.E., and Leigh, H. (1988) The relationship between repressive and defensive coping styles and monocyte, eosinophile, and serum glucose levels: Support for the opioid peptide hypothesis of repression. *Psychosom. Med.*, **50**, 567–575.

Jankovic, B.D., Markovic, B.M. and Spector, N.H. (eds) (1987) Neuroimmune interactions: Proceedings of the second international workshop on neuroimmunomodulation, *Ann. NY Acad. Sci.*, **496** (special issue).

Jasmin, C., Lê, M.G., Marty, P., Herzberg, R. and the Psycho-Oncologic Group (1990) Evidence for a link between certain psychological factors and the risk of breast cancer in a case control study. *Ann. Oncol.*, **1**, 22–29.

Jemmott, J.B., Hellman, C., McClelland, D.C., Locke, S.E., Kraus, L., Williams, R.M. and Valeri, C.R. (1990) Motivational syndromes associated with Natural Killer cell activity. *J. Behav. Med.*, **13**, 53–73.

Justice, A. (1985) Review of the effects of stress on cancer in laboratory animals: Importance of time of stress application and type of tumor. *Psychol. Bull.*, **98**, 108–138.

Kaplan, G.A. and Reynolds, P. (1988) Depression and cancer mortality and morbidity: Prospective evidence from the Alameda County Study. *J. Behav. Med.*, **11**, 1–13.

Kennedy, S., Kiecolt-Glaser, J.K. and Glaser, R. (1988) Immunological consequences of acute and chronic stressors: Mediating role of interpersonal relationships. *Br. J. Med. Psychol.*, **61**, 77–85.

Khansari, D.N., Murgo, A.J. and Faith, R.E. (1990) Effects of stress on the immune system. *Immunol. Today*, **11**, 170–175.

Kiecolt-Glaser, J.K. and Glaser, R. (1988) Methodological issues in behavioral immunology research with humans. *Brain Behav. Immunity*, **2**, 67–78.

Kiecolt-Glaser, J.K., Ricker, D., George, J., Messick, G., Speicher, C.E., Garner, W. and Glaser, R. (1984a) Urinary cortisol levels, cellular immunocompetency, and loneliness in psychiatric inpatients. *Psychosom. Med.*, **46**, 15–23.

Kiecolt-Glaser, J.K., Garner, W., Speicher, S., Pennk, G.M., Holliday, J. and Glaser, R. (1984b) Psychosocial modifiers of immunocompetence in medical students. *Psychosom. Med.*, **46**, 7–14.

Kiecolt-Glaser, J.K., Stephens, R.E., Lipetz, P.D., Speicher, C.E. and Glaser, R.

(1985) Distress and DNA repair in human lymphocytes. *J. Behav. Med.*, **8**, 311–320.

Kiecolt-Glaser, J.K., Glaser, R., Strain, E.C., Stout, J.C., Tarr, K.L., Holliday, J.E. and Speicher, C.E. (1986) Modulation of cellular immunity in medical students. *J. Behav. Med.*, **9**, 5–21.

Kiecolt-Glaser, J.K., Fisher, L.D., Ogrocki, P., Stout, J.C., Speicher, C.E. and Glaser, R. (1987a) Marital quality, marital disruption, and immune function. *Psychosom. Med.*, **49**, 13–34.

Kiecolt-Glaser, J.K., Glaser, R., Shuttleworth, E.C., Dyer, C.S., Ogrocki, P. and Speicher, C.E. (1987b) Chronic stress and immunity in family care givers of Alzheimer's disease victims. *Psychosom. Med.*, **49**, 523–535.

Klein, H.G. and Leitman, S.F. (1989) Adoptive immunotherapy in the treatment of malignant disease. *Transfusion*, **29**, 170–178.

Knapp, P.H., Giorgi, R., Levy, E. and Heeren, T. (1990) Short term immunologic effects of induced emotion. *Psychosom. Med.*, **52**, 246 (Abstract).

Kropiunigg, U., Hamilton, G., Roth, E. and Simmel, A. (1989) Selektive Wirkung von Persönlichkeitsmerkmalen und psychosozialem Stress auf die T-Lymphozyten-Subpopulationen. *Psychother. Med. Psychol.*, **39**, 18–25.

Krown, S.E., Pinsky, C.M., Wanebo, H.J., Braun, D.W., Wong, P.P. and Oettgen, H.F. (1980) Immunologic reactivity and prognosis in breast cancer. *Cancer*, **46**, 1746–1752.

Landmann, R.M., Müller, F.B., Perini, C., Wesp, M., Erne, P. and Bühler, F.R. (1984) Changes in immunoregulatory cells induced by psychological and physical stress: Relationship to plasma catecholamines. *Clin. Exp. Immunol.*, **58**, 127–135.

Lennox, E.S. (1985) What are tumor antigens? In Reif, A.E. and Mitchel, M.S. (eds) *Immunity to Cancer*. Academic Press, Orlando, pp. 17–27.

Levy, S.M., Herberman, R.B., Maluish, A.M., Schlien, B. and Lippman, M. (1985) Prognostic risk assessment in primary breast cancer by behavioral and immunological parameters. *Health Psychol.*, **4**, 99–113.

Levy, S., Herberman, R., Lippman, M. and d'Angelo, T. (1987) Correlation of stress factors with sustained depression of Natural Killer cell activity and predicted prognosis in patients with breast cancer. *J. Clin. Oncol.*, **5**, 348–353.

Levy, S.M., Herberman, R.B., Whiteside, T., Sanzo, K., Lee, J. and Kirkwood, J. (1990) Perceived social support and tumor estrogen/progesterone receptor status as predictors of Natural Killer cell activity in breast cancer patients. *Psychosom. Med.*, **52**, 73–85.

Lewis, J.W., Shavit, Y., Terman, G.W., Nelson, L.R., Martin, F.C., Gale, R.P. and Liebeskind, J.C. (1985) Involvement of opioid peptides in the analgesic, immunosuppressive and tumor-enhancing effects of stress. *Psychopharmacol. Bull.*, **21**, 479–484.

Linn, M.W., Linn, B.S. and Jensen, J. (1984) Stressful events, dysphoric mood and immune responsiveness. *Psychol. Rep.*, **54**, 219–222.

Locke, S.E. and Gorman, J.R. (1989) Behavior and immunity. In Kaplan, H.I. and Sadock, B.J. (eds) *Comprehensive Textbook of Psychiatry*, 5th edition. Williams and Wilkins, Baltimore, pp. 1240–1249.

Locke, S.E., Kraus, L., Leserman, J., Hurst, M.W., Heisel, J.S. and Williams, R.M. (1984) Life change stress, psychiatric symptoms, and natural killer cell activity. *Psychosom. Med.*, **46**, 441–453.

Lysle, D.T., Cunnick, J.E., Fowler, H. and Rabin, B. (1988) Pavlovian conditioning of shock-induced suppression of lymphocyte reactivity: Acquisition, extinction, and preexposure effects. *Life Sci.*, **42**, 2185–2194.

Marty, P. (1983) *L'Ordre Psychosomatique*. Payot, Paris.

Morley, J.E., Kay, N., Allen, J., Moon, T. and Billington, C.J. (1985) Endorphins, immune function and cancer. *Psychopharmacol. Bull.*, **21**, 485–488.

Moss, R.B., Moss, H.B. and Peterson, R. (1989) Microstress, mood, and natural killer-cell activity. *Psychosomatics*, **30**, 279–283.

Nathanson, L. (1977) Immunology and immunotherapy of human breast cancer. *Cancer. Immunol. Immunother.*, **2**, 209–224.

Neale, J.M., Cox, D.S., Vladimarsdottir, H. and Stone, A.A. (1988) The relationship between immunity and health: Comment on Pennebaker, Kiecolt-Glaser, and Glaser. *J. Consult. Clin. Psychol.*, **56**, 636–637.

North, R.J. (1985) Suppressor cells: T-cells and macrophages. In Reif, A.E. and Mitchel, M.S. (eds) *Immunity to Cancer*. Academic Press, Orlando, pp. 239–249.

Penn, I. (1986) The occurrence of malignant tumors in immunosuppressed states. *Prog. Allergy*, **37**, 259–300.

Pennebaker, J.W., Kiecolt-Glaser, J.K. and Glaser, R. (1988) Disclosure of traumas and immune function: Health implications for psychotherapy. *J. Consult. Clin. Psychol.*, **56**, 239–245.

Persky, V.W., Kempthorne-Rawson, J. and Shekelle, R.B. (1987) Personality and risk of cancer: 20-year follow-up of the Western Electric Study. *Psychosom. Med.*, **49**, 435–449.

Pettingale, K.W. (1985) Towards a psychobiological model of cancer: Biological consideration. *Soc. Sci. Med.*, **20**, 779–787.

Pettingale, K.W., Greer, S. and Tee, D.E.H. (1977) Serum IgA and emotional expression in breast cancer patients. *J. Psychosom. Res.*, **21**, 395–399.

Pierce, G.E. (1978) Tumor immunity as related to the clinical course of cancer. In Waters, H. (ed.) *The Handbook of Cancer Immunology*, Volumes 3–4. Garland, New York, pp. 71–106.

Plaut, M. (1987) Lymphocyte hormone receptors. *Ann. Rev. Immunol.*, **5**, 621–669.

Plotnikoff, N.P. (1985) The ying–yang hypothesis of opioid peptide immunomodulation. *Psychopharmacol. Bull.*, **21**, 489.

Prehn, R.T. and Prehn, L.M. (1989) The flip side of tumor immunity. *Arch. Surg.*, **124**, 102–106.

Ramirez, A.J., Craig, T.K.J., Watson, J.P., Fentiman, I.S., North, W.R.S. and Rubens, R.D. (1989) Stress and relapse of breast cancer. *Br. Med. J.*, **298**, 291–293.

Rayner, A., Grimm, E.A., Lotze, M.T., Chu, E.V. and Rosenberg, S.A. (1985) Lymphokine-activated Killer (LAK) cells. Analysis of factors relevant to immunotherapy of human cancer. *Cancer*, **55**, 1327–1333.

Razavi, D. and Holland, J.C. (1990) Behavioral factors in cancer risk and survival. In Holland, J.C. and Zittoun, R. (eds) *Psychosocial Aspects of Oncology*. Monographs/European School of Oncology. Springer, Berlin, pp. 83–90.

Razavi, D., Farvacques, C., Delvaux, N., Befort, T., Paesmans, M., Leclercq, G., van Houtte, P. and Paridaens, R. (1990) Psychosocial correlates of oestrogen and progesterone receptors in breast cancer. *Lancet*, **335**, 931–933.

Redd, W.H. and Jacobsen, P.B. (1988) Emotions and cancer. New perspectives on an old question. *Cancer*, **62**, 1871–1879.

Reif, A.E. and Mitchel, M.S. (eds) (1985) *Immunity to Cancer*. Academic Press, Orlando.

Riley, V. (1981) Psychoneuroendocrine influences on immunocompetence and neoplasia. *Science*, **212**, 1100–1109.

Roitt, I. (1988) *Essential Immunology*, 6th Edition. Blackwell Scientific Publications, Oxford.

Rosenberg, S.A., Longon, D.L. and Lotze, M.T. (1989) Principles and applications of biologic therapy. In DeVita, V.T., Hellman, S. and Rosenberg, S.A. (eds) *Cancer: Principles and Practice of Oncology*. J.B. Lippincott Company, Philadelphia, pp. 301–347.

Roszman, T.L., Cross, R.J., Brooks, W.H. and Markesbery, W.R. (1985) Neuroimmunomodulation: Effects of neural lesions on cellular immunity. In Guillermin, R., Cohn, M. and Melnechuk, T. (eds) *Neural Modulation of Immunity*. Raven Press, New York, pp. 95–109.

Sabbioni, M. and Hürny, C. (1990) Psychoneuroimmunological studies. In Holland, J.C. and Zittoun, R. (eds) *Psychosocial Aspects of Oncology*. Monographs/European School of Oncology. Springer, Berlin, pp. 127–132.

Schleifer, S.J., Keller, S.E., Camerino, M., Thornton, J.C. and Stein, M. (1983) Suppression of lymphocyte stimulation following bereavement. *JAMA*, **250**, 374–377.

Schleifer, S.J., Keller, S.E., Meyerson, A.T., Raskin, M.J., Davis, K.L. and Stein, M. (1984) Lymphocyte function in major depressive disorder. *Arch. Gen. Psychiatry*, **41**, 484–486.

Schleifer, S.J., Keller, S.E., Siris, S.G., Davis, K.L. and Stein, M. (1985) Depression and immunity. Lymphocyte function in ambulatory depressed patients, hospitalized schizophrenic patients and patients hospitalized for herniorrhaphy. *Arch. Gen. Psychiatry*, **42**, 129–133.

Schleifer, S.J., Keller, S.E., Bond, R.N., Cohen, J. and Stein, M. (1989) Major depressive disorder and immunity. Role of age, sex, severity, and hospitalization. *Arch. Gen. Psychiatry*, **46**, 81–87.

Smith, E.M. (1988) Hormonal activities of lymphokines, monokines, and other cytokines. *Prog. Allergy*, **43**, 121–139.

Spiegel, D., Bloom, J.R., Kraemer, H.C. and Gottheil, E. (1989) Effect on psychosocial treatment on survival of patients with metastatic breast cancer. *Lancet*, **ii**, 888–891.

Stanton, M.E. and Levine, S. (1988) Pavlovian conditioning of endocrine responses. In Ader, R., Weiner, H. and Baum, A. (eds) *Experimental Foundations of Behavioral Medicine: Conditioning Approaches*. Lawrence Erlbaum, Hillside, New Jersey, pp. 25–46.

Stein, M., Keller, S. and Schleifer, S. (1981) The hypothalamus and the immune response. In Weiner, H., Hofer, M.A. and Stunkard, A.J. (eds) *Brain, Behavior, and Bodily Disease*. Raven Press, New York, pp. 45–65.

Stutman, O. (1985) Immunological surveillance revisited. In Reif, A.E. and Mitchell, M.S. (eds) *Immunity to Cancer*. Academic Press, Orlando, pp. 323–345.

Tartter, P.I., Steinberg, B., Barron, D.M. and Martinelli, G. (1987) The prognostic significance of natural killer cytotoxicity in patients with colorectal cancer. *Arch. Surg.*, **122**, 1264–1268.

Temoshok, L. (1985) Biopsychosocial studies on cutaneous malignant melanoma: psychosocial factors associated with prognostic indicators, progression, psychophysiology and tumor–host response. *Soc. Sci. Med.*, **20**, 833–840.

Temoshok, L. and Fox, B.H. (1984) Coping styles and other psychosocial factors related to medical status and to prognosis in patients with cutaneus malignant melanoma. In Fox, B.H. and Newberry, B.H. (eds) *Impact of Psychoendocrine Systems in Cancer and Immunity*. C.J. Hogrefe, Lewiston, pp. 258–287.

Vánky, F., Willems, J., Kreicbergs, A., Aparisi, T., Andréen, M., Broström, L.Å., Nilsonne, U., Klein, E. and Klein, G. (1983a) Correlation between lymphocyte-

26   *Psychobiological Mechanisms*

mediated auto-tumor reactivities and the clinical course. I. Evaluation of 46 patients with sarcoma. *Cancer Immunol. Immunother.*, **16**, 11–16.

Vánky, F., Péterffy, A., Böök, K., Willems, J., Klein, E. and Klein, G. (1983b) Correlation between lymphocyte-mediated auto-tumor reactivities and the clinical course. II. Evaluation of 69 patients with lung carcinoma. *Cancer Immunol. Immunother.*, **16**, 17–22.

Williams, J.M. and Felten, D.L. (1981) Sympathetic innervation of murine thymus and spleen. A comparative histofluorescence study. *Anat. Rev.*, **199**, 531–542.

Williams, J.M., Peterson, R.G., Shea, P.A., Schmedtje, J.F., Bauer, D.C. and Felten, D.L. (1981) Sympathetic innervation of murine thymus and spleen. Evidence for a functional link between the nervous and immune systems. *Brain Res. Bull.*, **6**, 83–84.

Woloski, B.M.R.N.J., Smith, E.M., Meyer, W.J., Fuller, G.M. and Blalock, J.E. (1985) Corticotropin-releasing activity of monokines. *Science*, **230**, 1035–1037.

Zonderman, A.B., Costa, P.T. and McCrea, R.R. (1989) Depression as a risk for cancer morbidity and mortality in a nationally representative sample. *JAMA*, **262**, 1191–1195.

2

Animal Studies of Stress and Cancer

BENJAMIN H. NEWBERRY, TIMOTHY L. GORDON
and SUSANNE M. MEEHAN
Department of Psychology, Kent State University, Kent, Ohio, USA

The notion that stressful conditions can alter the development of cancer has been confirmed repeatedly by experiments on animal models. In contrast, studies relating human cancer to stress (or to stress-relevant personality factors) are almost necessarily less definitive (e.g. Fox, 1988; Newberry *et al.*, 1991). However, the animal research indicates that *stressful conditions can inhibit neoplastic processes as well as promote them.* Reviews and discussions of the literature have made this point repeatedly (e.g., Justice, 1985; LaBarba, 1970; Newberry, 1981a; Newberry *et al.*, 1985; Newberry *et al.*, 1984; Peters and Mason, 1979; Riley, 1979; Sklar and Anisman, 1981). Once it is clear that stressful conditions can either exacerbate or inhibit cancer (and it has been clear for at least 20 years; LaBarba, 1970), this disparity becomes a major issue for the field. Until we know why stress can both inhibit and promote experimental neoplasms, the animal literature provides little more than a rather obvious warning to be wary of simple generalizations about psychological factors in human cancer.

BACKGROUND

Before we describe recent animal studies, we need to summarize the situation as it existed around 1980. For our present purposes there are logically three major classes of variables to consider: (1) stressor characteristics;

Cancer and Stress: Psychological, Biological and Coping Studies
Edited by C. L. Cooper and M. Watson. © 1991 John Wiley & Sons Ltd

(2) mediating variables; and (3) tumor system characteristics. We shall consider these in turn, but will do so very briefly.

Stressor characteristics

Two thoughtful papers published within the last decade have emphasized stressor characteristics as influencing whether stress will enhance, inhibit, or fail to affect the development of experimental cancers (Justice, 1985; Sklar and Anisman, 1981).

Sklar and Anisman (1981) saw stressor chronicity and controllability as crucial. Broadly, their view was as follows: Acute, uncontrollable stress is likely to stimulate tumor development, whereas otherwise similar, but controllable, stress is much less likely to have such an effect; chronic exposure to a stressor is less likely to enhance tumor development and can in fact have an inhibitory effect.

Sklar and Anisman's own studies of transplanted P815 mouse mastocytoma illustrate the types of findings which show the importance of stressor variables. Regarding controllability, they found that inescapable, but not escapable, shock stimulated tumor development (Sklar and Anisman, 1979) and that spontaneous fighting – which might be regarded as a coping attempt – was associated with a reduction in the tumorigenic effect of a change from social isolation to group housing (Sklar and Anisman, 1980). As for chronicity, Sklar and Anisman (1979) demonstrated that, although one session of shock following tumor cell transplantation stimulated P815 development, five or 10 daily sessions did not. Sklar *et al.* (1981) found that adapting animals to the shock regimen prior to tumor transplantation served to keep a single post-transplantation shock session from affecting tumor growth. Thus more extended shock exposure can either undo (Sklar and Anisman, 1979) or prevent (Sklar *et al.*, 1981) the effect of the single post-transplantation shock session.

Sklar and Anisman's (1980) studies of social conditions provide an additional illustration of the complexity of environmental influences. Stimulation of P815 by shock stress occurred only in group-housed animals. In animals housed individually, shock actually inhibited development of the tumors.

Justice (1985) also emphasized stressor timing, but his emphasis was on the possibility of cross-baseline rebounds following the termination of a stressor regimen. Justice explicitly incorporated opponent process theory into his thinking. Thus tumors whose growth is stimulated by stressful circumstances should be inhibited by opponent processes, which will dominate when the stressor is no longer present; and neoplasms which are inhibited by stress are expected to be stimulated following termination of stressor exposure. Justice's review of the data suggested to him that virally induced cancers will tend to behave according to the first pattern and that non-viral tumors will follow the second. He also noted that the opponent process might become dominant during adaptation to the stressor and before stressor exposure ends.

The Sklar and Anisman viewpoint (and possibly, but less obviously, the Justice viewpoint) implies that opposite effects can occur at different points on a single continuum (in this case time or opportunity for adaptation). If this is so, there must be a point on the continuum at which tumor development would not differ from control values (Newberry *et al.*, 1984).

Mediation

We cannot discuss mediating mechanisms in detail, but we do need to mention a few general points. One difficulty in studying mediation is that lengthy chains (or networks) of events are usually involved, and therefore identifying some process as part of the mediating chain/network need not indicate where that process fits. As an example, the identification of a hormone as a mediator will not by itself tell one whether it is acting directly on tumor cells or indirectly via effects on something like immune function, energy substrates or the nervous system.

Something that may need more emphasis than it usually receives is the variety of plausible mechanisms. The most often mentioned possibility is that stress-induced reduction in lymphoid or reticuloendothelial system function may exacerbate cancer (see for example Fitzmaurice, 1988; Riley, 1981). It would be surprising if this could not occur, but there are reasons to doubt that it is the only mediating sequence of importance, one reason being the very existence of tumor inhibition by stress. We can list some of the other possibilities which have been mentioned (Fitzmaurice, 1988; Justice, 1985; Newberry *et al.*, 1984; Pettingale, 1985; Sklar and Anisman, 1981).

The stress–immune–cancer connection may not be simple. There is reason to believe that stress can enhance immune function, and also that immune function can sometimes stimulate neoplastic processes. Moreover, there are several mediational possibilities that do not involve the immune system in any obvious way. There is evidence that stress or stress-responsive hormones can interfere with DNA repair, alter the metabolism of carcinogens or procarcinogens, modulate the expression of viral genes, affect the proliferation rates of hormone-responsive tumor cells, stimulate growth factor production, reduce the release of vitamin A from the liver, alter the availability and distribution of energy substrates, retard angiogenesis and reduce secretion of collagenase by tumor cells. Note that among the seemingly plausible mechanisms for stress effects are several that might inhibit cancer development.

There has been little precise information regarding which mediating sequences are actually responsible for stress effects on experimental cancers. One reason for this lack is the difficulty of obtaining convincing evidence. The most useful data would demonstrate that a stress effect fails to occur under a blockade of the proposed mediator. However, the blockade can be difficult or impossible to carry out with precision, and the results can present problems of interpretation.

Tumor system characteristics

By "tumor system" we must mean a particular combination of induction procedure, tumor and host, because variations in any of these could alter response of the cancer to stress and because often they cannot be studied independently. One reason for suspecting tumor system differences in tumor stress response is that different mediating processes are likely to be operating. When cancer is induced by the inoculation of oncogenic virus particles, for example, host antiviral defenses may be important, but proximal processes which alter the metabolism of chemical carcinogens are irrelevant. When transplanted cells are utilized tumor initiation, and probably many aspects of progression, do not take place in the host being studied and so cannot be affected by the host's exposure to stressful conditions.

Other relevant differences are largely independent of the general method of tumor induction. If a tumor does not metastasize, such factors as the susceptibility of vascular walls to penetration by tumor cells are relatively unimportant. Alterations in angiogenesis are important only for solid tumors. Modulation of antitumor immune function is irrelevant for tumors which the lymphoreticular system cannot recognize. Hormonal changes which occur under stress could have different direct effects on different types of tumors. Effects which are peculiar to chronic postinduction stress cannot occur with tumors which quickly kill their hosts.

Up to the early 1980s few clear comparisons of tumor systems in terms of tumor response to stress were available. One of the best examples was by Albert (1967), who reported that crowding strongly inhibited the development of spontaneous mammary tumors in mice but strongly stimulated the development of mesenchymal cancers. Riley and colleagues (Riley, 1966; Riley *et al.*, 1982) found that infection of mice with lactate dehydrogenase elevating virus failed to affect a transplanted histocompatible melanoma, stimulated development of a similar but partially histoincompatible melanoma and a lymphoma, and inhibited the development of mammary tumors. Such results provide at least some basis for thinking that tumor system differences contribute to the diversity of outcomes under stress (Newberry *et al.*, 1985).

In summary, the earlier studies and discussions taken as a whole suggested (1) that stress can promote, inhibit or fail to affect cancer, (2) that stressor differences, particularly differences in stressor timing, are partly responsible for these divergent outcomes, (3) that, although there are a variety of plausible mediators for stress effects, none of them had clear empirical support, and (4) that the characteristics of tumor systems probably help to determine what, if any, effect stress will have.

STUDIES OF STRESS AND EXPERIMENTAL CANCERS

The discussion below is organized by tumor systems, beginning with chemically induced tumors and turning to transplanted tumors. When two types of tumor induction were used in the same article we discuss them together. All relationships mentioned below were reported by the original authors to be statistically significant at the 0.05 level or better unless indicated otherwise, although that does not mean that the statistical tests utilized were the most appropriate ones.

Although we used a systematic literature search, we doubt that we discovered all of the relevant research, and we were unable to obtain a few articles. We found no articles relating stress to cancers induced by the inoculation of oncogenic virions into the hosts. We eliminated from consideration studies of stress and *in vitro* cytotoxicity using tumor cell lines as target cells. We did not search for studies of exercise and cancer. Exercise can certainly be considered physiologically stressful, particularly in poorly conditioned organisms. However, it is usually considered an anomalous stressor at best because it has been associated with health benefits and psychological wellbeing. Exercise experiments have been performed and have tended to show an inhibition of tumor by exercise (for example, Kritchevsky, 1990).

Chemically induced cancers

The DMBA rat mammary tumor (DMBA-RMt), induced by feeding or intravenous injection of 7,12-dimethylbenz(a)anthracene, seems to be the most common chemically induced tumor used in stress studies. Earlier research typically reported inhibition of these tumors by stressful conditions (Newberry, 1981b).

Goldman and Vogel (1984) investigated mild restraint, beginning approximately midway through a five-week series of DMBA instillations. Tumor development was assessed after three months. Restraint significantly reduced tumor weight but did not affect tumor incidence (percentage of positive animals) or number of tumors per animal. Earlier studies using longer restraint durations have found restraint to reduce the incidence and number of DMBA-RMt (Newberry, 1978; Newberry *et al.*, 1976). Goldman and Vogel also assessed the adenylate cyclase response of corpus striatum tissue to stimulation by dopamine. They found that the stressed animals had stronger adenylate cyclase responses in addition to lower tumor weights. In a second experiment, they compared strains and substrains of rats on both DMBA-RMt development and the cyclase response. Long–Evans rats were resistant to tumor development and showed the strongest adenylate cyclase responses. They speculated that stress acts through neural controls on hormones to which the DMBA-RMt is sensitive.

Newberry and Mactutus (unpublished results) compared the response of the DMBA-RMt to mild predictable restraint (Newberry, 1978) with the response to a varied, unpredictable regimen in which the type of stimulation, its time of onset and its duration all varied. (The study was undertaken partly in response to a suggestion by Henry *et al.* (1975) that unpredictable stress would enhance tumor development generally and referred specifically to the inhibition of the DMBA-RMt by predictable stressors.) Newberry and Mactutus found that the unpredictable treatment and the predictable restraint both reduced tumor counts, and did so to an equal degree. A parallel experiment was performed under very similar conditions with the much more slowly developing spontaneous (viral) C3H/HeJ mouse mammary tumor. This experiment gave a different pattern of results: predictable restraint had no effect, and the varied unpredictable regimen enhanced tumor development.

Later studies followed up on the failure of unpredictable stress to promote the DMBA-RMt and lead us to conclude that conditions known to promote cancer in other systems will inhibit the development of this tumor. Boyle (1984) varied the severity of restraint stress. He compared a no-stress condition to the 12 h daily restraint used by Newberry and Mactutus and to a mixture of 12, 24, and 36 h restraint periods which pilot work suggested was as severe as could be used. Tumor counts declined with increased restraint severity (by about 90% in the most severe condition). As glucocorticoids have frequently been mentioned as mediators of stress-induced tumor enhancement and because adaptation to long-term stressor exposure could prevent chronic glucocorticoid elevations from occurring, Gerstenberger (1985) studied the effects of dexamethasone beginning five days after DMBA administration. Dexamethasone from 5 to 75 μg/kg/day reduced tumor counts. All doses were sufficient to reduce weight gain, and the higher doses reduced leukocyte counts.

Gerstenberger's findings suggest that glucocorticoid-induced immunosuppression is probably not a factor in the DMBA-RMt. Data from Madden *et al.*(1988) supports this. They found that 33 days of restraint reduced DMBA-RMt development but did not affect thymocyte or splenocyte responses to mitogens. Parenthetically, they also found that 33 days of aerobic training had no effect on DMBA-RMt despite being sufficient to increase cardiac size.

Chang *et al.* (1986) studied the effects of superior cervical ganglion-ectomy, surgical blinding-plus-anosmia, and their combination on DMBA-RMt. Their intent was to investigate the role of the pineal gland in mammary tumorigenesis, but no sham surgery was performed. Both ganglionectomy and the three-way surgery reduced tumor counts. The three-way surgery also reduced tumor incidence and weight. The treatments seemed to be effective in altering pineal function, but it appears that the effect of surgical stress outweighed any influence of those changes.

Effects of housing were investigated by Steplewski *et al.* (1987) using both DMBA-RMt and a transplanted mammary adenocarcinoma. Some animals (group G/I) were switched from group housing to individual housing (apparently at the time of tumor induction) and developed larger tumors than did animals maintained in groups from weaning. Additionally, in the DMBA study, animals housed individually from weaning (group I) had dramatically lower tumor weights than did the others. The absence of tumor inhibition in the I condition with the transplanted tumor suggests that these systems differ with respect to some aspect of cancer psychobiology.

There are studies of chemically induced tumors other than mammary: Andrianopoulos *et al.* (1988) provided evidence that 1,2-dimethyl-hydrazine (DMH) colon carcinogenesis can be inhibited by a severe "activity stress" in which animals are allowed food for only 1 h per day and are simultaneously given access to a running wheel. Activity stress, either after 10 weeks of DMH or both during and after that period, reduced the proportion of animals developing colon tumors. A second experiment demonstrated that activity stress can moderate some of the early cytologic and histologic changes occurring after a single DMH administration.

The development of estrogen-induced pituitary prolactinoma was inhibited by stress in an experiment by Gottesfeld and Liehr (1987). Restraint (1 h daily at random times of day, beginning the day after implantation of estradiol pellets) significantly reduced pituitary hyperplasia. It also reduced serum prolactin levels, but not significantly. Both restraint and estradiol dramatically reduced animal body weights.

Not all studies of chemically induced neoplasia have produced evidence for stress modulation of tumor development. Cohen *et al.* (1984) investigated neoplasms induced by N-methyl-N'-nitro-N-nitrosoguanidine (MNNG) given in drinking water. They were interested in the possibility that agents which affect the gastric lining might alter gastric carcinogenesis. The stressor was restraint (24 h, twice per week for up to 80 weeks). Overall tumor incidence did not differ in the MNNG + stress and MNNG-alone groups. (No statistical analyses were reported.) Aspirin seemed to stimulate tumor development; thus a stressor having severe gastric effects might have potentiated MNNG carcinogenesis. Additionally, stress and aspirin reduced water consumption, and therefore the doses of MNNG received by animals in those conditions were lower than those received by animals in the MNNG-only condition.

Another negative result was reported by Sotelo *et al.* (1989), who investigated stress and brain tumors produced by prenatal exposure to ethyl nitrosourea (ENU). One group of rats was exposed to daily sessions of signalled footshock in a group cage. The dependent variable was the age at which clinical signs (unspecified) of CNS tumors appeared. Those ages were virtually identical for the stress and no-stress groups.

We found one study involving spontaneous tumors of unknown etiology (Wozniak *et al.*, 1982). We include it here because the tumors were not transplanted. Using C57BL/6J mice, Wozniak *et al.* crossed frontal pole transection with cold stress given on five occasions from 2.5 to 25 months of age. Longevity was not affected by either treatment. However, loglinear analyses suggested that cold stress influenced the cause of death. Stress was negatively related to reticulum cell sarcomas but positively related to pulmonary metastatic tumors originating from them. This study suggests that stress effects on cancer need not have implications for longevity. It also suggests that stress effects on primary tumors can be opposite to those on metastasis.

Transplanted cancers

As was the case with chemically induced cancers, mammary tumors are well represented among those investigated using transplantation models. We have already mentioned the transplanted mammary tumor experiment performed by Steplewski *et al.* (1987); another report (Steplewski *et al.*, 1985) concerned the possibility that recovery from stress is protective. Female Lewis rats received mammary adenocarcinoma cells subcutaneously. Animals were restrained for 11 days post-transplantation; one group was then sacrificed and a second was left undisturbed for 12 additional days. No-restraint controls were sacrificed at the same times. Restraint delayed the appearance of palpable tumors. Tumor weight did not differ significantly immediately after the 11 days of restraint, but after 12 days of recovery the stressed animals had lower tumor weights than the controls. No group was restrained for the full 23 days, and it is thus not possible to tell whether stress or recovery from it produced the ultimately smaller tumors of the restrained rats. Steplewski *et al.* (1985) also examined several aspects of immune function. Among their findings were higher neutrophil and suppressor cell numbers in recovered stressed animals and lower NK cell activity among controls at the second sampling time.

Two reports concerned surgical stress and metastases from transplanted mammary cancers. Takekoshi *et al.* (1984) used MRMT-1 cells in young Sprague–Dawley rats. The treatment conditions were tumor excision 14 days postinoculation, and the same excision plus laparotomy. Parallel groups received no tumor. Some animals from each of the six groups were sacrificed after three days. The rest were followed for 80 days or until death. At three days post-transplantation, laparotomy reduced PHA response even in comparison to tumor excision. Evidence favoring a role for stress immunodepression was found in Winn's assay, in which spleno-cytes from the study animals were inoculated into irradiated recipients along with fresh tumor cells. Tumor takes in this assay were higher with spleen cells from laparotomized animals than with spleen cells from unstressed or tumor-excised animals. Of the tumor-bearing animals followed until death or 80 days, a higher percentage of the laparotomized rats had lung metastases. A similar study (Tanemura *et al.*, 1982) incorporated a non-specific immunostimulant (OK-432) as well as laparotomy. OK-432 given before tumor excision and laparotomy prevented the increase in lung metastasis produced by laparotomy alone. Importantly from the standpoint of drawing conclusions about the mechanisms of stress effects, OK-432 did not affect metastasis incidence in the absence of laparotomy.

Lewis *et al.* (1983), who used the rat 13762B ascites mammary tumor, crossed subcutaneous implantation of naltrexone pellets and, 10 days after pellet implantation, four daily sessions of a footshock schedule known to induce opioid-mediated analgesia. Tumor inoculation was carried out on the day of the last shock session. Shock reduced survival time, and this effect was blocked by naltrexone. Moreover, naltrexone had no effect in non-shock animals. In another study by this group (Lewis *et al.*, 1983/84) morphine influenced 13762B in a manner similar to footshock, except that tolerance developed only to the morphine. The fact that opportunity for adaptation to footshock did not alter its tumor-enhancing effect is in contrast to some other findings (see Sklar and Anisman, 1981).

We located two reports on the rat Walker 256 tumor. One study (Visintainer *et al.*, 1982) compared the effects of escapable and inescapable shock. One shock session was given, the day after tumor transplantation. Tumor rejection was lower in the inescapable shock group than in the escapable shock group or no-shock controls. These results, with those of Sklar and Anisman (1979), suggest that controllability can be an important variable. It is worth remembering, however, that many findings of tumor inhibition by stress have been with uncontrollable stressors.

Simon *et al.* (1980) introduced Walker 256 cells intravenously to simulate metastasis. Surgical stress increased lung metastases. Stimulation of the midbrain periaqueductal gray (PAG) also promoted metastases, but the effect was not antagonized by naloxone given shortly before the stimulation. Since PAG stimulation activates opioid systems, its stimulation of tumor would be consistent with the results of Lewis *et al.* (1983), but the fact that naloxone failed to block the Simon *et al.* effect makes the situation unclear.

Two reports by Hattori *et al.* dealt with immunostimulants and laparothoracotomy in rats given intravenous injections of Sato lung cancer cells. In Hattori *et al.* (1982a), the surgical stress seemed clearly to increase lung metastases, although no statistical tests of this effect were reported. Two immunostimulants, lentinan and levamisole, inhibited metastasis formation in comparison with surgery alone. In a second group of experiments (1982b), the dependent variables related to survival time. It again seemed clear that laparothoracotomy had an adverse effect, but only one drug – this time OK-432 – mitigated the effect. It is of interest that the immunostimulant with the clearest effect on survival was not the one with the clearest effect on metastasis.

Pollock *et al.* (1984) studied the effect of amputation on lung metastases from mouse 3LL cells injected into a hind footpad. Amputation of the non-tumor-bearing hind limb at seven days postinoculation increased the incidence of metastasis significantly. Amputation of the tumor-bearing limb at seven days reduced the incidence, presumably because it reduced the release of metastatic cells or the secretion of tumor-promoting substances by the primary. Pollock *et al.* also reported studies on *in vitro* NK cell activity in which amputation and 3LL reduced cytotoxicity.

Giraldi *et al.* (1989) studied various combinations of protective housing, rotation (Riley, 1981), and intraperitoneal (i.p.) saline injection as these affected the size of a primary Lewis lung tumor and lung metastases. A total of 10 treatment conditions was used. Their piecemeal statistical analysis is confusing because of the number of treatment combinations. Protective housing had no effect on the primary but retarded metastasis. Rotation stress stimulated both primary growth and metastasis in animals which lived in protective housing and were not given the stress of saline injections. Saline injections stimulated metastasis, but not the primary, in protected housing animals not subject to rotation stress. The most interesting result of this study is that the stressors which affect primary tumors can be different from those which affect metastasis.

Temoshok *et al.* (1987) took the approach of examining behavioral individual differences. Female hamsters acclimatized to social housing were subjected to mechanical shaking beginning 13 days before tumor transplantation. This stressor hastened the appearance of tumors. A measure of behavioral activation taken eight days after stressor onset was positively correlated with delay in tumor appearance among the stressed animals but not among no-stress controls. The possibility of interactions between psychological individual differences and stressors in predicting disease has been prominent in the human literature (Newberry *et al.*, 1991) and is worth further investigation in animal models.

A study of metastases from mouse melanoma was undertaken by Stoll and Chadha (1989). They found no effect of sham splenectomy or actual splenectomy on lung metastases from cells injected intravenously two weeks after the surgery. The "sham" animals may have recovered from surgery too completely for any effect to occur, but the absence of a splenectomy effect is more surprising. The authors suggested that it might be because the balance of immune system suppressor, helper, and effector functions was unchanged.

In a study by Turney *et al.* (1986) one session of footshock, apparently rather similar to that used by Sklar and Anisman (1979), failed to affect development of P815 mastocytoma in DBA/2j mice. However, although the statistical analyses were not the most appropriate, the data did suggest that footshock blocked the antitumor effect of killed *Corynebacterium parvum* in group-housed mice. Tourney *et al.* noted that their *C. parvum* findings raise questions about the relationship of psychological variables to the success of immunotherapies.

Zöller *et al.* (1989) found that laparotomy hastens death from BSp73 pancreatic cancers. It appears to decrease the latency to palpability of primary tumors (footpad) and increase the incidence of metastases. Accompanying data on immune function (cell numbers and cytotoxicity) provided evidence for both immunodepression and, usually beginning some days after surgery, immunoenhancement. *C. parvum* had antitumor effects, even in surgically stressed animals, but the pattern was consistent with the possibility of an independent effect rather than a blocking of the stress effect.

Four strains of Morris hepatoma, inoculated into BUF rats, were studied by Blatteis *et al.* (1980). Heat and simulated high altitude reduced the weights of all four tumors at 32–40 days post transplantation. Cold stress did not affect tumor mass but did reduce survival time with one of the slowly growing tumor lines. Data on food consumption, body weight growth, and tumor growth suggested to Blatteis *et al.* that differences in energy substrate availability and utilization might have contributed to their findings.

Greenberg *et al.* (1984) reported a series of studies on tailshock, stress hormones, and host ability to clear radiolabeled mouse tumor cells. They provided evidence that the clearance of label reflected death of tumor cells and was NK-mediated. Several of their specific findings are of interest: a 15 min shock session retarded elimination of NK-sensitive YAC 1.3 and SL2-5 lymphomas, but not of NK-insensitive P815-16 mastocytoma; opioid antagonists increased SL2-5 elimination in shocked animals; lengthening the shock session to 60 min eliminated the shock effect, and three days of restraint sessions prior to shock enhanced host elimination of SL2-5. Treatment with ACTH over two days also improved the hosts' response to these cells.

Six days of rotation stress, presumably initiated just before tumor transplantation, enhanced development of allogeneic 6C3HED lymphosarcoma (Kandil and Borysenko, 1988). Rotation also reduced *in vitro* cytolytic activity against 6C3HED cells over the first two weeks of the experiment. Interleukin-2 activity (tumor-free animals) was affected similarly by rotation. Corticosterone levels were increased in rotated mice (tumor-free), but the increase appeared to occur only during the 10 days following termination of the stress regimen. Plasma β-endorphin was not affected. (We should note that specific statistical comparisons were not provided in this report.)

Two reports on transplanted sarcomas failed to suggest a general effect of surgical stress. Radosevic-Stasic *et al.* (1989) studied allogeneic Sarcoma I in mice. Laparotomy (under 3 min halothane anesthesia) served as the stressor. Some animals with or without surgery were given 1 h of halothane anesthesia. Tumor rejection was delayed in the halothane-only condition but not by surgery or surgery-plus-halothane. Keller (1983) found in rats with D-12 fibrosarcoma that, although removal of the tumor-bearing leg increased the incidence of lymph node metastases, removal of the other leg did not. Neither splenectomy, sham splenectomy, nor sham hepatectomy influenced metastasis incidence, but partial hepatectomy increased it. Keller mentioned growth factor production by regenerating liver as a possible mechanism for the hepatectomy effect.

Sapolsky *et al.* (1985) implicated aging in stress-induced tumor enhancement. They injected virus-transformed fetal cells into young and aged Fischer rats. The stressor was seven days of widely varying treatments given several times per day. One group of young rats was given corticosterone after each stressor to stimulate the slower poststress return of corticosterone to baseline in aged animals. Stress increased tumor take rates in both young and old rats, and greatly increased tumor weight in old rats. Poststressor corticosterone in young stressed animals produced the same large tumor sizes that occurred in aged stressed animals.

CONCLUSIONS

There is still much confusion in this area. The research does not seem focused enough to get at critical issues effectively. It sometimes seems as though the reviews by LaBarba (1970), Peters and Mason (1979), Riley (1979), Sklar and Anisman (1981) and Justice (1985) had never been written. Another source of ambiguity (and frustration) is the poor quality of statistical analysis. The absence of and piecemeal use of statistics prevent readers from learning enough about the results of many of the experiments we read. Therefore, the research itself and the way it was reported means that any attempt to draw systematic conclusions can reflect little more than guesswork.

That having been said, we proceed with our guesses. Our overall view, as summarized at the beginning of this chapter, is largely unchanged. We find no reason to abjure our contention that stressor variables and tumor system variables are important, and that mediating mechanisms are poorly understood – even though a few things do seem slightly clearer.

With regard to stressor characteristics, we see little progress. There is evidence in the recent research for differential effects of different stressor regimens, but there is too little of it and as a whole it is not very systematic. Visintainer *et al.* (1982) confirmed the importance of shock controllability (cf. Sklar and Anisman, 1979). Greenberg *et al.* (1984) supplied additional evidence that opportunity for adaptation can eliminate or reverse the tumorigenic effects of acute stress. Studies suggesting more qualitative stressor differences include those by Blatteis *et al.* (1980), Giraldi *et al.* (1989), Radosevic-Stasic *et al.* (1989) and Wozniak *et al.* (1982), but their methods were too different to allow general conclusions.

As far as tumor system differences are concerned, one thing stands out – that chemically induced cancers are more likely to be inhibited, and transplanted tumors and metastasis are more likely to be promoted, by stress. Of course, this difference could reflect the particular systems that happened to be studied or such factors as the length of stressor exposure (usually longer with the chemically induced tumors). Data from Newberry and Mactutus (unpublished), Steplewski *et al.* (1987) and Blatteis *et al.* (1980) suggest that whether cancer is stimulated, inhibited, or unaffected in relation to controls may depend non-additively on both the tumor system and the stress regimen used. Blatteis *et al.* (1980) and Greenberg *et al.* (1984) reported differences between transplanted tumors in responses to the same stressors. Data suggesting that primary tumors and metastasis may respond differently were to be found in the reports by Wozniak *et al.* (1982) and Giraldi *et al.* (1989). The fact that removal of a tumor-bearing limb stimulated metastases from rat D-12 fibrosarcoma (Keller, 1983) and inhibited those from mouse 3LL (Pollock *et al.*, 1984) may also be relevant. A role for host differences was demonstrated by Sapolsky *et al.* (1985) and Temoshok *et al.* (1987).

Our belief that stress-induced immunodepression can mediate tumor enhancement is growing, albeit slowly. Among the important data are those of Tanemura *et al.* (1982) in which an immunostimulant prevented a stress effect without having an effect alone. Also significant are the findings of Greenberg *et al.* (1984), in which NK mediation was strongly suggested, and of Takekoshi *et al.* (1984) in which an *in vivo* assay showed lower cytotoxicity against the type of tumor cells used in the main study when the effector cells came from stressed animals.

Another good lead favors the involvement of endogenous opioids (Greenberg *et al.*, 1984; Lewis *et al.*, 1983; Simon *et al.*, 1980). There is also some evidence for the involvement of other neuro-hormonal systems (Goldman and Vogel, 1984) and of gastrointestinal changes (Andrianopoulos *et al.*, 1988; Cohen *et al.*, 1984).

A chapter this brief can do little more than sensitize readers to the issues and direct them to a few references. We could not undertake to relate stress studies to the detailed tumor biology of particular systems, or to speculate at length on the meaning of every experiment in relation to every other. Nearly everything about relationships between stress and cancer is cloudy, and the seeming complexity of the phenomena will probably preclude its clearing up soon.

REFERENCES

Albert, Z. (1967) Effect of number of animals per cage on the development of spontaneous neoplasms. In Conalty, M.L. (ed.) *Husbandry of Laboratory Animals*. Academic Press, New York.

Andrianopoulos, G.D., Nelson, R.L., Misumi, A., Bombeck, C.T. and Lloyd, M.N. (1988) Effect of activity stress on experimental rat colon carcinogenesis: early histopathologic changes and colon tumor induction. *Cancer Det. Prev.*, **13**, 31–39.

Blatteis, C.M., Cardoso, S.S., Narayanan, T.J., Hughes, M.H. and Morris, H.P. (1980) Depressed growth of Morris hepatomas in altitude- and heat-stressed but not in cold-stressed Buffalo rats. *JNCI*, **64**, 1451–1458.

Boyle, D.A. (1984) *Stress Severity and Development of the 7,12-Dimethylbenz(a)anthracene-induced Rat Mammary Tumor*. Master of Arts Thesis, Kent State University.

Chang, N., Tseng, M.T. and Spaulding, T.S. (1986) Induction and growth of mammary tumors after superior cervical ganglionectomy in sighted and blind-anosmic rats. *Life Sci.*, **38**, 1821–1826.

Cohen, A., Geller, S.A., Horowitz, I., Toth, L.S. and Werther, J.L. (1984) Experimental models for gastric leiomyosarcoma: the effects of N-methyl-N'-nitro-N-nitrosoguanidine in combination with stress, aspirin, or sodium taurocholate. *Cancer*, **53**, 1088–1092.

Fitzmaurice, M.A. (1988) Physiological relationships among stress, viruses, and cancer in experimental animals. *Intern. J. Neurosci.*, **39**, 307–324.

Fox, B.H. (1988) Psychogenic factors in cancer, especially its incidence. In Maes, S., Spielberger, C.D., Defares, P.B. and Sarason, I.G. (eds) *Topics in Health Psychology*. Wiley, New York.

Gerstenberger, T.J. (1985) *The Effects of Dexamethasone and Deoxycorticosterone Acetate on 7,12-Dimethylbenz(a)anthracene-induced Rat Mammary Tumor*. Master of Arts Thesis, Kent State University.

Giraldi, T., Perissin, L., Zorzet, S., Piccini, P. and Rapozzi, V. (1989) Effects of stress on tumor growth and metastasis in mice bearing Lewis lung carcinoma. *Eur. J. Cancer Clin. Oncol.*, **25**, 1583–1588.

Goldman, P.R. and Vogel, W.H. (1984) Striatal dopamine-stimulated adenylate cyclase activity reflects susceptibility of rats to 7,12-dimethylbenz(a) anthracene-induced mammary tumor development. *Carcinogenesis*, **5**, 971–973.

Gottesfeld, Z. and Liehr, J.G. (1987) Chronic exposure to random restraint stress retards the development of estrogen-induced pituitary prolactinoma. *Neurosci. Lett.*, **80**, 44–48.

Greenberg, A.H., Dyck, D.G. and Sandler, L.S. (1984) Opponent processes, neurohormones and natural resistance. In Fox, B.H. and Newberry, B.H. (eds) *Impact of Psychoendocrine Systems in Cancer and Immunity*, C.J. Hogrefe, Lewistown, New York.

Hattori, T., Hamai, Y., Ikeda, T., Takiyama, W., Hirai, T. and Miyoshi, Y. (1982a) Inhibitory effects of immunopotentiators on the enhancement of lung metastases induced by operative stress in rats. *Gann*, **73**, 132–135.

Hattori, T., Hamai, Y., Ikeda, T., Takiyama, W., Hirai, T. and Miyoshi, Y. (1982b) Survival time of tumor-bearing rats as related to operative stress and immunopotentiators. *Jpn. J. Surg.*, **12**, 143–147.

Henry, J.P., Stephens, P.M. and Watson, F.M. (1975) Force breeding, social disorder, and mammary tumor formation in CBA/USC mouse colonies: a pilot study. *Psychosom. Med.*, **37**, 277–283.

Justice, A. (1985) Review of the effects of stress on cancer in laboratory animals: importance of time of stress application and type of tumor. *Psychol. Bull.*, **98**, 108–138.

Kandil, O. and Borysenko, M. (1988) Stress-induced decline in immune responsiveness in C3H/HeJ mice: relation to endocrine alterations and tumor growth. *Brain Behav. Immun.*, **2**, 32–49.

Keller, R. (1983) Elicitation of macroscopic metastases via surgery: various forms of surgical intervention differ in their induction of metastatic outgrowth. *Invasion Metastasis*, **3**, 183–192.

Kritchevsky, D. (1990) Influence of caloric restriction and exercise on tumorigenesis in rats. *Proc. Soc. Exp. Biol. Med.*, **193**, 35–38.

LaBarba, R.C. (1970) Experiential and environmental factors in cancer: a review of research with animals. *Psychosom. Med.*, **32**, 259–276.

Lewis, J.W., Shavit, Y., Terman, G.W., Nelson, L.R., Gale, R.P. and Liebeskind, J.C. (1983) Apparent involvement of opioid peptides in stress-induced enhancement of tumor growth. *Peptides*, **4**, 635–638.

Lewis, J.W., Shavit, Y., Terman, G.W., Gale, R.P. and Liebeskind, J.C. (1983/84) Stress and morphine affect survival of rats challenged with a mammary ascites tumor (MAT 13762B). *Nat. Immun. Cell Growth Reg.*, **3**, 43–50.

Madden, J.E., Baldwin, D.R., Chu, E., Gerstenberger, T.J., Noorbakhsh, H., Steele, J.H., Stevenson, J.R. and Newberry, B.H. (1988) Stress, mammary tumors, mitogen response and cardiac size. In Lobo, A. and Tres, A. (eds) *Psicosomatica y Cancer*. Ministerio de Sanidad y Consumo, Madrid.

Newberry, B.H. (1978) Restraint-induced inhibition of 7,12-dimethylbenz(a)-anthracene-induced mammary tumors: relation to stages of tumor development. *JNCI*, **61**, 725–729.

Newberry, B.H. (1981a) Effects of presumably stressful stimulation (PSS) on the development of animal tumors: some issues. In Weiss, S.M., Herd, J.A. and Fox, B.H. (eds) *Perspectives on Behavioral Medicine*. Academic Press, New York.

Newberry, B.H. (1981b) Stress and mammary cancer. In Bammer, K. and Newberry, B.H. (eds) *Stress and Cancer*. C.J. Hogrefe, Toronto.

Newberry, B.H., Gildow, J., Wogan, J. and Reese, R.L. (1976) Inhibition of Huggins tumors by forced restraint. *Psychosom. Med.*, **38**, 155–162.

Newberry, B.H., Liebelt, A.G. and Boyle, D.A. (1984) Variables in behavioral oncology: overview and assessment of current issues. In Fox, B.H. and Newberry, B.H. (eds) *Impact of Psychoendocrine Systems in Cancer and Immunity.* C.J. Hogrefe, Lewiston, New York.

Newberry, B.H., Gerstenberger, T.J., Madden, J.E. and Newberry, D.L. (1985) Evidence for tumor system specificity in experimental tumor response to "stress". In Lindfors, O., Lehvonen, R., Vauhkonen, M.-J. and Achté, K. (eds) *Psychosomatics of Cancer*, Psykiatrian Tutkimussaatio, Helsinki.

Newberry, B.H., Jaikins-Madden, J.E. and Gerstenberger, T.J. (1991) *A Holistic Conceptualization of Stress and Disease.* AMS, New York.

Peters, L.J. and Mason, K.A. (1979) Influence of stress on experimental cancer. In Stoll, B.A. (ed.) *Mind and Cancer Prognosis*. Wiley, Chichester.

Pettingale, K.W. (1985) Towards a psychobiological model of cancer: biological considerations. *Soc. Sci. Med.*, **20**, 779–787.

Pollock, R.E., Babcock, G.F., Romsdahl, M.M. and Nishioka, K. (1984) Surgical stress-mediated suppression of murine natural killer cell cytotoxicity. *Cancer Res.*, **44**, 3888–3891.

Radosevic-Stasic, B., Udovic-Sirola, M., Stojanov, L., Ribaric, L. and Rukavina, D. (1989) Growth of allogeneic sarcoma in mice subjected to halothane anesthesia and/or surgical stress. *Anesth. Analg.*, **69**, 570–574.

Riley, V. (1966) Spontaneous mammary tumors: decrease in incidence of mice infected with an enzyme-elevating virus. *Science*, **153**, 1657–1658.

Riley, V. (1979) Cancer and stress: overview and critique. *Cancer Det. Prev.*, **2**, 163–195.

Riley, V. (1981) Psychoneuroendocrine influences on immunocompetence and neoplasia. *Science*, **212**, 1100–1109.

Riley, V., Fitzmaurice, M.A. and Spackman, D.H. (1982) Immunocompetence and neoplasia: role of anxiety stress. In Levy S.M. (ed.) *Biological Mediators of Behavior and Disease: Neoplasia*. Elsevier, New York.

Sapolsky, R.M. and Donnelly, T.M. (1985) Vulnerability to stress-induced tumor growth increases with age in rats: role of glucocorticoids. *Endocrinology*, **117**, 662–666.

Simon, R.H., Lovett, E.J. III, Tomaszek, D. and Lundy, J. (1980) Electrical stimulation of the midbrain mediates metastatic tumor growth. *Science*, **209**, 1132–1133.

Sklar, L.S. and Anisman, H. (1979) Stress and coping factors influence tumor growth. *Science*, **205**, 513–515.

Sklar, L.S. and Anisman, H. (1980) Social stress influences tumor growth. *Psychosom. Med.*, **42**, 347–365.

Sklar, L.S. and Anisman, H. (1981) Stress and cancer. *Psychol. Bull.*, **89**, 369–406.

Sklar, L.S., Bruto, V. and Anisman, H. (1981) Adaptation to the tumor-enhancing effects of stress. *Psychosom. Med.*, **43**, 331–342.

Sotelo, J., Palencia, G., Rosas, N. and Perez, R. (1989) Effect of chronic stress on ENU-induced tumors. *Biol. Psychiatry*, **26**, 690–694.

Steplewski, Z., Vogel, W.H., Ehya, H., Poropatich, C. and Smith, J.M. (1985) Effects of restraint stress on inoculated tumor growth and immune response in rats. *Cancer Res.*, **45**, 5128–5133.

Steplewski, Z., Goldman, P.R. and Vogel, W.H. (1987) Effect of housing stress on the formation and development of tumors in rats. *Cancer Lett.*, **34**, 257–261.

Stoll, H.L. III and Chadha, K.C. (1989) Effect of splenectomy upon the growth of B16-F10 melanoma and its relation to the interferon system. *J. Surg. Oncol.*, **40**, 79–84.

Takekoshi, T., Sakata, K., Kunieda, T., Saji, S., Tanemura, H. and Yamamoto, S. (1984) Facilitation of tumor metastasis by operative stress and participation of cell-mediated immunity. *Oncology*, **41**, 245–251.

Tanemura, H., Sakata, K., Kunieda, T., Saji, S., Yamamoto, S. and Takekoshi, T. (1982) Influences of operative stress on cell-mediated immunity and on tumor metastasis and their prevention by nonspecific immunotherapy: experimental studies in rats. *J. Surg. Oncol.*, **21**, 189–195.

Temoshok, L., Peeke, H.V.S., Mehard, C.W., Axelsson, K. and Sweet, D.M. (1987) Stress–behavior interactions in hamster tumor growth. *Ann. N.Y. Acad. Sci.*, **496**, 501–509.

Turney, T.H., Harmsen, A.G. and Jarpe, M.A. (1986) Modification of the antitumor action of *Corynebacterium parvum* by stress. *Physiol. Behav.*, **37**, 555–558.

Visintainer, M.A., Volpicelli, J.R. and Seligman, M.E.P. (1982) Tumor rejection in rats after inescapable or escapable shock. *Science*, **216**, 437–439.

Wozniak, D., Finger, S., Blumenthal, H. and Poland, R. (1982) Brain damage, stress, and life span: an experimental study. *J. Gerontol.*, **37**, 161–168.

Zöller, M., Heumann, U., Betzler, M., Stimmel, H. and Matzku, S. (1989) Depression of nonadaptive immunity after surgical stress: influence on metastatic spread. *Invasion Metastasis*, **9**, 46–68.

Section II

PSYCHOSOCIAL AND PERSONALITY FACTORS

3

Psychological Factors in Cancer Prognosis

MAGGIE WATSON* and AMANDA RAMIREZ†
*Cancer Research Campaign, Psychological Medicine Group,
The Royal Marsden Hospital and Institute of Cancer Research, London and
Surrey, UK and †Imperial Cancer Research Fund, Clinical Oncology Unit and
Division of Psychiatry, Guy's Hospital, London, UK

He made her melancholy, sad, and heavy;
and so she died; had she being light like you,
of such a merry, nimble, stirring spirit,
she might ha' been a grandma ere she died;
and so may you, for a light heart lives long.
                                        Love's Labour's Lost *(V.ii, 14–18)*
                                        William Shakespeare

In Fox's excellent review (Fox, 1983) he suggests that it is more plausible to expect that psychological factors influence the course rather than the onset of disease. Examining psychological factors in prognosis, after the diagnosis is known, also represents a more manageable route to answering questions about their importance, or otherwise, in cancer. Examination does not require large-scale prospective studies and it is feasible to obtain answers over a relatively short period of time. The biology of carcinogenesis may not be very amenable to influence by psychological variables (Pettingale, 1985; Waterfield *et al.*, 1983). By taking already diagnosed patients and following their progress, prospectively, the possible influence of psychological factors, and coping in particular, may be determined. The main question posed by such studies is not who is at risk of cancer but who does best, or worst, once the disease is diagnosed.

Cancer and Stress: Psychological, Biological and Coping Studies
Edited by C. L. Cooper and M. Watson. © 1991 John Wiley & Sons Ltd

IS THERE A CANCER PERSONALITY?

In the film *Manhattan* the character played by Woody Allen confesses that he never shows his anger, just "grows a tumor", reflecting the popular idea that cancer patients are emotionally inhibited. The idea that the person most likely to get cancer is somehow emotionally suppressed is by no means new. A great deal of anecdotal evidence has been cited to support the notion of mental states influencing disease course by either direct or indirect methods. When considering the role of psychological factors in cancer an analogy can be drawn with the heart disease literature.

We know that there is a coronary-prone behaviour type, and although there may be disagreement about what constitute important behavioural elements and underlying biological mechanisms, it is nevertheless acknowledged that there exists something called a Type A or coronary-prone individual. So, is there a Type C or cancer-prone individual? One of the earliest observations of the King's College Research Group was that women with breast cancer were more likely to control feelings of anger than an age-matched group with benign breast disease (Morris *et al.*, 1981). These findings have been independently replicated (Grassi *et al.*, 1986; Watson *et al.*, 1984). A recent review (Gross, 1989) indicated that some 18 separate studies existed in which emotional control was implicated as a risk factor in either carcinogenesis or disease prognosis. Most of these studies have involved some comparison between cancer patients and controls, and there is increasing evidence to suggest that breast cancer patients in particular show a behavioural type characterised by suppression of emotions. It is likely, but by no means certain, that this represents a pre-existing disposition and is not simply a reaction to having cancer. However, only a very small number of studies have looked at this behavioural type in relation to survival (Blumberg *et al.*, 1954; Derogatis *et al.*, 1979; Stavraky, 1968; Temoshok, 1985): it is not at all clear that patients showing the behaviours described will relapse and die more quickly. What *is* clear, is that emotional control in particular is linked to more symptoms of depression and anxiety among breast cancer patients (Watson *et al.*, 1991). This may be true of other disease groups because it is quite widely acknowledged that effective coping involves some ventilation of emotions. At the same time, there is insufficient evidence to support the notion that having a Type C personality contributes in any way to decreased survival. Although there is an increasing literature which suggests that the Type C behaviour pattern exists, further research is needed to clarify what constitute the important elements of this typology and any underlying physical mechanisms.

COPING

Does the patient's method of coping with cancer affect length of survival? This issue has been the focus of much research. The fact that this may be considered to be a legitimate area for scientific investigation stems from recent evidence that human endocrine and immunological responses are conditionable and reactive to stress (Ader, 1981). Evidence to support the notion of the conditionability of the immune system is dealt with in more detail elsewhere (see Chapter 1).

Given the increasing literature on the possible role of coping responses in cancer prognosis it is quite reasonable to attempt an evaluation of the evidence, in order to glean ideas about what might constitute productive areas for further research and to determine whether there is support for this notion. Studies on coping can be divided into three different overlapping topics.

(1) Those studies which examine the issue of whether psychological responses are associated with degree of disease at presentation;
(2) prospective studies which look at whether earlier psychological responses can be related to subsequent disease status;
(3) studies making a direct psychological intervention in order to test its effect on survival.

Disease status at presentation

A few studies have looked at associations between psychological measures and the extent of disease at initial diagnosis. Antoni and Goodkin (1988) found that the extent of cervical intraepithelial neoplasia could be related to psychological response, with more advanced invasiveness being found in those women showing passive, pessimistic, conforming, avoiding and somatically anxious responses. Women whose disease was more contained (i.e. evidence of less disease promotion) were optimistic and employed more active coping styles. The study by Levy and colleagues (1985) suggested however that the relationship between psychological responses and disease status might be more complex than a simple association. The authors found that Natural Killer (NK) cell activity was associated with the extent of cancer spread to the axillary lymph nodes in breast cancer patients and that low levels of NK activity were found in those patients who were rated as being well adjusted to their illness. Patients who had higher NK activity appeared to be distressed or maladjusted and had more advanced spread of the disease. Psychological responses have also been associated with the degree of tumor thickness in patients with malignant melanoma (Temoshok, 1985). Younger patients showing a coping style consisting of strong defensiveness in conjunction with high anxiety were more likely to have thicker and more invasive tumors. More recently, Razavi and colleagues (1990) were able to observe an association between psychosocial variables and oestrogen and progesterone receptor status. They concluded that "The fact that a given psychosocial variable correlates with another prognostic factor could indicate that the correlation is mediated through a third factor". Studies of psychosocial variables and either extent of disease at presentation or prognostic variables assessed at presentation may provide some interesting insights into mechanisms, but their cross-sectional nature limits the findings and, unlike prospective studies, gives no indication of causal mechanisms.

Coping and subsequent disease status

This topic represents the area most frequently examined and Table 1 gives details of some of the studies. Any evaluation of the role of coping in cancer prognosis from these studies is extremely limited because of a number of problems. For some studies the length of follow-up between psychological assessment and the survival end point is quite short. However, a very long follow-up is not necessarily an indication of merit, as length of follow-up will depend on the initial disease stage of the sample being studied. Five years or greater for patients with advanced disease at study entry is probably not necessary. Furthermore, the length of follow-up required to make an acceptable survival analysis depends on the type of cancer being studied, for example, breast tumours are known to be slow growing and one would anticipate that a longer follow-up would be required for such a group. It seems unlikely that any group of cancer patients would require a follow-up of longer than 10 years from initial assessment as this is unlikely to provide further useful information. Other factors which are more crucial in deciding whether or not psychological responses are important relate to the types of survival analyses used. Some studies have divided patients, in a somewhat arbitrary fashion, into long- and short-term survivors and then compared these two groups on the psychological variables assessed. Fashions in statistical analyses change, however, and more recent techniques involve the use of multiple regression and similar survival models as they represent a more fastidious approach to analysing survival data. Comparisons between studies are also made more difficult by the different survival end-points used and the starting point from which survival is analysed. It is unacceptable to analyse survival only from the point at which a psychological assessment occurred, yet one still sees analyses being made from the point of psychological assessment, rather than from the time of original diagnosis. The latter clearly represents the most accurate point from which any assessment of survival can be made, and if all studies adopted this protocol comparisons between them might be easier.

Studies vary in terms of whether they measure the relapse-free interval, the length of time to death, or the number of patients still alive with or without commenting on disease status. Studies in this area clearly need to follow the protocol used in treatment trials in terms of the statistical methods used to analyse survival and the survival end points.

Turning away from these issues, one of the most difficult elements in studies in this area and in evaluating their results concerns the methods of psychological assessment used. Glancing through Table 1, there appears to be little consensus about the methods employed for measuring psychological responses. A substantial number of studies have used standardised and reliable questionnaire methods, but very few studies have used the same methods. It is not uncommon to find highly idiosyncratic assessment methods used, where authors make no comment about the reliability or validity of their approach (for example, Cassileth et al., 1985; Hislop et al., 1987). Where the assessment involves a compilation of items drawn from a series of other questionnaires there is a responsibility on the part of the authors to provide some data on the validity or reliability of these revised assessments. A number of other studies have used non-standardised interview techniques (Greer et al., 1979; Dean and Surtees, 1989; DiClemente and Temoshok, 1985). It is incumbent upon investigators to provide data indicating that these assessments were reliable (which is not always done – see, for example, Dean and Surtees, 1989). The assessment of coping responses, even if standardized between studies, presents further difficulties as discussed elsewhere (see Chapter 9). Most studies are cross-sectional, in the sense that psychological responses were assessed at one stage and were not then reassessed later. Coping responses are likely to be variable and although there can be immense practical difficulties in reassessing patients it would be useful if this could be undertaken. However, it is not entirely clear from the literature when one ought to make these assessments and whether there is any critical period following which coping responses have less impact upon survival. As Derogatis and colleagues (1983) have demonstrated, a substantial proportion of newly diagnosed patients show evidence of psychological morbidity. It seems likely that the period immediately following diagnosis is one of flux. Many patients accommodate to the stress of their diagnosis over the four to six weeks immediately afterwards and, if the investigators' main concern was to measure more stable coping responses it seems reasonable that this period would be best avoided.

Quite a few of the studies suffer from small sample size, sometimes making it difficult to control for other factors which may affect survival such as the type of medical treatment the patient has received. It is also important to control for biological prognostic variables in some way. One of the studies with the longest follow-up (Pettingale et al., 1985) did not include details of lymph node status among breast cancer patients because

Table 1. Studies of coping and cancer prognosis

Authors	Patients	Standardised psychological assessment method	Length of follow-up	Survival end point	Outcome
Achterberg et al., 1977	$n = 126$ Mainly advanced (90%) Range of diagnoses	MMP1 Locus of control FIRO-B SRI POMS	2 months	Disease status at follow up: 1 = no evidence of tumour 2 = tumour size significantly diminished 3 = tumour stabilised 4 = significant tumour growth	Poor prognosis related to: denial little ability to fight the disease significantly dependent on others
Buddeberg et al., 1990	$n = 107$ Early Breast	ZKV	3.5 years	Survival status	No relationship
Cassileth et al., 1985	$n = 359$ Unresectable $(n = 204)$ Stage I or II melanoma $\}$ $(n = 155)$ Stage II breast	Compilation questionnaire	3–8 years	Time to relapse Length of survival	No relationship
Davies et al., 1973	$n = 46$ Advanced Solid tumours $(n = 22)$ Lymphoma/leukaemia $(n = 24)$	Only on subsample $n = 18$ WAIS, MAACL Cornell Medical Index Locus of control L-K Personality Inventory	Up to 1.3 years (450 days)	Length of survival Length of diagnosed illness	Poorer prognosis related to: apathetic given-up, greater dysphoric feelings of anxiety, depression and hostility

Study	Sample	Measures	Follow-up	Outcome	Findings
Dean and Surtees, 1989	$n = 121$ Early Breast	PSE–Spitzer RDC GHQ EPI	6–8 years	Relapse Death	Better prognosis related to: denial expression of emotion
Derogatis et al., 1979	$n = 35$ Advanced Breast	SCL-90R ABS GAIS PAIE	1 year (retrospective)	Survival ≦1 year	Better prognosis related to: hostility psychoticism depression guilt
DiClemente and Temoshok, 1985	$n = 117$ Mainly early (86% Stage I) Malignant melanoma		2.2 years (26 months)	Any form of disease recurrence	Poorer prognosis related to: stoicism (females only) helpless/hopeless (males only)
Edwards et al., 1985	$n = 26$ Advanced Non-seminomatous testicular	POI DSFI BSI MMPI	7 years	Short < 1 year Long – alive and free of disease at follow up	Better progress related to: more introverted expressed more symptomatic distress lower self-regard
Hislop et al., 1987	$n = 133$ Mainly early (79%) Breast	Compilation questionnaire	4 years (approx.)	Length of disease-free survival Time to death and first relapse	Better prognosis related to: internal locus of control extrovert socially active Poorer prognosis related to: high anger anxiety depression

(continued)

Table 1. (*continued*)

Authors	Patients	Standardised psychological assessment method	Length of follow-up	Survival end point	Outcome
Holland *et al.*, 1986	*n* = 346 Stage II Breast	SCL-90	Not stated	Disease-free survival	No relationship
Jamison *et al.*, 1987	*n* = 49 Advanced Breast		Not stated	Long *vs* short survivors (median split)	No relationship
Levy *et al.*, 1988	*n* = 36 Recurrent disease Breast	ABS	7 years	Time to death Length of survival at follow up	Better prognosis related to: positive mood Poorer prognosis related to: negative mood (at baseline)
Morris *et al.*, 1991	*n* = 168 Breast (early) (*n* = 107) Lymphoma (all stages) (*n* = 61)	Wakefield DI STAI MHLC CECS	5 years	Length of recurrence-free survival Time to death	Poorer prognosis related to: suppression of anger powerful others (MHLC) (male lymphoma patients only)
Neuser, 1988	*n* = 35 Transplant patients	Personality Research Form	2 years (754 days)	Length of survival from BMT	Better prognosis related to: strive for recognition and help

Study	Sample	Instruments	Follow-up	Outcome measure	Findings
Pettingale et al., 1985	n = 57 Early Breast	HDS HDHQ EPI	10 years	Survival Relapse	Better prognosis related to: fighting spirit denial. Poorer prognosis related to: helpless/hopeless
Greer et al., 1979 – 5 year follow-up on same sample as Pettingale, 1985					
Rogentine et al., 1979	n = 64 Early Malignant melanomas	RLCQ SCL-90R LDC	1 year	Relapse rate at 1 year from assessment	Better prognosis related to: high "adjust-ment" score
Shrifte, 1961	n = 22 Stage not clearly specified Cervical		2 years	Number of patients recurrence free, dead or relapsed	Poor prognosis related to: "unproductive wasted vitality"
Stavraky, 1968	n = 204 All stages Breast (n = 83) Cervix (n = 36) Lung (n = 28) Others (n = 57)	MMPI	3.3–5.5 years (40–66 months)	Length of survival	Better prognosis related to: more frequently hostile
Weisman and Worden, 1975	n = 163 All stages Various diagnoses	MMPI POMS	1.5 years	Patients divided into long or short survivors on the basis of a "sur-vival quotient"	Poorer prognosis related to: more frustration vulnerability poor resolution more suicide themes in TAT "uncooperative"

lymph node sampling was not available routinely at the initiation of the study. It has been consistently shown that axillary lymph node status is an important prognostic variable and more recent studies (Dean and Surtees, 1989; Buddeberg *et al.*, 1990) have shown this to be the most important prognostic factor. As the numbers in the Pettingale study were quite small the effects observed may also be due, as Hürny and Bernhard (1989) point out, to "unequal distribution of lymph node-positive patients within the four categories of responses".

If we ignore these methodological problems for the moment, and simply look at those coping responses which have been related to prognosis, can we find any trends? Denial has been related to both poor (Achterberg *et al.*, 1977) and good (Dean and Surtees, 1989; Greer *et al.*, 1979) prognosis. Levels of depression and anxiety have also been related to both short (Davies *et al.*, 1973) and long (Derogatis *et al.*, 1979) survival times. If there is any trend it appears to be that those patients with shorter duration of survival are characterised by a passive and helpless response to their diagnosis and those who do better appear to be more likely to express an internal locus of control or a fighting attitude toward their disease.

These coping responses may not, of course, act directly on the disease but may influence other behaviours which can affect survival. Neuser's (1988) study, for instance, suggests that those with a survival advantage beyond one year after bone marrow transplant seemed more able to muster help and resources from outside themselves and among their support systems. Spiegal and colleagues (1989) suggest that social support may be an important factor in survival because "social support is important in mediating how individuals cope with stress". Patients who are helpless and passive as opposed to assertive and resilient may differ on a number of variables, such as the type of treatment they receive, the amount of financial and social support they receive and their ability to make use of a host of other resources, which could in theory affect survival. It may be these factors rather than the actual coping responses themselves which act to influence survival, if it is influenced at all.

In looking at the weight of the data in this area the ratio of studies finding no relationship between psychological responses and survival to those which do find some relationship is in the order of 1:3. Such a preponderance of studies supporting the issue of coping response affecting cancer prognosis cannot be ignored – there appears to be a phenomenon. However, studies need to use replicable psychological assessment methods on reasonably large sample sizes, using survival analyses with clearly described starting and end-points, and including important prognostic and treatment variables. Careful and fastidious research may help to clarify the exact nature of the phenomenon. Last, but by no means least, in analysing any effects of coping response upon survival it would be important to determine what *proportion* of risk it contributes to prognosis in order to determine whether it is important or trivial.

Intervention

Although a number of authors have suggested that the intervention or psychotherapy they provided to patients has brought about miraculous cures there are few well-controlled studies, yet this would be a useful approach to examining the possible role of coping in cancer prognosis. It does, however, involve an experimental manipulation (a psychothera-peutic intervention) which cannot always be guaranteed to work, but does provide the neatest kind of experimental design. To date only two well-controlled studies appear to exist; one showing an effect of the intervention (Spiegal *et al.*, 1989) and the other showing no difference (Linn *et al.*, 1982). The study by Linn and colleagues was on male patients, with the largest diagnostic group being lung cancer patients, and all patients had advanced disease. This sample was followed up for 12 months and survival was assessed in terms of number of days from study entry to death and number of days from diagnosis to death. A number of standardised psychological assessment questionnaires were used and patients were divided at random into intervention or control groups. Important clinical and prognostic variables were also included in the survival analysis. A counselling intervention was used, with patients being seen several times a week, although it was not clearly stated how long this intervention lasted. The authors could find no differences between the groups in relation to survival, although they observed a non-significant trend for depression to be significantly associated with mortality. The Spiegal study (1989) was also on patients with advanced disease, but these were women with breast cancer. Patients were randomly assigned to the intervention which in this case continued over a period of one year. A survival advantage was observed for those women who had experienced the group psychotherapy, although this was not apparent until approximately eight months after therapy had ended. These two studies are not directly comparable as one used male and the other female patients and they had differing forms of psychotherapy lasting, apparently, for different lengths of time. Both studies appear to have been carefully conducted but replication is required. The study by Morgenstern and colleagues (1984) is interesting because, although they observed a beneficial effect of the support programme in terms of increased survival for the intervention group compared with the controls, this was explained largely by a selection bias with a failure to match the samples in terms of duration of lag period between cancer diagnosis and programme entry. This highlights the difficulties of conducting this kind of intervention study and shows how easy it is to make fallacious statements about psychotherapy and survival. More recently it has been suggested that some types of psycho-logical support contribute to a poor prognosis (Bagenal *et al.*, 1990). The Bristol Cancer Help Centre offers various alternative therapies for patients with cancer, although much of what they offer could, in fact, be described as counselling. A comparison between 334 breast cancer patients attending this centre and 461 case-matched controls was made approximately 8–12 months following study entry. Although the groups were matched this was not a randomised design. It was found that patients attending the centre did not gain any substantial survival benefit and in fact appeared to do less well. The authors suggest however, that "the difference in sur-vival amongst patients with metastatic disease could be the result of a difference in severity of disease at time of entry to the BCHC (Bristol Cancer Help Centre)", and a subsequent analysis (Chilvers *et al.*, 1990) has shown that BCHC attenders were likely to have more severe disease. Patients attending the BCHC had two options: they could attend for one day or for one full week – this was not accounted for in the analysis of survival. No measures of the psychological make-up of those women attending or of the effect of intervention upon either psychological responses or quality of life were included, which requires further investigation. A follow-up of this study which will take account of some of these variables is planned. At present the issue of whether psychothera-peutic intervention affects survival is an open book.

Taking together all three areas described above, it would appear first that some psychological responses are associated with biological prognostic factors when these are assessed at initial diagnosis. Whether this is a causal relationship is unclear and as Razavi and colleagues (1990) suggest, some third moderating factor may hold the key to these relationships. Sec-ondly, the way in which patients cope with cancer may influence survival and the increasing number of studies supporting this notion (even though many are flawed) cannot be ignored. Whether the coping responses have a direct or indirect effect on survival is not clear. More collaborative research, with standardisation of techniques and fastidious statistical ana-lyses, might provide some real progress in this area. Finally, psychological intervention, in the form of counselling or supportive psychotherapy, might provide some survival advantage but, more importantly, may improve quality of survival.

STRESSFUL LIFE EXPERIENCES AND CANCER

Early reports

The observations of 18th- and 19th-century clinicians suggest an associ-ation between stressful life experiences and cancer. These include the anecdotes and descriptive work of Richard Guy, James Paget, Deshaies Gendron and Herbert Snow. Gendron reported in 1701 a series of cases, including that of Mrs Emerson, who "upon the death of her daughter, underwent great affliction and perceived her breast to swell ... it broke out in a most inveterate cancer ... she had always enjoyed a perfect state of health".

Lawrence LeShan (1959) in a comprehensive review of 75 studies of psychological factors in the development of cancer, concluded that "the most consistently recorded relevant psychological factor had been the loss of a major emotional relationship prior to the first noted symptoms of the neoplasm". Many of these early studies were clearly subjective and poorly designed with small sample sizes and inadequate controls. More equivocal findings have emerged from recent systematic research looking at the role of stressful life experiences in the onset of tumour growth.

STRESSFUL LIFE EXPERIENCES AND THE ONSET OF CANCER

Epidemiological and clinical studies

Epidemiological studies have failed to demonstrate a strong correlation between one type of severely stressful life experience – death of a spouse – and subsequent cancer morbidity and mortality. Using data from the longitudinal study of the Office of Population Censuses and Surveys in the UK, Jones and his colleagues (1984) found little evidence of an increase in registration of cancer after conjugal bereavement and only a slight suggestion of increased mortality. Such excesses in cancer mortality as did occur were to be seen six months or more after the bereavement. The authors comment that "this could be taken as weak evidence in support of the stress of bereavement causing excess mortality from cancer, with a relatively long interval between widowerhood and death from cancer of the widower" (Jones and Goldblatt, 1986). Similar negative findings emerge from other large epidemiological studies (Ewertz, 1986; Kaprio *et al.*, 1987; Helsing *et al.*, 1982). Acknowledged weaknesses in these investigations include the small numbers of people in the population with the combination of events of interest and the limited length of follow-up after widow(er)hood. The nature and circumstances surrounding the conjugal bereavements may be important but cannot be examined in this type of study.

A number of controlled clinical studies have examined the relationship between stressful life experiences and the onset of breast cancer. Muslin and his colleagues (1966) showed that women who had malignant breast tumours were no more likely to have had a significant separation experience in the three years prior to diagnosis than those who had benign breast disease. "Significant separation experience" was defined as the permanent loss of a first degree relative or other person whom the subject specifically stated was emotionally important to her. This information was obtained using a self-report questionnaire at the time of breast biopsy, when the patients were unaware of their diagnosis. The cancer and benign breast disease patients were matched in pairs according to demographic data.

Events and situations causing severe or prolonged distress were recorded for a series of women undergoing breast tumour biopsy (Greer and Morris, 1975). Again no differences were found between women with malignant and benign pathology in the number or type of stressful experiences they reported for the five years prior to the appearance of the breast lump. The data were collected using an unstructured interview. Unfortunately the authors provided no numerical details of their results.

Several studies have compared the experience of life events in patients with malignant and benign breast lumps, using life events questionnaires which measure patients' reports of the number of different types of life events they have experienced and a summed score of the tendency of those events to cause change in their lives. Despite using similar life events inventories, the findings of these studies are inconsistent. Schonfield (1975) found that patients with cancer experienced significantly less change due to life events in the three years prior to biopsy than patients with benign tumours. In contrast, Priestman and his colleagues (1985) found no difference in the type of events or the amount of disruption they caused in women with benign and malignant tumours over the same time period. They did, however, find that an apparently healthy control group reported significantly higher levels of stress. Cooper and his colleagues had differing findings in two of their studies. In a study of 121 women undergoing breast biopsy, patients with cancer reported significantly more life events in the two years preceding disease onset than those with benign disease or well women (Cheang and Cooper, 1985). A subsequent study looked at 2163 patients who underwent breast examination, either because their GPs referred them with breast problems or as part of a general medical examination (Cooper *et al.*, 1986). Patients diagnosed as having cancer reported significantly fewer life events overall than those with benign breast disease or no breast disease in the two-year period prior to the breast examination. The cancer patients did, however, rate their events as more upsetting or stressful on a 10-point Likert-type scale. The actual events recorded by the cancer group tended to be loss- or illness-related events; most notably death of husband, death of a close friend, retirement and surgery.

Snell and Graham (1971) compared patients with breast cancer and those with other types of cancer and non-neoplastic disease of organs other than breast and genitalia. They found no difference between the groups for the experience of single life events or the cumulative number of life events. Using an interview, they enquired about specific experiences including death, divorce, illness, economic hardship, residential mobility and feelings of being upset.

Less attention has been paid to the relationship between stressful life experiences and other types of cancer. Horne and Picard (1979) interviewed patients with undiagnosed chest X-ray lesions. Patients found to have lung cancer were significantly more likely than patients who had benign lesions to have experienced a major loss (including death of a loved one, loss of employment, and loss of prestige) in the five years prior to diagnosis.

A comparison of patients with gastric and colorectal carcinoma and normal controls showed that those with gastric cancer had experienced significantly more life changes in the two years prior to the onset of symptoms. This was a small study using a self-report life events inventory (Lehrer, 1980). Lehrer speculated that whilst the development of colorectal cancer may be related to dietary habits, gastric cancer could be more stress related. He thus highlights the general possibility that the effect of stressful life experiences on tumour growth may not be ubiquitous and could vary according to the type of tumour.

Jacobs and Charles (1980) ascertained life events for the two years before the onset of cancer in children. The cancer group experienced significantly more life events and change associated with those events than children with non-malignant diseases.

Antecedent life events and the onset of haematological malignancies were studies in pairs of monozygotic twins who were discordant for the cancer. Using a self-report life events inventory the healthy twins were found to have had increased or equivalent life changes compared with their sick twin (Smith *et al.*, 1984).

All these studies fulfil the basic requirement of analytical investigation. They compare patients who have documented malignant disease with controls. Furthermore they use recognised or adequately described psychosocial assessments and subject their data to statistical analyses. They do, however, have limitations in their design and methodology which undermine the validity and reliability of their results and which may explain the inconsistent nature of their findings.

The main weakness of these studies is the inability to date the onset of tumour growth. It is important to be able to do this accurately in order to ensure that the life events recorded do precede tumour initiation. In reality the correlations observed in these studies are between life events and the clinical presentation of cancer and it is possible that many of the ascertained life events in fact occurred in the context of early clinically undetected, malignant, disease. It is also possible that those life events which did genuinely antedate the onset of tumour growth were not ascertained because they occurred outside the time period under scrutiny. Typically these studies examined life events in the 1–5 years prior to clinical presentation of cancer: it is known, however, that malignant transformation can occur many years before presentation of the cancer (Shackney *et al.*, 1978). In an extreme example, extrapolation from the growth rate of a colonic adenosarcoma observed by Spratt and Ackerman (1961) put its origins 52 years before diagnosis!

Another important methodological weakness common to these studies is the nature of the control groups – mainly derived from patient populations, most having organic pathology. In the breast cancer studies the controls were chiefly women with benign breast disease which may itself represent a premalignant state (Davis *et al.*, 1964). Snell and Graham's study of breast cancer patients (Snell and Graham, 1971) included women with other malignant disease in the control group. The lung cancer patients in Horne and Picard's study (Horne and Picard, 1979) were compared with patients with non-neoplastic chest disease.

Stressful life events increase the rate of consultation with a physician (Mechanic, 1974; Miller *et al.*, 1976), physical symptoms and some physical diseases (Brown and Harris, 1989). It is therefore likely that the patients in the control populations would themselves have increased experience of life events, prior to their physical presentation, compared with the general population. As a result, their use as controls might mask any correlation between antecedent life experiences and cancer in the study group.

An important aspect of any investigation examining the relationship between life events and the development of cancer is the use of a valid and reliable measure of those life events. Most of the studies reviewed have used self-report questionnaires, either the Holmes and Rahe Schedule of Recent Experiences (1967) or variants of it. The use of these inventories in life events research has been extensively criticised (Craig and Brown, 1984; Creed, 1985). Those shortcomings most relevant to the study of life events and cancer will be discussed here. These inventories are designed to measure life events according to their propensity to produce *change or disruption* in a person's life. Each broad type of event is given a weighted score assigned by a body of judges according to its tendency to produce change and disruption. One of the assumptions of this approach is that events such as childbirth are comparable in all subjects because they are all likely to involve the same amount of change and adjustment. Scrutiny of the early literature concerning life events and cancer suggest that it is the undesirable or threatening nature of an event which is important, rather than its propensity to cause change *per se*. Furthermore, there is a growing consensus in stress research in general that the specific meaning for the individual of life events needs to be taken into account, rather than assigning arbitrary scores without regard to the circumstances surrounding particular events.

Self-report questionnaires are further limited by their inclusion of vague and general items that leave it to the subject to decide upon the criteria for inclusion of an event. The general inaccuracy and insensitivity resulting from this tends to lead to a low association between life events and onset of cancer in studies in which patients do not yet know their diagnosis (Cooper *et al.*, 1986; Priestman *et al.*, 1985). Such an approach also introduces serious potential for bias from subjects who know they have cancer (as in the study of Jacobs and Charles, 1980). They may overreport events in an attempt to make sense of their illness. For example, in response to the question "have any relatives been seriously ill in the last six months" a patient with a diagnosis of stomach cancer might include a relatively trivial but related illness, such as gastritis occurring in a distant cousin.

More controversially, the emotional suppression that has been described as typical of cancer patients (Greer and Watson, 1985; Temoshok, 1985) may be a systematic source of underreporting of adverse life events using this method of data collection.

The validity of self-report life event inventories is further undermined by the assumption that the impacts of different events are additive. There is little evidence to support this view and one of the consequences of this approach is that it is possible to accrue a higher stress score based on a number of minor, potentially positive, events such as Christmas and going to university, than from a single severely stressful experience such as a divorce.

STRESSFUL LIFE EXPERIENCES AND CANCER PROGNOSIS

The studies purporting to examine the role of stressful life experiences in the onset of cancer are sufficiently flawed that they cannot provide good evidence for such a relationship. Until the onset of tumour growth can be accurately dated, the possible aetiological influence of life experiences cannot be investigated. Their influence on the prognosis of an already established cancer is more amenable to study, mainly because disease progression is more amenable to measurement. This is particularly so in specialised oncology units where patients are subject to regular clinical, biochemical and radiological scrutiny. There is accumulating evidence that psychological factors influence neurological, endocrinological and immunological functions, which may in turn influence tumour prognosis. It is thus possible to envisage a physiological mechanism whereby psychological factors exert an effect on tumour growth. Despite this, the relationship between stressful life experiences and disease prognosis in cancer has received relatively little attention. Recently it has been examined in two studies of women with breast cancer. Breast cancer is an eminently suitable tumour type for such investigation. Although biological factors (such as axillary lymph node involvement by tumour and histological grade of the primary cancer) are well known to influence prognosis, they are insufficient to account for the variable outcome. Host factors may well explain differences in outcome and these could include psychological and social variables.

Marshall and Funch (1983) at Roswell Park Memorial Institute examined the relationship between stressful life events occurring before diagnosis of breast cancer and subsequent survival. They used data, originally collected by Snell and Graham (1971), which looked at the relationship between prediagnosis life events and the onset of cancer. High prediagnosis life events scores were associated with decreased survival, whilst social involvement was associated with increased survival. In this study the most powerful predictor of survival was the stage of disease at diagnosis. This accounted for 15–20% of the variance of survival time. Stressful life events and social involvement accounted for 9% of the variance, but only in women aged less than 46 years. Social indicators accounted for none of the variance of survival among the older age groups analysed. The authors acknowledged the limitations of their study: it was restricted to women from the original cohort who were known to have died. Thus 20% of the women originally interviewed were not included in the analysis; they were either alive or their death had not been recorded in the cancer registry. The social indicators looked at in this study were crude, and may underestimate the effects of social variables upon survival. Despite these caveats this study demonstrates a relationship between stressful life events and survival from breast cancer.

The influence of stressful life experiences on the development of relapse in operable breast cancer has been examined in a case control study at Guy's Hospital, London (Ramirez *et al.*, 1989). Adverse life events and ongoing difficulties occurring during the postoperative disease-free interval were recorded in 50 women who had developed a first recurrence following a diagnosis of operable breast cancer, and during the equivalent follow-up time of 50 women whose operable breast cancer was in remission. The cases and controls were matched on a pairwise basis for the main physical and pathological factors known to be prognostic in breast cancer and those sociodemographic variables which influence the frequency of life events and difficulties. The incidence and nature of the stressful experiences were measured using the Bedford College Life Events and Difficulties Schedule (Brown and Harris, 1978), an instrument that has overcome many of the problems of low validity and reliability which have plagued this area of research (Craig and Brown, 1984). It measures life experiences according to how threatening and undesirable they are to the individual. A semistructured interview is used to gather as coherent and full an account as possible of any incident which might be relevant to the research enquiry. A set of previously developed rules and detailed questioning is used to decide whether or not an event is to be included. The nature and severity of the stressful experiences are subsequently rated by a panel of independent judges, who are unaware of the patients' self report of the adversity of the experience and whether or not the experience was followed by disease recurrence. This attempts to minimise any bias from the patient or the interviewer. The threat rating is based on a judgement about how the average person would be expected to react to the experience, given the patients' biography and the particular circumstances surrounding the experience. This approach allows accurate dating of life events and difficulties to ensure that they precede disease progression.

Severely threatening adverse life events and difficulties were shown to be associated with first relapse of breast cancer. These included death of loved ones, but more particularly severe non-health events such as divorce and a son receiving a seven-year prison sentence for grevious bodily harm. Non-severe life experiences such as a routine varicose vein operation or minor road traffic incident showed no association with relapse.

For those women who relapsed there appeared to be a relationship between the time of last severe life event they experienced and the date of relapse. The average time between these severe life events and recurrence was 17.5 months.

There was some preliminary evidence that the impact of the severely stressful life experiences was confined to those patients with oestrogen receptor positive tumours (Ramirez *et al.*, 1990), suggesting that the effect on relapse is mediated via a hormonal mechanism.

The findings of this small retrospective study suggest that the experience of a severe life event of difficulty represents a risk factor for recurrence of breast cancer.

DEPRESSION AS A RISK FACTOR

The studies which have looked at the association between depression and cancer morbidity and mortality have been reviewed by Bernard Fox (1989). He concludes that the combined evidence is "not consistent with a strong relationship between depressive symptoms and cancer among major segments of the population". He suggests however, that more detailed analysis of existing and new data may shed further light on the question. An interesting aspect to pursue is the possibility that affective states as part of a reaction to severe events may predispose to cancer. LeShan (1959) commented on the frequency with which psychological distress consequent upon a major loss preceded the development of cancer. George Engel (1967) subsequently developed his well-known "giving up – given up" hypothesis which argues that stress-related feelings of helplessness and hopelessness contribute to the development of physical disease. These feelings involve loss of self confidence and an overwhelming sense of failure and are expressed in terms of "it's too much, it's no use, I can't take it any more, I give up".

Schmale and Iker's classic study (1971) of women with dysplastic cervical cells found at routine cervical examination supports Engel's hypothesis by showing that hopelessness predicted cervical cancer. The women were interviewed prior to the results of cone biopsy. The presence or absence of cervical cancer was significantly predicted on the basis of the presence or absence of a "hopelessness prone personality" and/or recently experienced hopelessness in response to an event. These findings were largely replicated by Goodkin *et al.* (1986) using self-report life events and behavioural questionnaires. They found a modest correlation between negative life events scores and severity of cervical cell dysplasia, which was enhanced by high levels of premorbid pessimism and despair.

The role of depression in the prognosis of cancer has in general been examined as an integral part of studies looking at coping and disease progression (see Table 1). As such their interpretation is complicated by the same methodological problems, in particular the multiplicity of measures of depression used and variability in the criteria applied to define depressive states.

There is some support for a relationship between certain cognitive, behavioural and psychological symptoms of depression and poor prognosis in cancer. These include helplessness (Pettingale *et al.*, 1985; Levy and Wise, 1988) and depressed mood (Levy and Wise, 1988; Temoshok, 1985). Levy has also shown a relationship between listlessness and apathy and natural killer cell activity in women undergoing treatment for early stage breast cancer (Levy *et al.*, 1987). These clinical states could correspond to Engel's "given up" formulation.

There is less evidence to suggest that clinically significant depression in patients with cancer is associated with poor prognosis. Dean and Surtees (1989) have recently conducted a survival analysis in breast cancer patients which showed that women who had enough symptoms to fulfil the criteria for a psychiatric illness (according to Research Diagnostic Criteria (RDC) and the General Health Questionnaire (GHQ)) before operation were *less* likely to have a recurrence during the follow-up. They also showed that women who had persistent psychiatric symptoms and who were classified as cases according to the GHQ three months after operation were *more* likely to die. These data suggest that the timing of episodes of depression may be of importance in relation to cancer prognosis.

CONSIDERATIONS FOR FUTURE RESEARCH

The studies of Marshall and Funch (1983) and Ramirez *et al.* (1989) provide some support for the influence of stressful life experiences on disease prognosis in breast cancer. The nature of this influence requires clarification. The main determinants of cancer prognosis are biological. Stressful life experiences are not necessary for tumour growth nor are they sufficient by themselves to cause disease progression. Presumably they interact with biological variables in a multifactorial process. Their influence on a cancer may be restricted to a physical subpopulation as suggested in the Guy's study; equally their impact may be confined to patients who have particular cognitive and behavioural coping responses to their disease or who subsequently develop depressive states. For example, stressful life experiences may exert their influence only in those cancer patients who display helplessness or who suppress negative emotions. It is interesting that both the Guy's and the Roswell Park studies suggest that the stressful experiences which influence disease progression are those which carry lasting implications for coping and adjustment. Such experiences may mediate their impact through neuroendocrine or immune pathways, or by behavioural changes which involve exposure to physical risk factors. Large prospective studies are required to corroborate the Roswell Park and Guy's findings. These would also allow the study of interactions between stressful life experiences and other psychosocial variables which may modify their impact on relapse. Such variables include coping responses, social support and psychiatric morbidity; all of which have been suggested as prognostic factors in themselves. Putative neuroendocrine and immune intermediaries could also be examined in a longitudinal study.

REFERENCES

Achterberg, J. and Lawlis, G.F. (1977) Psychological factors and blood chemistries as disease outcome predictors for cancer patients. *Multivariate Exp. Clin. Res.*, **3**, 107–122.

Ader, R. (1981) *Psychoneuroimmunology*. Academic Press, New York.

Antoni, M.H. and Goodkin, K. (1988) Host moderator variables in the promotion of cervical neoplasia – I. Personality facets. *J. Psychosom. Res.*, **32**, 327–338.

Bagenal, F.S., Easton, D.F., Harris, E., Chilvers, C.E.D. and McElwain, T.J. (1990) Survival of patients with breast cancer attending Bristol Cancer Help Centre. *Lancet*, **336**, 606–610.

Blumberg, E.M., West, P.M. and Ellis, F.W. (1954) A possible relationship between psychological factors and human cancer. *Psychosom. Med.*, **16**, 277–286.

Buddeberg, C., Wolf, C., Sieber, M., Riehl-Emde, A., Bergant, A., Steiner, R., Landolt-Ritter, C. and Richter, D. (1990) *Coping strategies and course of disease of breast cancer patients*. Paper presented at the 18th European Conference on Psychosomatic Research, Helsinki, Finland.

Brown, G.W. and Harris, T. (1978) *Social Origins of Depression. A Study of Psychosocial Disorder in Women*. Tavistock Publications, London.

Brown, G.W. and Harris, T. (1978) *Social origins of depression. A Study of Psychosocial Disorder in Women*. Tavistock Publications, London.

Cassileth, B.R., Lusk, E.J., Miller, D.S., Brown, L.L. and Miller, C. (1985) Psychosocial correlates of survival in advanced malignant disease? *New Eng. J. Med.*, **312**, 1551–1555.

Cheang, A. and Cooper, C.L. (1985) Psychosocial factors in breast cancer. *Stress Med.*, **1**, 11–24.

Chilvers, C.E.D., Easton, D.F., Bagenal, F.S., Harris, E. and McElwain, T.J. (1990) Bristol Cancer Help Centre. *Lancet*, **336**, 1186–1188.

Cooper, C.L., Davies-Cooper, R.F. and Faragher, B. (1986) A prospective study of the relationship between breast cancer and life events, type of behaviour, social support and coping skills. *Stress Med.*, **2**, 271–277.

Craig, T.J.K. and Brown, G.W. (1984) Life events meaning and physical illness a review. In Mathews, A. and Steptoe, A. (ed.) *Public Health Care and Human Behaviour*. Academic Press, London, pp. 7–39.

Creed, F. (1985) Life events and physical illness. *J. Psychosom. Res.*, **29**(2), 113–125.

Davies, R.K., Quinlan, D.M., McKegrey, F.P. and Kimball, C.P. (1973) Organic factors and psychological adjustment in advanced cancer patients. *Psychosom. Med.*, **35**, 464–471.

Davies, H.H., Simons, N. and Davis, J.B. (1964) Cystic disease of the breast: relationships to carcinoma. *Cancer*, **17**, 957–978.

Dean, C. and Surtees, P.G. (1989) Do psychological factors predict survival in breast cancer? *J. Psychosom. Res.*, **33**, 561–569.

Derogatis, L.R., Abeloff, M.D. and Melisaratos N. (1979) Psychological coping mechanisms and survival time in metastatic breast cancer. *JAMA*, **242**, 1504–1508.

Derogatis, L.R., Morrow, G.R., Fetting, J., Penman, D., Piasetsky, S., Schmale, A.M., Henricks, M. and Carnicke, C. (1983) The prevalence of psychiatric disorders among cancer patients. *JAMA*, **249**, 751–757.

DiClemente, R.J. and Temoshok, L. (1985) Psychological adjustment to having cutaneous malignant melanoma as a predictor of follow-up clinical status. *Psychosom. Med.*, **47**, 81.

Edwards, J., Di Clemente, C. and Samuels, M.L. (1985) Psychological characteristics: A pre-treatment survival marker of patients with testicular cancer. *J. Psychosocial Oncol.*, **3**, 79–94.

Engel, G.L. (1967) A psychological setting of somatic disease: the giving up – given up complex. *Proc. Roy. Soc. Med.*, **60**, 553–555.

Ewertz, M. (1986) Bereavement and breast cancer. *Br. J. Cancer*, **53**, 701–703.

Fox, B.H. (1983) Current theory of psychogenic effects on cancer incidence and prognosis. *J. Psychosocial Oncol.*, **1**(1), 17–31.

Fox, B.H. (1989) Depressive symptoms and risk of cancer. *JAMA*, **262**(9), 1231.

Gendron, D. (1701) *Enquiries into the Nature, Knowledge and Cure of Cancers*. London.

Goodkin, K., Antoni, M.H. and Blaney, P.H. (1986) Stress and hopelessness in the promotion of cervical intra-epithelial neoplasia to invasive squamous cell carcinoma of cervix. *J. Psychosom.*, **30**, 67–76.

Grassi, L., Nappi, G., Susa, A. and Molinari, S. (1986) Eventi stressanti supporto sociale e caratteristiche psicologiche in pazienti affecte da carcinoma della mammella *Rivista di Psichiatria*, **21**, 315–328.

Greer, S. and Morris, T. (1975) Psychological attributes of women who develop breast cancer: a controlled study. *J. Psychosom. Res.*, **19**, 147–153.

Greer, S. and Watson, M. (1985) Towards a psychobiological model of cancer: psychological considerations. *Soc. Sci. Med.*, **20**(8), 773–777.

Greer, S., Morris, T. and Pettingale, K.W. (1979) Psychological response to breast cancer: effect on outcome. *Lancet*, **ii**, 785–787.

Gross, J. (1989) Emotional suppression in cancer onset and progression. *Soc. Sci. Med.*, **12**, 1239–1248.

Helsing, K.J., Comstock, T.W. and Szklo, M. (1982) Causes of death in the widowed population. *Am. J. Epidemiol.*, **116**, 524–532.

Hislop, T.G., Waxler, N.E., Coldman, W.J., Elwood, J.M. and Kan L. (1987) The prognostic significance of psychosocial factors in women with breast cancer. *J. Chron. Dis.*, **40**, 729–735.

Holland, J.C., Korzun, A.H., Tross, S., Cella, D.F., Norton, L. and Wood, W. (1986) Psychosocial factors and disease free survival (DFS) in Stage II breast carcinoma. *Proc. ASCO*, **5**, 237 (Abstract only).

Holmes, T.H. and Rahe, R.H. (1967) Social readjustment scale. *J. Psychosom. Res.*, **11**, 213–218.

Horne, R.L. and Picard, R.S. (1979) Psychosocial risk factors for long cancer. *Psychosom. Med.*, **41**, 503–514.

Hürny, C. and Berhard, J. (1989) Coping and survival in patients with primary breast cancer: A critical analysis of current research strategies and proposal of a new approach integrating biomedical, psychological, and social variables. *Recent Results in Cancer Research*, **115**, 255–271.

Jacobs, T.J. and Charles, E. (1980) Life events and occurrence of cancer in children. *Psychosom. Med.*, **42**(1), 11–24.

Jamison, R.N., Burish, T.G. and Wallston, K.A. (1987) Psychogenic factors in predicting survival of breast cancer patients. *J. Clin. Oncol.*, **5**, 768–772.

Jones, D.R. and Goldblatt, P.O. (1986) Cancer mortality following widow(er)hood: Some further results from the OPCS longitudinal study. *Stress Med.*, **2**, 129–140.

Jones, D.R., Goldblatt, P.O. and Leon, D.A. (1984) Bereavement and cancer, some data on death of spouses from the longitudinal study of the Office of Population Censuses and Surveys. *Br. Med. J.*, **289**, 461–464.

Kaprio, J., Koskenbvuo, M. and Rita, H. (1987) Mortality after bereavement: A prospective study of 95,647 widowed persons. *Am. J. Pub. Health.*, **77**, 283–287.

Lehrer, S. (1980) Life change and gastric cancer. *Psychosom. Med.*, **42**(5), 499–502.

LeShan, L. (1959) Psychological states as factors in the development of malignant diseases; A critical review. *J. Natl. Cancer Inst.*, **22**, 1–18.

Levy, S.M. and Wise, B.D. (1988) Psychosocial risk factors in cancer prognosis. In Cooper, C.R. (ed.) *Stress and Breast Cancer*. John Wiley, London, pp. 77–97.

Levy, S.M., Herberman, R.B., Maluish, A.M., Schlein, B. and Lippman, M. (1985) Prognostic risk assessment in primary breast cancer by behavioural and immunological parameters. *Health Psychol.*, **4**, 99–113.

Levy, S.M., Lee, J., Bagley, C. and Lippman, M. (1988) Survival hazards analysis in first recurrent breast cancer patients: Seven-year follow-up. *Psychosom. Med.*, **50**, 520–528.

Linn, M.W., Linn, B.S. and Harris, R. (1982) Effects of counseling for late stage cancer patients. *Cancer*, **49**, 1048–1055.

Marshall, J.R. and Funch, D.P. (1983) Social environment and breast cancer: A cohort analysis of patient survival. *Cancer*, **52**, 1546–1550.

Mechanic, D. (1974) Discussion of research programmes and relations between stressful life events and episodes of physical illness. In Dohrenwend, B.S. and Dowhrenwend, B.P. (eds) *Stressful Life Events; their nature and effects*. John Wiley, New York, pp. 87–97.

Miller, P., Ingham, J.G. and Davison, S. (1976) Life events, symptoms and social support. *J. Psychosom. Res.*, **20**, 515–522.

Morganstern, H., Gellert, G., Walter, S.D., Ostfeld, A.M. and Siegal, B.S (1984) The impact of a psychosocial support program on survival with breast cancer: The importance of selection bias in program evaluation. *J. Chron. Dis.*, **37**, 273–287.

Morris, T., Greer, S., Pettingale, K. and Watson, M. (1981) Patterns of expression of anger and their psychological correlates in women with breast cancer. *J. Psychosom. Res.*, **25**, 111–117.

Morris, T., Pettingale, K. and Haybittle, J. (1991) Psychological response to cancer diagnosis and outcome in patients with breast cancer and lymphoma. Submitted for publication.

Muslin, H.L., Gyarfas, K. and Pieper, W. (1966) Separation experience and cancer of the breast. *Ann. NY Acad. Sci.*, **125**, 802–806.

Neuser, J. (1988) Personality and survival time after bone marrow transplantation. *J. Psychosom. Res.*, **32**, 451–455.

Pettingale, K.W. (1985) Towards a psychobiological model of cancer: Biological considerations. *Soc. Sci. Med.*, **20**, 779–787.

Pettingale, K.W., Morris, T., Greer, S. and Haybittle, J.L. (1985) Mental attitudes to cancer: An additional prognostic factor. *Lancet*, **i**, 750.

Priestman, T.J., Priestman, S.G. and Bradshaw, C. (1985) Stress and breast cancer. *Br. J. Cancer*, **5**, 493–498.

Ramirez, A.J., Craig, K.J., Watson, J.P., Fentiman, I.S., North, W.R.S. and Rubens, R.D. (1989) Stress and relapse of breast cancer. *Br. Med. J.*, **298**, 291–293.

Ramirez, A.J., Richards, M.A., Gregory, W. and Craig, T.K.J. (1990) Psychological correlates of hormone receptor status in breast cancer. *Lancet*, **335**, 1408.

Razavi, D., Farvacques, C., Delvaux, N., Beffort, T., Paesmans, M., Leclercq, C., van Houtte, P. and Paridaens, R. (1990) Psychosocial correlates of oestrogen and progesterone receptors in breast cancer. *Lancet*, **335**, 931–933.

Rogentine, G.N., van Kammen, D.P., Fox, B.H., Docherty, J.P., Rosenblatt, J.E., Boyd, S.C. and Bunney, W.E. (1979) Psychological factors in the prognosis of malignant melanoma: A prospective study. *Psychosom. Med.*, **41**, 647–655.

Schonfield, J. (1975) Psychological and life experience differences between Israeli women with benign and cancerous breast lesions. *J. Psychosom. Res.*, **43**, 117–125.

Schmale, A. and Iker, H. (1971) Hopelessness as a predictor of cervical cancer. *Soc. Sci. Med.*, **5**, 95–100.

Shackney S.C., McCormack, G.W. and Cuchural, G.J. (1978) Growth patterns of solid tumours and their relation to responsiveness to therapy. *Ann. Int. Med.*, **89**, 107–121.

Shrifte, M.L. (1961) Toward identification of a psychological variable in host resistance to cancer. *Psychosom. Med.*, **24**, 390–397.

Smith, C.K., Harrison, S.D., Ashworth, C., Montiano, D., Davis, A. and Fefer, A. (1984) Life change and onset of cancer in identical twins. *J. Psychosom. Res.*, **28**, 525–532.

Snell, L. and Graham, S. (1971) Social trauma as related to cancer of the breast. *Br. J. Cancer*, **25**, 721–734.

Spiegal, D., Bloom, J.R., Kraemer, H.C. and Gottheil, E. (1989) Effect of psychosocial treatment on survival of patients with metastatic breast cancer. *Lancet*, **ii**, 888–891.

Stavraky, K.M. (1968) Psychological factors in the outcome of human cancer. *J. Psychosom. Res.*, **12**, 251–259.

Spratt, J.S. and Ackerman, L.A. (1961) The growth of a colonic adenosarcoma. *Am. Surgeon.*, **27**, 23–28.

Temoshok, L. (1985) Biopsychological studies on cutaneous malignant melanoma: Psychosocial factors associated with prognostic indicators, progression, psychophysiology and tumor-host response. *Soc. Sci. Med.*, **20**, 833–840.

Waterfield, M.D., Scrace, G.T., Whittle, N., Stroobant, P., Johnsson, A., Wasteson, A., Westermark, B., Heldin, C.H., Huang, J.S. and Devel, T.F. (1983) Platelet-derived growth factor is structurally related to the putative transforming protein p28[sis] of simian sarcoma virus. *Nature*, **304**, 35–39.

Watson, M., Pettingale, K.W. and Greer, S. (1984) Emotional control and automatic arousal in breast cancer patients. *J. Psychosom. Res.*, **28**, 467–474.

Watson, M., Greer, S., Rowden, L., Gorman, C., Robertson, B., Bliss, J. and Tunmore, R. (1991) Relationships between emotional control, adjustment to cancer and depression and anxiety in breast cancer patients. *Psycholog. Med.*, **21**, 51–57.

Weisman, A.D. and Worden, J.W. (1975) *Coping and vulnerability in cancer patients. Research Report*. Private Publication, Boston.

4

Cancer and Personality

HANS J. EYSENCK
Institute of Psychiatry, University of London, UK

The theory that cancer is more likely to develop in certain types of person-ality than in others goes back a long time; "melancholia", in particular, has usually been associated with cancer, although the meaning of that term is not always clear (Schwarz, 1987). Quite generally, such theories stem from an even older belief emphasizing the existence of a body–mind continuum, rather like the notion of a space–time continuum in physics, and opposed to cartesian ideas and notions of complete body–mind discontinuity. Such a view was expressed 4000 years ago in the Indian *Mahabharata* (Santi Parva, XVI 8–9): "There are two classes of disease – bodily and mental. Each arises from the other, and neither can exist without the other. Thus mental disorders arise from physical ones, and likewise physical disorders arise from mental ones". Such a holistic view is clearly opposed to the high degree of specialization characteristic of modern medicine and its aim to "cure the disease"; a more holistic aim would be to "cure the person who has the disease". This is a longstanding argument in medicine, but recent studies have indicated that there might be some truth in the belief that there exists a "cancer-prone" personality – and also a rather different "coronary heart disease-prone" personality (Eysenck, 1989, 1991).

What makes up the cancer-prone personality? The two characteristics most usually emphasized in the past, on the basis of detailed observation, were (1) the suppression of emotion, lack of outlets for strong feelings, and failure to express such emotion; and (2) the inability to cope with interpersonal stress, leading to feelings of hopelessness and helplessness, and finally depression, and a tendency to give up easily rather than fight. Kissen and Eysenck (1962) and Bahnson and Bahnson (1960) attempted to

Cancer and Stress: Psychological, Biological and Coping Studies
Edited by C. L. Cooper and M. Watson. © 1991 John Wiley & Sons Ltd

put these rather vague theories on a more objective basis (Pohler, 1989), and a large amount of work has been carried out to discover to what extent these theories might have a factual basis. A detailed account of these studies is given elsewhere (Eysenck, 1985).

By and large, there is now a good deal of evidence concerning the existence of a cancer-prone personality. Baltrusch *et al.* (1988) have described this type of personality as overcooperative, appeasing, unassertive, overpatient, avoiding conflict, seeking harmony, compliant, defensive in response to stress, and unexpressive of negative emotions such as anger and anxiety. Temoshok (1987) has used the notion of the "Type C" personality, first described by Morris (1980), to distinguish it from the "Type A" coronary heart disease-prone type or the "Type B" healthy type of personality introduced by Friedman and Rosenman (see Chesney and Rosenman, 1985; Eysenck, 1990). The major characteristic of Type A has turned out to be an inclination to easy anger, hostility and aggression (Booth-Kewley and Friedman, 1987; Friedman and Booth-Kewley, 1987).

There is one obvious objection to any strong conclusion which might be derived from all this work. In the first place there is the possibility that the disease process might change pre-existing personality patterns in the direction found in these studies, rather than that personality predisposes towards disease. In the second place, the results obtained lack a causal mechanism that might give verisimilitude to an otherwise implausible relationship. There is now sufficient evidence on the former point from large-scale prospective studies to make this criticism inapplicable (Eysenck, 1987, 1988a, b; Grossarth-Maticek *et al.*, 1985, 1988a, b). There is now also in existence a theory, supported by many experimental studies, which can explain in a satisfactory manner the observed relationship between personality, stress and cancer (Eysenck, 1986).

PROSPECTIVE STUDIES

Space limits this discussion to only the three major prospective studies which have been undertaken in an effort to link personality and cancer. The first of these was in Yugoslavia (Grossarth-Maticek *et al.*, 1985); the second and third in Heidelberg, Germany (Grossarth-Maticek *et al.*, 1988a; Eysenck, 1988a). In all cases healthy subjects were approached on a randomized basis to take part in the study; age and sex composition were imposed to eliminate young people (with a long life expectancy) in order to increase chances of finding adequate numbers of deaths from cancer and coronary heart disease (CHD).

In addition to medical information on such variables as cholesterol level, blood pressure, blood sugar, etc., and on behavioural variables like smoking, drinking, sport activity, etc., interviewers elicited details concerning personality characteristics hypothesized to be relevant to cancer-proneness. Several different approaches to personality measurement have been used; details (including the actual inventories employed) will be found elsewhere (Grossarth-Maticek *et al.*, 1988a; Grossarth-Maticek and Eysenck, 1990). The three main instruments used were:

(1) a personality inventory containing seven scales, each of about 12 items, measuring different components of the cancer-prone personality;
(2) a holistic questionnaire assigning each subject to one of four types: Type 1 (cancer-prone); Type 2 (CHD-prone); Type 3 (hysterical); Type 4 (healthy, autonomous). Type 3 may be liable to drug addiction, but not prone to cancer or CHD;
(3) a psychometric inventory covering the same four types, but also Type 5 (rational, antiemotional), and Type 6 (egocentric, psychopathic). Type 5 goes with Types 1 and 2 as being disease prone, Type 6 with Types 3 and 4 as not being disease prone. Here our interest is in the verification of the hypothesis that Type 1 is cancer-prone, Type 2 CHD-prone and Types 3 and 4 relatively healthy and unlikely to develop either cancer or CHD. Statistical details concerning these studies are given elsewhere in the references already cited; the results given here are not altered in any significant way if corrections are made for differences in smoking behaviour, or any of the medical variables.

The results obtained 10 years after the beginning of the project differ, depending on the characteristics of the populations studied. The Yugoslav population was on average 60 years old at the commencement of the study; the two Heidelberg groups on average 10 years younger. Hence we would expect a much higher number of deaths in the Yugoslav group. The first ("normal") Heidelberg group was a random sample of the population; the second ("stressed") Heidelberg group was selected on the basis of being nominated as being severely stressed by the members of the first ("normal") Heidelberg group. As the two Heidelberg groups show minimal differences in age and sex, smoking, or any other disease-relevant variables measured in this study, the comparison constitutes a severe test of the proposition that stress may be a risk factor in cancer and CHD. We put forward the hypothesis that the "stressed" group would show a much higher level of mortality than the "normal" group, and might indeed rival the (older) Yugoslav sample in that respect.

Figure 1 shows the results for the Yugoslav group, and the number of subjects in each type group. It would appear that Type 1 subjects, as expected, tended to die of cancer rather than of CHD, while Type 2 subjects, as expected, tended to die of CHD rather than of cancer. Type 3 and Type 4 subjects showed a much lower mortality than Type 1 and Type 2.

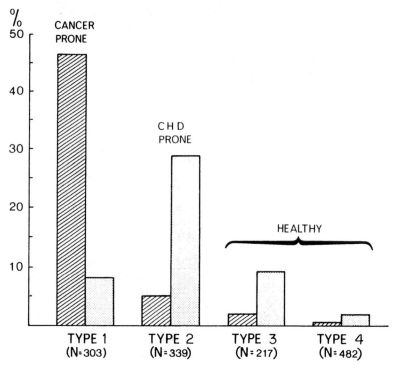

Figure 1. Prospective studies investigating link between personality and cancer. Ten-year results of the Yugoslav study comparing personality types 1–4 and mortality from cancer or CHD. ▨ death from cancer; ▨ death from infarct or stroke. For details see text. (From Grossarth-Maticek *et al.*, 1985)

These comparisons are fully significant statistically, at a high level ($P < 0.001$).

The Heidelberg "normal" group (Figure 2) shows a much lower mortality than the Yugoslav group, being much younger. Nevertheless, here too Type 1 has a higher death rate for cancer, Type 2 for CHD, while deaths among Types 3 and 4 are almost entirely absent. These data too are in line with expectation.

Finally, turning to Figure 3. As expected, the stress suffered by this "stressed" group has increased mortality levels very much above those of the "normal" group, and almost up to those of the much older Yugoslav group. Type 1 again shows greater mortality for cancer, Type 2 for CHD. Types 3 and 4 show little mortality. Clearly, stress is a killer, but it kills selectively, dependent upon personality disposition.

Figures 1–3 give the results derived from the holistic type assessment, that is, they are based on an ipsative method of measurement. Normative

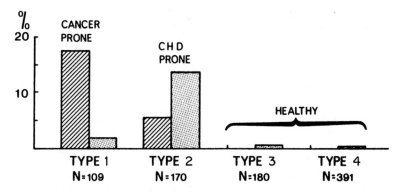

Figure 2. Results of the Heidelberg study "normal" group comparing personality types 1–4 and mortality from cancer or CHD. ▨ Death from cancer; ▦ death from infarct or stroke. For details see text. (From Grossarth-Maticek *et al.*, 1988)

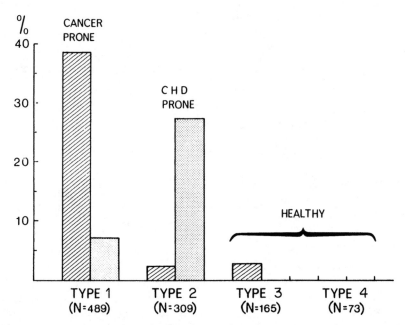

Figure 3. Results of the Heidelberg study "stressed" group comparing personality types 1–4 and mortality from cancer or CHD. ▨ Cancer; ▦ infarct or stroke. For details see text. (From Grossarth-Maticek *et al.*, 1988)

measures described above give equally striking results. Using the seven scales mentioned, we can construct a path model with cancer as the dependent variable, and the seven scales as the independent variables. The results, in the form of standardized partial repression coefficients, are given in Figure 4. (These data are from the Yugoslav study.) The explained variance (R^2) for these variables is 0.55, with an error term denoting the unexplained variance of 0.45; this is indicated in Figure 4 as e ($e = R$). Actually the R^2 for the first three predictors is 0.49, so that little is gained by including the other four predictors (Eysenck, 1988a).

The two major contributors to successful prediction are clearly X_1 and X_3, which are very similar to the two major traditional hypotheses mentioned in the introduction – suppression of emotion (X_3) and failure to cope with interpersonal stress, resulting in chronic hopelessness (X_1). It is interesting that X_2 (anger and excitement, largely as a result of stress) has a negative regression coefficient, but has a positive value for CHD, illustrating the opposite direction taken by stress reactions of probands of Type 1 and Type 2 respectively (Eysenck, 1988a).

Schmidt, 1984 (unpublished data) has pointed out some weaknesses in the statistical treatment, particularly the assumption that the dependent variable (cancer) is dichotomous; in addition, the items of the psychosocial scales are also used in a dichotomous form. Using more appropriate statistics, Schmidt found higher correlations with cancer incidence throughout (except for the anger/excitement scale), suggesting that something like 60% of the total variance for cancer incidence could be accounted for in terms of the personality variables chosen. It is interesting to note

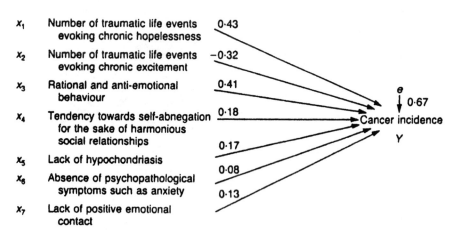

Figure 4. Results of normative measures of assessment of comparison of mortality from cancer/CHD with personality type, in the form of standardized partial regression coefficients. Data from Grossart-Maticek *et al.*, 1985. For details see text

that the inclusion of other variables (blood cholesterol, incidence of herpes, hepatitis, liver cirrhosis, vitamin A and vitamin C intake, and lymphocyte percentage) do not do much to increase the accuracy of the prediction of cancer incidence in this sample (Grossarth-Maticek *et al.*, 1983). This is an important finding, demonstrating the importance of personality and stress compared with the other risk factors.

One final prospective study may be mentioned because it used a psychometrically more sophisticated scale, and because it used a method of test administration which is novel and of some promise. In this method the test is administered twice, with six months intervening. During this time the subjects may succeed in dealing with the stressful situation; this will be shown by a *decrease* in their disease-prone scores. Such a change is a favourable development, and will be denoted "D" for development. If the subject fails to show such a development, or gets worse, their disease-prone scores will stay the same or increase, and will be marked "S" for stagnation. We would expect "D" probands of a given type to survive better than "S" probands at the end of the follow-up.

In the questionnaire used in this study, two further personality types were added to the four already encountered, as mentioned on page 75. Type 5 is rational–antiemotional, and hence also likely to develop cancer

Table 1. Incidence of cancer and CHD in six personality types, when stress response is improving (D) or worsening (S)

Type		Cancer	CHD	Other causes	Still living
1	S(82)	35	11	15	21
	D(71)	3	4	5	59
2	S(104)	17	49	25	13
	D(84)	1	10	7	66
3	S(56)	8	9	10	29
	D(72)	0	1	0	71
4	S(46)	5	2	3	36
	D(85)	0	1	0	84
5	S(57)	18	9	27	3
	D(91)	1	0	1	89
6	S(57)	6	9	34	8
	D(63)	1	2	3	57
	868	95	107	130	536

From Grossarth-Maticek and Eysenck, 1990.
S, stagnant; no change or worse score on second administration of questionnaire; D, development; change of score showing improvement on second administration of questionnaire.

(see Figure 4). Type 6 is egocentric and psychopathic, and predicted to be unlikely to develop cancer or CHD. Table 1 shows the results of a study using 868 subjects (Grossarth-Maticek and Eysenck, 1990). It will be seen that again Type 1 is most likely to develop cancer, Type 2 to develop CHD, with Type 5 also disease-prone. Of particular importance is the difference between the S and D subjects. Of the 38 Type 1 subjects to die of cancer, 35 are S and only three are D. Similarly for Type 2, of 59 to die, 49 are S, and only 10 D. Overall, of all those who died of any cause, 292 are S, and only 40 are D. This clearly is an important new variable to assess the development of stress as a risk factor in cancer, CHD and other death-causing diseases. (The questionnaire used in this study is printed in Grossarth-Maticek and Eysenck, 1990.)

SYNERGISTIC COMBINATION OF RISK FACTORS

It is known that personality and stress are not the only risk factors for cancer and CHD; smoking, drinking, blood pressure, cholesterol, and above all heredity are well known to play an important part. These risk factors do not act additively but synergistically (Kleinbaum *et al.*, 1982; Kooperman, 1981; Perkins, 1989; Rothman, 1974; Saracci, 1987; Walker, 1981). None of these authors have looked at personality in this context, and it may be useful to quote some data to illustrate the synergistic action of this variable when paired with others.

Table 2 shows the number of lung cancer deaths, other deaths and total deaths for non-smokers and smokers of Type 1, compared with individ-

Table 2. Percentage of deaths from lung cancer and other causes in group of Type 1 compared with Types 2, 3 and 4, and in smokers and non-smokers

	Yugoslavia			Heidelberg (stressed)		
	Deaths from			Deaths from		
	Lung cancer	Other causes	Total	Lung cancer	Other causes	Total
Non-smokers						
Type 1	1 (0.8%)	118	119	9 (3.8%)	227	236
Others	0	550	550	3 (1.0%)	297	300
Smokers						
Type 1	31 (16.9%)	153	184	37 (14.6%)	216	253
Others	6 (1.2%)	482	488	0	247	247

From Grossarth-Maticek *et al.*, 1988.

uals of Types 2–4 (Eysenck, 1988a). (These are data from our Yugoslav and Heidelberg (stressed) studies, already discussed.) Among non-smokers, as expected, there are very few deaths from lung cancer, but of the 13 that occur, 10 occur in persons of Type 1. For smokers, there are 74 deaths, only six of which occur in persons other than Type 1. These results give rise to an association between Type 1 and lung cancer of $P = 0.0001$ for both the samples considered. It is clear that quite independent of smoking, individuals of Type 1 are cancer-prone compared with individuals of Types 2, 3 and 4. (See also Grossarth-Maticek et al., 1988a, who used the Mantel–Haenszel (1959) formula to eliminate the differential effects of smoking.)

Table 2 also makes clear that there is a *synergistic interaction* between smoking and typology. The only group with a high proportion of deaths from lung cancer is that of smokers of Type 1: smokers not of Type 1 and non-smokers either of Type 1 or of the other types have negligible rates of death from cancer. Of the two factors smoking and personality, personality seems to be the stronger (Grossarth-Maticek et al., 1988a). Of 735 smokers not of Type 1, only six were found to have died of lung cancer; this figure is not very different from three non-smokers of Type 1 who died out of the 850 non-smokers. Clearly, smoking appears to represent a danger to health as far as lung cancer is concerned only for individuals of Type 1.

The data may deserve a slightly more formal analysis, following the traditional methods of epidemiology (Perkins, 1989). The background factor (non-smokers, not of Type 1) for the two populations (Yugoslav and Heidelberg stressed) taken together is 0.35% for lung cancer mortality ($n = 850$). For personality in non-smokers it is 2.82% giving an excess of 2.47% (2.82 – 0.35), which may be called the personality effect. For smoking in personality other than Type 1 the effect is 0.45% (0.80 – 0.35), i.e. about one-fifth of that of personality. The combined effect of smoking and personality is 15.21% (15.56 – 0.35) which is five times the effect expected from simple addition of the smoking and personality effects (0.45 + 2.47 = 2.92%). Thus synergism produces a 500% increase in cancer mortality from smoking and personality.

This calculation is taken over 2377 people, giving 78 cases of lung cancer mortality; the numbers are clearly not large enough to take the resulting calculations as anything but a very rough and ready guideline. Also it may be objected that the calculation brings together two rather unlike populations (Yugoslav and German), differing in age and stress. However, both groups give similar results when analysed independently, and hence may not be too dissimilar for the purpose of analysis. (The Heidelberg normal group had too few cases of lung cancer to be included.) Other studies, giving identical results, are discussed by Eysenck (1991).

We have carried out similar analyses for other risk factors (blood pressure, blood cholesterol) and compared these with personality as a risk factor. Details and figures are given elsewhere (Grossarth-Maticek *et al.*, 1988a). These analyses were carried out for all three samples – the Yugoslav, the Heidelberg normal and the Heidelberg stressed. The results are quite similar, no matter which dependent variable, which organic variable and which place of investigation is considered.

(1) The organic variable has different relevance for mortality depending on the psychosocial type. Its relevance is greatest with that type which itself has the greatest specific mortality, i.e. Type 1 for cancer, and Type 2 for coronary heart disease. In other words, the psychosocial types are relevant, not only for mortality, but in a similar way for sensitivity to organic risk factors.

(2) The psychosocial types do show differences with respect to the organic variables, but these differences cannot explain away the relevance of the types for mortality; according to the figures for mortality, type-specific mortality differences when adjusted for differences of the organic variables are still highly significant.

These data suggest several conclusions. Psychosocial variables, and particularly personality type and stress, are important in mediating deaths from cancer and coronary heart disease. These personality variables are more influential than physical factors like smoking, blood pressure, and cholesterol.

Finally, personality and physical factors interact in a synergistic fashion. These are important findings for any attempt to prevent deaths from cancer and coronary heart disease.

The finding that risk factors in cancer and coronary heart disease act synergistically is so important that they may be amplified by two further studies (Eysenck, 1991). One of these is summarized in Table 3.

In Table 3 we are dealing with the results of a study in which we compare death rates of subjects having one, two, three, or all four of four different risk factors. The risk factors were:

(1) smoking (more than 20 cigarettes per day, for over 10 years);
(2) heredity (at least one first-degree relative suffering from or died of lung cancer);
(3) chronic bronchitis;
(4) stress, i.e. subjects of Type 1 or 2.

Not all combinations of risk factors could be found in sufficient numbers, but the data show very clearly the synergistic effects of multiplying risks.

It will be seen that in these subjects, who were on average between 51 and 54 years old at the beginning of the study, 13 years later *none* had died

Table 3. Different combinations of risk factors for lung cancer and other causes of death

Combination of risks	N	Lung cancer	%	Other causes of death	%	Average age
Only H	50	0	0	5	10	51
Only C	100	0	0	12	12	52
Only S	59	0	0	16	27	52
H + C	50	1	2	4	8	53
H + B	52	0	0	8	15	51
C + B	55	0	0	11	20	52
C + S	100	2	2	21	21	53
H + S	49	0	0	9	18	54
B + S	50	0	0	8	16	53
C + H + B	26	2	8	5	19	51
C + H + S	50	10	20	14	28	51
C + B + S	51	5	10	10	20	51
H + C + B + S	26	8	31	8	31	52
(H + C + B + S + BT)	26	3	12	4	15	52

H, heredity; C, smoking; B, chronic bronchitis; S, personality/stress
From Eysenck, 1991.

of lung cancer of those who only showed *one* risk factor. Of those showing two risk factors, only about 1% died of lung cancer. Combinations of three risk factors showed quite elevated death rates for lung cancer, varying from 8 to 20%. Combinations of four risk factors raised the death rate from lung cancer to 31%, demonstrating the strong synergistic effect of multiplying risk factors.

Of particular interest is the group of four risk factor subjects put in parentheses; they had received prophylactic behaviour therapy (BT), and accordingly had a death rate from lung cancer only about one-third as high as the group of four risk factor subjects who received no therapy. Thus even for those most exposed to lung cancer prophylactic treatment is possible, and can be efficacious. The prophylactic action of behaviour therapy in this connection has been discussed at length elsewhere (Grossarth-Maticek and Eysenck, 1991; Eysenck and Grossarth-Maticek, 1989, 1991).

Table 4 shows the synergistic interaction between smoking and personality/stress as risk factors for lung cancer. In each case other risk factors (e.g. heredity – number of close family members who died of lung cancer) have been equated. Groups with and without stress are *matched* for age and sex, as well as for heredity. Stress is defined as having a higher point total for Types 1 + 2 + 5, as compared with 3 + 4 + 6. These follow-up data show that:

(1) non-smokers have very little risk of lung cancer, regardless of stress;

Table 4. Lung cancer deaths among smokers and non-smokers according to presence or absence of stress

Number of cigarettes smoked daily	Died of lung cancer			
	Without stress (n)		With stress (n)	
Non-smoker	1 (0.2%)	512	1 (0.2%)	512
10–20	1 (0.4%)	271	2 (0.7%)	271
21–35	3 (1.1%)	271	8 (2.9%)	271
36–40	5 (4.9%)	101	11 (10.9%)	101
41–60	7 (6.9%)	101	17 (16.8%)	101

(2) subjects without stress run much less risk (less than half) of lung cancer with stress, when equated for smoking;

(3) risk of lung cancer increases monotonically with amount smoked, both in with and without stress subjects (dose-response curve);

(4) the interaction factor is indicated by the fact that among non-stress subjects, the smoking increases the risk tenfold, among stressed subjects, twenty-sixfold. This is a clear indication of the importance of synergistic action.

Results of comparing subjects of differing genetic disposition to lung cancer, with or without stress, are similar, and are given in Table 5. It will be seen that the proportion of deaths from lung cancer increases monotonically with increase in the number of close relatives who died of lung cancer, or were suffering from lung cancer; this is equally true for subjects with or without stress. Equally, subjects suffering from stress are roughly twice as likely to die of lung cancer than no-stress subjects, when equated for genetic risk. Finally, there is a clear synergistic interaction. For no-

Table 5. Lung cancer deaths among stressed and non-stress subjects depending on genetic predisposition

Number of close relatives died or are suffering from lung cancer	Died of lung cancer			
	Without stress		With stress	
	n	%	n	%
1	191	2 (1.1)	191	2 (0.5)
2	98	2 (2.2)	98	4 (4.1)
3	33	2 (6.7)	33	5 (15.2)
4	33	3 (9.1)	33	6 (19.4)
5	25	4 (16.0)	25	8 (40.0)

From Eysenck, 1991.

stress subjects, high genetic risk increases the risk factor eight times, for stressed subjects, 30 times. Thus genetic risk factors interact with stress in a very similar fashion to smoking. Stress and personality as risk factors increase dramatically (roughly doubling) the risk attending smoking, or having close relatives die of lung cancer.

It will be clear that personality and stress act in a synergistic fashion as risk factors in cancer and CHD, very much as do the other risk factors mentioned. None is of great importance by itself and in isolation; it is when risk factors combine that they become deadly. The ease with which Type 1 and Type 2 behaviours and attitude can be altered in the direction of autonomous, health-giving behaviour would seem to single them out for such prophylactic treatment, using the methods of behaviour therapy (Grossarth-Maticek and Eysenck, 1991; Eysenck and Grossarth-Maticek, 1991). Eysenck (1990) has attempted to summarize earlier findings along these lines, and to demonstrate their social importance for disease prevention. It is important to note that although attempts to reduce mortality by decreasing cigarette consumption have not on the whole been very successful (Eysenck, 1991), intervention along psychological lines using a form of behavioural therapy has, this would seem, strengthened the claims for a *causal* role for such psychological factors.

PERSONALITY AND CANCER: CAUSAL LINKS

In science, pure description in the absence of causal links is not very persuasive; at least the possibility of a testable theory concerning the connection between the variables found to be correlated should be apparent. In suggesting such a theoretical link between cancer and personality I am well aware of the complexity of the issues involved, and of the paucity of supporting data. Nevertheless, I believe that the theory in question does at least point us in the right direction, however much change there must be in details once it is subjected to rigorous testing (Eysenck, 1986). The theory will not be discussed in great detail, but some of the supporting evidence will be cited (Eysenck, 1991).

Figure 5 illustrates the assumed causal pathway. Personality (Type 1) and stress combine and interact to produce feelings of helplessness, hopelessness and depression; these in turn produce hormonal and other reactions, of which cortisol is here given as the representative (others are the endogenous opiates, ACTH, etc.). These in turn produce immune deficiency, which allows budding cancers to develop. The well-established fact that immune reactions can be conditioned along classical lines suggests one possible way in which such reactions may be learned (Ader and Cohen, 1975; Solvasan et al., 1988). There is a good deal of evidence to support such a model.

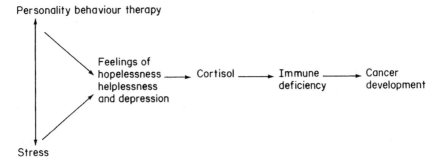

Figure 5. Assumed causal pathway connecting personality, stress and development of cancer

The model owes much to a similar one by Solomon (Solomon, 1987; Solomon and Moos, 1964; Solomon et al., 1968) who has argued powerfully for the concept of an "immunosuppression-prone" personality (Solomon, 1985), which may correspond to "Type 1". Having surveyed the literature, he produced first 35, and later another 30 postulates, many of which are relevant to our discussion. The main postulates of interest here are given below, numbered in sequence.

Solomon's postulates, 1987

(1) Enduring coping style and personality factors (trait characteristics) should influence the susceptibility of an individual's immune system to alteration by exogenous events, including reactions to events. (Thus, an "immunosuppression-prone" behavioral pattern is hypothesized.)

(2) Emotional upset and distress (state characteristics) should alter the incidence, severity, and/or course of diseases that are immunologically resisted (infectious and neoplastic) or are associated with aberrant immunologic function (allergic and autoimmune).

(3) Severe emotional disturbance and mental dysfunction should be accompanied by immunologic abnormalities.

(4) Experimental behavioral manipulation (for example, stress, conditioning) should have immunologic consequences.

(5) Experimental manipulation of appropriate parts of the central nervous system should have immunologic consequences.

(6) Hormones and other substances regulated or elaborated by the central nervous system should influence immune mechanisms.

(7) Biochemical and functional similarities might be expected between the substances modulating the function and reactivity of the central nervous system (neuropeptides) and the substances with comparable effects on the immune system (cytokines).

(8) Behavioral interventions (such as psychotherapy, relaxation techniques, imagery, biofeedback and hypnosis) should be able to enhance or optimize immune function.

(9) Altered CNS neurotransmitter receptor site sensitivities felt to be associated with mental illnesses should be reflected in lymphocyte receptors.

(10) The "functional" modes of expression of CNS and immune system should be similar.

Linn et al. (1981) have shown that stress and anxiety are associated with depressed immunological response. Levy et al. (1985, 1987) found that natural killer (NK) cell activity in breast cancer patients was strongly correlated with psychosocial stress indicators which accounted for 51% of the baseline NK activity variance. Green and Green (1987) reported that relaxation increases salivary immunoglobin A_1. Bandura et al. (1988) found that perceived self-inefficacy in exercising control over cognitive stressors activated endogenous opioid systems. Kiecolt-Glaser et al. (1984) found that distressed and lonely subjects had significantly higher cortisol levels and a lower level of NK cell activity. Glaser et al. (1986) discovered stress-related impairments in cellular immunity, and Glaser and Kiecolt-Glaser (1985) found that even "relatively mild stress" depressed cellular immunity in healthy adults. Kiecolt-Glaser et al. (1984) found that high scores on stressful life events and loneliness had significantly lower levels of NK cell activity. Herberman (1986), Irwin et al. (1987), Nemeroff et al. (1984) and Rou et al. (1988) found impaired immune reaction in depressed groups, and Linn et al. (1988), Arnetz et al. (1987), Glaser et al. (1985) and Shavit et al. (1989) found impaired immune reactions to stress. Jemmott and Magloine (1988) found that stress lowered salivary concentrations of S-IgA, while social support increased them. Grossarth-Maticek and Eysenck (1989) found that behaviour therapy significantly increased the percentage lymphocyte count in terminally ill women suffering from cancer, and also increased their survival time. Pennebaker et al. (1988) found that self-disclosure improved cellular immune functioning. Kiecolt-Glaser et al. (1985) found an enhancement of immunocompetence by relaxation and social contact.

Irwin et al. (1987) have shown that life events can cause depression and reduce the effectiveness of the immune function. Similarly, Murphy et al. (1987), in a prospective study of 1003 adults, found a significant correlation between depression and mortality. Rodin (1980, 1986) showed that appropriate psychotherapy reduced depression and cortisol level through psychotherapy. Dabbs and Hopper (1991) showed that cortisol level correlated with anxiety, depression and high heart rate.

Finally, the relationship between mood and the immune system response has been established in a series of studies (Baker, 1987; Dillon and Baker, 1985; Linn *et al.*, 1984; McClelland *et al.*, 1980, 1985; Stone *et al.*, 1987). Animal studies, too, have contributed to the formulation of the model (e.g. Glaser *et al.*, 1985; Laudenslager *et al.*, 1983; Borysenko and Borysenko, 1982; and for a review, Justice, 1985).

The studies quoted are only among the most recent; for reviews of the older and perhaps less convincing materials the following are suggested: Jemmett and Locke (1984); Miller (1983, 1985); Baker (1987); Kennedy *et al.* (1988); Teshima (1986); Plotnikoff *et al.* (1986); Korneva *et al.* (1985); Antoni (1987); Steptoe (1989). Taking all the published data together, they do seem to support the sort of model suggested by Dilman and Ostronmova (1984) and Eysenck (1986), briefly outlined above. There is evidence that: (1) personality and stress produce immunodestructive substances in the bloodstream; (2) that these substances have an immunodestructive function; and that (3) behavioural manipulations can reverse this process. Thus there appears to exist a preliminary model to explain along causal lines the effectiveness of behaviour therapy in prophylaxis for cancer, and in prolonging life in cancer sufferers.

There is one apparent objection to this argument. As Zonderman *et al.* (1989) have shown, there is no evidence in a nationally representative sample for any correlation between depressive symptoms and cancer morbidity. The answer to this is very simple. Depression is a multifaceted set of symptoms, like fever, which may have diverse causes and relate to different disorders; the difference between reactive and endogenous depression is perhaps the best known. The type of depression referred to in our theory is subclinical, and might be defined as "hopelessness depression" (Alloy *et al.*, 1988). This concept is largely based on the work of Seligman (1975) and Abramson *et al.* (1978), and is essentially a cognitive diathesis–stress theory of depression (Alloy *et al.*, 1985). According to this theory, "a proximal sufficient cause of depression is an expectation that highly desired outcomes are unlikely to occur, or that highly aversive outcomes are likely to occur, and that no response in one's repertoire will change the likelihood of occurrence of these outcomes" (Alloy *et al.*, 1988, p. 7). It is in this sense that the term has been used in our research. Other varieties of depression may or may not be relevant, and it is important to note that animal work has emphasized the importance of differentiating between escapable and inescapable shocks, and the vital contribution of predictability (Miller, 1981).

SUMMARY AND CONCLUSIONS

The data referred to here constitute only a small part of what is now available. In particular, the large literature now available on the effects of psychotherapy and behaviour therapy is only hinted at; the demonstration that intervention studies can actually change the probability of dying of cancer for Type 1 personalities very drastically is experimental proof for a causal, and not only a statistical, association between personality and cancer (Eysenck and Grossarth-Maticek, 1991).

One criticism sometimes presented of the conclusion that personality is an important risk factor for cancer should perhaps be mentioned. It is based on the possibility that early undiagnosed "minicancers" may affect personality; it is suggested that the slowly developing and undiagnosed cancer may distort the personality picture in the direction of Type 1. This is unlikely, for two reasons. First, the strong prophylactic influence of behaviour therapy (Eysenck and Grossarth-Maticek, 1989, 1991) suggests that no such early "minicancer" has influenced the data, or else that behaviour therapy can actually cure cancer – a claim we would be very chary to make. In the second place, the 10-year follow-up of the Heidelberg subjects has been followed by a further four-year follow-up, which has given essentially similar results. In this later follow-up the original ascertainment of personality and stress was undertaken 10 years ago or more, and it would strain credulity to assume that the cancer finally diagnosed influenced personality and behaviour over 10 years before being diagnosed! We are continuing the follow-up and will report on further developments (Eysenck, 1991).

What, then, has been accomplished? There can now be little doubt about the importance of personality reactions to stress for the development of cancer, or the involvement of interpersonal stress altogether. We have a good idea of what the cancer-prone personality is like, and instruments are available to measure it reliably. We have a theory which bridges the gap between a psychological variable (personality) and a physical one (cancer), and which has good support from a variety of experimental studies. Finally, we can *alter* the strength of the relationship between personality and cancer by behaviour therapy in predictable ways. All of this is only the beginning of an important quest, but it is an important beginning. We now have a much better idea of the right questions to ask, the right methods to use, and the anomalies and weaknesses in our theories which need research to clear up. These are important advances.

REFERENCES

Abramson, L.Y., Seligman, M.E.P. and Teasdale, H. (1978) Learned helplessness in humans: critique and reformulation. *J. Ab. Psychol.*, **87**, 49–474.

Ader, R. and Cohen, N. (1975) Behaviorally conditioned immunosuppression. *Psychosom. Med.*, **37**, 333–340.

Alloy, L.B., Clements, C. and Kolden, G. (1985) The cognitive diathesis – stress theories of depression: Therapeutic implications. In Reiss, S. and Bortzin, R.

(eds) *Theoretical Issues in Behavior Therapy*. Academic Press, New York, pp. 379–410.

Alloy, L.B., Abramson, L.Y., Metalsky, G.I. and Hartlage, S. (1988) The hopelessness theory of depression: Attributional aspects. *Br. J. Clin. Psychol.*, **27**, 5–21.

Antoni, M.H. (1987) Neuroendocrine influences in psychoimmunology and neoplasia: A review. *Psychology and Health*, **1**, 3–24.

Arnetz, B., Wanerman, J., Petrini, B., Brenner, F., Levi, L., Enerath, P., Solovaara, H., Hgelm, R., Thoerell, T. and Petterson, I. (1987) Immune function in unemployed women. *Psychosom. Med.*, **49**, 3–12.

Bahnson, C.B. and Bahnson, M.B. (1960) Role of ego defences: Denial and regression in the etiology of malignant neoplasms. *Ann. NY Acad. Sci.*, **125**(3), 827–895.

Baker, C. (1987) Psychological factors and immunity. *J. Psychosom. Res.*, **31**, 1–10.

Baltrusch, H., Stangel, W. and Waltz, M. (1988) Cancer from the behavioral perspective: The Type C pattern. *Activ. Nerv. Sup.*, **30**, 18–20.

Bandura, A., Cioffi, D., Taylor, C.B. and Brouillard, M.E. (1988) Perceived self-efficacy in coping with cognitive stress and opioid activation. *J. Person. Soc. Psychol.*, **55**, 479–488.

Booth-Kewley, S. and Friedman, H.S. (1987) Psychological predictors of heart disease: A qualitative review. *Psycholog. Bull.*, **101**, 343–362.

Borysenko, M. and Borysenko, J. (1982) Stress, behavior and immunity: Animal models and mediating mechanisms. *Gen. Hosp. Psych.*, **4**, 59–67.

Chesney, M. and Rosenman, R. (1985) *Anger and Hostility in Cardiovascular and Behavioral Disorders*. Hemisphere, Washington.

Dabbs, J.M. and Hopper, C.H. (1991) Cortisol, arousal, and personality in two groups of normal men. *Person. Indiv. Diff.*, in press.

Dillon, K.M. and Baker, K.N. (1988) Positive emotional states and enhancement of the immune system. *Int. J. Psychiat. Med.*, **15**, 13–18.

Dilman, V.M. and Ostroumova, M.V. (1984) Hypothalmic, metabolic, and immune mechanisms of the influence of stress. In Fox, B.H. and Newberry, B.H. (eds) *Impact of Psychoendrocrine Systems in Cancer and Immunity*. C.H. Hogrefe, New York, pp. 143–165.

Eysenck, H.J. (1985) Personality, cancer and cardiovascular disease: A causal analysis. *Person. Indiv. Diff.*, **5**, 535–557.

Eysenck, H.J. (1986) Smoking and Health. In Tollison, R.D. (ed.) *Smoking and Society*. Lexington Books, Lexington, pp. 17–88.

Eysenck, H.J. (1987) Anxiety, "learned helplessness", and cancer – a causal theory. *J. Anx. Dis.*, **1**, 87–104.

Eysenck, H.J. (1988a) The respective importance of personality, cigarette smoking and interaction effects for the genesis of cancer and coronary heart disease. *Person. Indiv. Diff.*, **9**, 453–464.

Eysenck, H.J. (1988b) Personality, stress and cancer: Prediction and prophylaxis. *Br. J. Med. Psychol.*, **61**, 57–75.

Eysenck, H.J. (1990) Type A behavior and coronary heart disease. The Third stage. *J. Soc. Behav. Person.*, **5**, 25–44.

Eysenck, H.J. (1991) *Smoking, Personality and Stress: Psychosocial factors in the prevention of cancer and coronary disease*. Springer-Verlag, New York.

Eysenck, H.J. and Grossarth-Maticek, R. (1989) Prevention of cancer and coronary heart disease and the reduction in the cost of the National Health Service. *J. Soc. Pol. Econ. Studies*, **14**, 25–47.

Eysenck, H.J. and Grossarth-Maticek, R. (1991) Creative novation behaviour therapy as a prophylactic treatment for cancer and coronary heart disease: II. Effects of treatment. *Behav. Res. Ther.*, **29**, 17–31.

Friedman, H.S. and Booth-Kewley, S. (1987) Personality, Type A behavior, and coronary heart disease: The role of emotional expression. *J. Person. Soc. Psychol.*, **53**, 783–792.

Glaser, R. and Kiecolt-Glaser, J. (1985) "Relatively mild stress" depresses cellular immunity in healthy adults. *Behav. Brain Sci.*, **8**, 401–403.

Glaser, R., Kiecolt-Glaser, J., Speicher, C. and Halliday, J. (1985) Stress, loneliness and changes in herpes virus latency. *J. Behav. Med.*, **8**, 249–260.

Glaser, R., Thorn, B.E., Tarr, K.L., Kiecolt-Glaser, J. and D'Ambrosia, S. (1985) Effects of stress on methyltransferase synthesis: An important DNA repair enzyme. *Health Psychol.*, **4**, 403–412.

Glaser, R., Kiecolt-Glaser, J., Stout, J.C., Tarr, K.L., Speicher, C.E. and Halliday, J. (1986) Stress-related impairments in cellular immunity. *Psychiat. Res.*, **16**, 233–239.

Green, R.G. and Green, M.L. (1987) Relaxation increases salivary immunoglobulin "A". *Psychol. Rep.*, **61**, 623–629.

Grossarth-Maticek, R. and Eysenck, H.J. (1988) Personality type, smoking habit and their interaction as predictors of cancer and coronary heart disease. *Person. Indiv. Diff.*, **9**, 479–495.

Grossarth-Maticek, R. and Eysenck, H.J. (1989) Length of survival and lymphocyte percentage in women with mammary cancer as a function of psychotherapy. *Psychol. Rep.*, **65**, 315–321.

Grossarth-Maticek, R. and Eysenck, H.J. (1990) Personality, stress and disease: Description and validation of a new inventory. *Psychol. Rep.*, **66**, 355–373.

Grossarth-Maticek, R., Bastiaans, J. and Kanazir, D.T. (1985) Psychosocial factors as strong predictors of mortality from cancer, ischaemic heart disease and stroke: The Yugoslav prospective study. *J. Psychosom. Res.*, **29**, 167–176.

Grossarth-Maticek, R., Eysenck, H.J. and Vetter, H. (1988) Personality type, smoking and their interaction as a predictor in cancer and coronary heart disease. *Person. Indiv. Diff.*, **9**, 479–495.

Grossarth-Maticek, R., Eysenck, H.J., Vetter, H. and Schmidt, P. (1988) Psychosocial types and chronic diseases: Results of the Heidelberg Prospective Psychosomatic Intervention Study. In Maes, S., Spielberger, C., Defares, P. and Sarason, I.G. (eds) *Topics in Health Psychology*. John Wiley, London, pp. 57–75.

Grossarth-Maticek, R., Kanazir, D.T., Vetter, H. and Schmidt, P. (1983) Psychosomatic factors involved in the process of cancerogenesis. *Psychother. Psychosom.*, **40**, 191–210.

Grossarth-Maticek, R. and Eysenck, H.J. (1991) Creative novation behaviour therapy as a prophylactic treatment for cancer and coronary heart disease: I. Description of treatment. *Behav. Res. Ther.*, **29**, 1–16.

Herberman, R. (1986) Cancer, AIDS, chronic fatigue and NK cells. *UCLA Symposium on Behavioral Neuroimmunology*. April 13, 1986.

Irwin, M., Daniels, E.T., Bloom, T.L., Smith, H. and Weiner, H. (1987) Life events, depressive symptoms, and immune function. *Am. J. Psych.*, **144**, 437–441.

Irwin, M., Vale, W. and Britton, K. (1987) Central cortico-trapin-releasing factor suppresses natural killer cell cytotoxicity. *Brain Behav. Immun.*, **1**, 85–87.

Jemmott, J.B. III and Locke, S.E. (1984) Psychosocial factors, immunologic mediation, and human susceptibility to infectious diseases: How much do we know? *Psychol. Bull.*, **95**, 78–108.

Jemmot, J.B. III and Magloine, K. (1988) Academic stress, social support, and secretory immunoglobulin A. *J. Person. Soc. Psychol.*, **55**, 803–810.

Justice, A. (1985) Review of the effects of stress and cancer in laboratory animals: Importance of time of stress application and type of tumour. *Psychol. Bull.*, **98**, 108–138.

Kennedy, S., Kiecolt-Glaser, J. and Glaser, R. (1988) Immunological consequences of acute and chronic stressors: Mediating role of interpersonal relationships. *Br. J. Med. Psychol.*, **61**, 77–85.

Kiecolt-Glaser, J., Garner, W., Speicher, C., Penn, G., Halliday, J. and Glaser, R. (1984) Psychosocial modifiers of immunocompetence in medical students. *Psychosom. Med.*, **46**, 7–14.

Kiecolt-Glaser, J., Rickers, D., George, J., Monick, G., Speicher, C.E., Garner, W. and Glaser, R. (1984) Urinary cortisol levels, cellular incompetency, and loneliness in psychiatric inpatients. *Psychosom. Med.*, **46**, 15–23.

Kiecolt-Glaser, J., Glaser, R., Willinger, D., Stunt, J., Merrick, G., Sheppard, S., Ricker, D., Romisher, C., Briner, W., Bonnell, G. and Domerberg, R. (1985) Psychosocial enhancement of immunocompetences in a geriatric population. *Health Psychol.*, **4**, 25–41.

Kissen, D.M. and Eysenck, H.J. (1962) Personality in male lung cancer patients. *J. Psychosom. Res.*, **6**, 123–137.

Kleinbaum, D.G., Kupper, L.L. and Morganstern, H. (1982) *Epidemiological Research: Principles and Quantitative Methods*. Lifetime Learning Publications, Belmont, pp. 403–418.

Kooperman, J.S. (1981) Interaction between discrete causes. *Am. J. Epidemiol.*, **113**, 716–724.

Korneva, E.A., Klimenko, V.M. and Shkhinek, E.K. (1985) *Neurotumoral Maintenance and Immune Hameostasis*. University of Chicago Press, Chicago.

Laudenslager, M.L., Ryan, S.M., Dougan, R.C., Hyson, R.C. and Maier, S.F. (1983) Coping and immunosuppression: Inescapable but not escapable shock suppresses lymphocyte proliferations. *Science*, **221**, 568–570.

Levy, S., Herberman, R.B., Maluish, A.M., Schlien, B. and Lippman, M. (1985) Prognostic risk assessment in primary breast cancer behavioral and immunological parameters. *Health Psychol.*, **4**, 99–113.

Levy, S., Herberman, R., Lippman, M. and d'Angelo, T. (1987) Correlation of stress factors with sustained depression of natural killer cell activity and predicted prognosis in patients with breast cancer. *J. Clin. Oncol.*, **5**, 348–353.

Linn, B.S., Linn, M.W. and Jensen, J. (1981) Anxiety and immune responsiveness. *Psychol. Rep.*, **49**, 969–970.

Linn, B.S., Linn, M.W. and Klimas, N. (1988) Effects of psychophysical stress on surgical outcome. *Psychosom. Med.*, **50**, 230–244.

Linn, M.W., Linn, B.S. and Jensen, J. (1984) Stressful events, dysphoric mood, and immune responsiveness. *Psychol. Rep.*, **54**, 219–222.

McClelland, D.C., Floor, E., Davidson, R.J. and Saron, C. (1980) Stressed power motivation, sympathetic activation, immune function and illness. *J. Human Stress*, **6**, 11–19.

McClelland, D.C., Ross, G. and Patel, V. (1985) The effect of an academic examination on salivary norepinephrine and immunoglobulin levels. *J. Human Stress*, **11**, 52–59.

Miller, N. (1983) Behavioral medicine: Symbiosis between laboratory and clinic. *Am. Rev. Psychol.*, **34**, 1–31.

Miller, N. (1985) Effects of emotional stress on the immune system. *Pavlovian J. Biol. Sci.*, **20**, 47–52.

Miller, S.M. (1981) Predictability and human stress: Toward a clarification of evidence and theory. *Adv. Exp. Soc. Psychol.*, **14**, 203–256.

Morris, T. (1980) A "Type C" for cancer? *Cancer Detect. Prev.*, **3**, 102–106.

Murphy, J.A., Monson, R.P., Sobol, A.M. and Leighton, A.H. (1987) Affective disorders and mortality. *Arch. Gen. Psych.*, **44**, 473–480.

Neineroff, C., Widerloo, E., Bissente, G., Walleus, H., Karlsson, I., Eklund, B., Kitts, C., Loisen, P. and Vale, W. (1984) Elevated concentrations of cortico-tropin-releasing-factor-like activity in depressed patients. *Science*, **226**, 1342–1344.

Pennebaker, J.W., Kiecolt-Glaser, J. and Glaser, R. (1988) Disclosure of traumas and immune function: Health implication for psychotherapy. *J. Consult. Clin. Psychol.*, **56**, 235–245.

Perkins, D.A. (1989) Interaction among coronary heart disease risk factors. *Ann. Behav. Med.*, **11**, 3–11.

Pohler, G. (1989) *Krebs und seelischer Konflikt*. Nexus, Frankfurt.

Plotnikoff, N., Faith, R., Murgo, A. and Good, R.A. (eds) (1986) *Enkephalins and Endorphins: Stress and the Immune System*. Plenum Press, New York.

Rodin, J. (1980) Managing the stress of aging: The role of control and coping. In Levine, S. and Urwin, H. (eds) *Coping and Health*. pp. 171–202.

Rodin, J. (1986) Health, control and aging. In Baltes, M. and Baltes, P.B. (eds) *Aging and the Psychology of Control*. Lawrence Erlbaum, Hillsdale, pp. 214–236.

Rou, B., Rose, J., Sunderland, T., Moritisa, J. and Murphy, D. (1988) Antisomatostatin G in major depressive disorder. A preliminary study with implications for autoimmune mechanisms of depression. *Arch. Gen. Psych.*, **45**, 924–928.

Rothman, K.J. (1974) Synergy and antagonism in cause–effect relationships. *Am. J. Epidemiol.*, **99**, 385–388.

Saracci, R. (1987) The interaction of tobacco smoking and other agents in cancer etiology. *Epidemiol. Rev.*, **9**, 175–193.

Schwarz, R. (1987) Melancholie und Krebs: Wandel der psychosomatischen Deutung von Krebserkrankungen aus medizinisch-historischer Sicht. *Zeitschr. Psychosom. Med.*, **33**, 101–110.

Seligman, M.E.P. (1975) *Helplessness*. W.M. Freeman, San Francisco.

Shavit, Y., Lewis, J., Terman, G., Gale, R. and Leibeskind, J. (1989) Opioid peptides mediate the suppressive effects of stress on natural killer cell cytotoxicity. *Science*, **223**, 188–190.

Solomon, G. (1985) The emerging field of psychoneuroimmunology. *Advances*, **2**, 6–19.

Solomon, G. (1987) Psychoneuroimmunology: Interaction between central nervous system and immune system. *J. Neurosci. Res.*, **18**, 1–9.

Solomon, G. and Moos, R. (1964) Emotions, immunity and disease: A speculative theoretical integration. *Arch. Gen. Psych.*, **11**, 657–674.

Solomon, G., Levine, S and Kraft, J. (1968) Early experience and immunity. *Nature*, **220**, 821–822.

Solvasan, H., Ghauta, V. and Hiramoto, R. (1988) Conditioned augmentation of natural killer cell activity. Independence on interferon-beta. *J. Immunol.*, **140**, 661–665.

Steptoe, A. (1989) Coping and psychophysiological reaction. In Miller, S. (ed.) *Special Issue of Advances in Behaviour Research and Therapy*. Pergamon Press, Oxford, **11**(4), 259–270.

Stone, A.A., Cox, D.S., Valdimarsdottir, H., Jemdorf, L. and Neale, J.M. (1987) Evidence that secretory IgA antibody is associated with daily mood. *J. Person. Soc. Psychol.*, **52**, 988–993.

Temoshok, L. (1987) Personality, coping style, emotion, and cancer: Towards an integrative model. *Cancer Surveys*, **6**, 545–567.

Teshina, H. (1986) Recent biopsychosociological approaches to cancer study in Japan. In: Day, S.B. (ed.) *Cancer, Stress, and Death*. Plenum Press, New York, pp. 79–87.

Walker, A.M. (1981) Proportion of disease attributable to the combined effect of two factors. *Int. J. Epidemiol.*, **10**, 81–85.

Zonderman, A.B., Costa, P.T. and McCrae, R.R. (1989) Depression as a risk factor for cancer morbidity and mortality in a nationally representative sample. *JAMA*, **262**, 1191–1195.

5

Cancer and Stress: The Effect of Social Support as a Resource

JOAN R. BLOOM, SOO H. KANG and PATRICK ROMANO
School of Public Health, University of California, Berkeley, California, USA

Over 100 years ago, the French sociologist Durkheim (Durkheim and Simpson, 1951) first suggested that interpersonal relations between individuals had critical consequences for people's health. In this important work, he discovered that the suicide rates of individuals who were marginal to the society in which they lived were higher than those of individuals who had interpersonal ties to family and friends. This empirical observation has been noted repeatedly over subsequent years in other contexts. Several studies, for example, have reported high mortality rates among individuals who have recently lost a spouse, and higher mortality rates among single or divorced persons than among those who are married (Parkes, 1972).

More recently, the concept of social relationships was linked to physical health by both Cassel (1976) and Cobb (1976). Using an epidemiological framework guided by the stress theory of disease etiology, Cassel (1976) suggested that social activities and psychological coping styles reduce the deleterious effects of stress and the risk of disease in a non-specific way. Presumably, individuals experiencing a stressful life event who can mobilize strong supportive resources from within their networks of social relationships are better able to reduce the possible negative effects of stress on health (Brown and Gary, 1987).

The existing literature provides little information regarding the causal process through which support influences health outcomes. Cassel did

Cancer and Stress: Psychological, Biological and Coping Studies
Edited by C. L. Cooper and M. Watson. © 1991 John Wiley & Sons Ltd

explain a plausible psychophysiological pathway by which linkages to society come to affect health. Recent work on how changes in emotional state are related to the immunological system provide preliminary empirical confirmation of such pathways (Levy *et al.*, 1985); several chapters within this volume focus specifically on this issue.

Over the last decade, a number of reviews of the literature on the relationship between social support and health have been published. Some have taken an epidemiological approach, considering the lack of social support as a cause of ill health (Broadhead *et al.*, 1983; Cohen and Syme, 1985; Wortman, 1983). Generally, this perspective has defined social support in terms of the individual's ties within a social network. Measured outcomes include overall mortality and, less frequently, ill health. Others have conceptualized social support as a set of independent constructs, such as instrumental, informational, and emotional support (Schaefer *et al.*, 1981), which can be related to mental health outcomes (Cohen and Wills, 1985; Bloom, 1982a, 1986; Vernon and Jackson, 1989). The goal of this chapter is to bring these two perspectives together and relate these ideas to the study of cancer outcomes.

THE RELATIONSHIP BETWEEN SOCIAL SUPPORT AND HEALTH

In most of the epidemiological studies reviewed in this chapter, social support refers to formal and informal relationships among relatives and friends, or membership or attendance in voluntary organizations. In this context, social support may be defined as "support accessible to an individual through social ties to other individuals, groups and the larger community" (Lin *et al.*, 1979) and the term social support is used interchangeably with social relationships, social ties or social connectedness.

Social support and mortality

The association between social relationships and mortality and other health outcomes has been investigated in several studies. Most of these indicate that people who are married have lower mortality rates than those who are single, widowed or divorced (Berkson, 1962; Cox and Ford, 1964; Ward, 1976; Helsing, 1981). People with more interactions and larger networks with relatives or friends have lower mortality rates than people who are alone or isolated (Berkman and Syme, 1979; House *et al.*, 1982; Blazer, 1982; Schoenbach, 1986). Although the evidence is not as strong, some studies have indicated that social relationships may be related to the development of physical illness. The greater social ties that an individual has, in the form of close relationships with family members, friends, acquaintances, co-workers, and the larger community, the less likely that the individual will experience illness (Lin *et al.*, 1979).

The studies of social relationships and health have generated a great interest in the field of social epidemiology since the latter part of the 1970s. Berkman and Syme's Alameda County Study, published in 1979, looked prospectively at the association between social relationships and mortality. Their concept of social ties was operationalized by an index (Social Network Index) which included marital status, contacts with relatives and friends, church membership and membership in other community organizations. After nine years of follow-up, a strong negative relationship between social ties and mortality was found (Berkman and Syme, 1979). In the past decade, their study has been replicated in three other communities in the USA: the Tecumseh Community Health Study (House *et al.*, 1982), the Durham County Study (Blazer, 1982) and the Evans County Study in Georgia (Schoenbach, 1986). The results are consistent – social ties are negatively related to mortality, even after controlling for self-reported health status. The first replication (House *et al.*, 1982) was a particularly important contribution as it not only replicated earlier findings, but also validated self-reported health ratings with physiological measures. Interest in social ties and health has spread into the international community and studies similar to Berkman and Syme's have been carried out in Gothenburg (Welin *et al.*, 1985) and Malmo (Hanson *et al.*, 1989), Sweden; and in eastern Finland (Kaplan, 1988). These studies again confirmed that strong social ties are related to better health.

The effect of social support on mortality in these studies varied moderately according to demographic characteristics such as age, sex, race and socioeconomic status. Since demographic factors are strongly related to health outcomes, it is important to determine how each of them modify the relationship between social ties and health. Such interactions between social support and demographic characteristics may limit the generalizability of promising interventions designed to improve health. Unfortunately, only a few of the studies cited above include data on social ties and health for different age, gender and racial groups.

Subgroup findings: age

The Evans County Study (Schoenbach, 1986) and the Alameda County Study for the elderly (Seeman *et al.*, 1987) were able to compare network risk relationships in different age groups. Seeman's study suggests that different types of ties assume greater importance with respect to mortality at different ages. For those aged 70 years and older, contacts with friends and/or relatives were the strongest predictors, while marital status was more important for those under 60 years of age. The Evans County study

(Schoenbach, 1986) found that among African American men, being married was only advantageous under age 60. Among white men and women, however, marriage was associated with lower mortality irrespective of age. Participation in church activities was associated with lower mortality for persons aged 60 years and above (except among African American men), but not for younger persons. In separate proportional hazards models for subjects aged 60–80 years with and without chronic diseases, the overall effect of social ties was significant in those 70 to 80 years of age, but not in those of 60–69 years. Other analyses demonstrated elevated risk among white subjects aged 60–80 years with the fewest ties.

The reason for these age differences is not very clear from these two studies. One possibility may be that older subjects lose social contacts as they become ill. As a result, older subjects who were already ill and, therefore, at high risk of death may have had fewer social ties at the beginning of the study. Although these studies followed subjects for long periods and assessed some aspects of baseline health status, this possibility cannot be ruled out.

Subgroup findings: gender

In several of the studies mentioned above differences by gender were also noted. The association between social network and mortality does not seem to apply equally to men and to women. Four studies have compared risks among men and women (Alameda, Evans, Tecumseh and eastern Finland). Only the Alameda County study found a negative association between social ties and mortality risk for women (Berkman and Syme, 1979). The Evans County, Tecumseh Community, and eastern Finland studies reported substantially stronger network effects for men than for women. These results suggest that the social network may be less beneficial to women than to men.

Subgroup findings: ethnicity

To date, most research on this topic has focused on the white, middle- and working-class groups. Only a few epidemiological studies have had sufficient ethnic diversity in their samples to assess the interactive effects of race and social support on mortality. Among the seven studies which reported data on whites (Evans County, Alameda County, Tecumseh Community Health, Durham County, Gothenburg, eastern Finland and Malmo), lack of social support was consistently associated with increased mortality risk among white men. Two studies (Alameda and Evans County) have explored the associations between social ties and mortality in non-white groups. The association of social integration with mortality among Evans County African American males is weaker than among white males (Schoenbach, 1986). The relative risk ratio for African American females in Evans County, although greater than that for white females in Evans County, is smaller than the relative risk for white females in all other studies (House *et al.*, 1988). This finding may be due to the relatively small number of African Americans in that study, despite a large total sample (Schoenbach, 1986).

The weaker effects of social ties on health among African Americans may also be due to inappropriate measurement instruments. The instruments measuring social ties in the previous studies were developed mainly for the general population, and they may not address issues important for minority groups. The concepts of social isolation, social bonds and support may have different meanings within different ethnic groups (Reed *et al.*, 1983). Different measures may therefore be necessary to assess the importance of social support in minority groups; for example, the importance of church attendance among African Americans may be different from its importance in the white population. The kind of support African Americans receive from their church may be more important than the frequency of their church visits. Measures incorporating these differences may be needed to clarify the relationship between social ties and health in minority groups.

Studies of social relationships and health among other ethnic groups are scarce. Only a few of these studies have found that social support, ties and relationships affect health outcomes. Perhaps the best known is Reed's study of Japanese living in Hawaii, which reported a strong relationship between social support and incidence of coronary heart disease (Reed *et al.*, 1983).

Subgroup findings: socioeconomic status

So far, the relationship between socioeconomic status (SES), social ties and health is not very clear. Numerous studies have documented that the level of health is positively related to SES (Moore *et al.*, 1962; National Center for Health Statistics, 1963; Ellis, 1958). Although there is evidence that lower SES persons score lower on structural support measures (Bell *et al.*, 1982; Warheit, 1979), SES does not seem to be important in discriminating between persons who are or are not affected by support (Bell *et al.*, 1982; Turner and Noh, 1983; Warheit, 1979). However, none of these studies used measures that described the functions or characteristics of social support; hence the data on the role of SES as a modifier of support effects are insufficient (Cohen and Wills, 1985).

In conclusion, the social support indexes used for general populations may not apply to specific gender, race or socioeconomic status subgroups. More research is necessary, using samples not derived from the general population and covering a wide range of ethnic groups.

Social support and disease outcomes

The epidemiological studies we have discussed thus far have focused mainly on the relationship between social ties and mortality. Other investigators have used different end points such as morbid outcomes and quality of life. For example, low social support has been implicated as a predictor of pregnancy complications (Nuckolls *et al.*, 1972). A substantial body of research now supports the hypothesis that social ties are related to the prevalence of and mortality from coronary heart disease. Coronary heart disease rates have been linked to a variety of psychosocial factors including geographic and sociocultural mobility, rapid cultural change, stressful life situations and certain behavioral characteristics (Jenkins, 1971, 1976).

Among the epidemiological studies mentioned above, the Finland study examined the effect of social support on cardiovascular disease (Kaplan, 1988). Kaplan reported a relative risk of cardiovascular death of 2.42 for men in the lowest quintile of social connections compared with those in the highest quintile. A strong relationship between social connections and cardiovascular disease risk was *not* found in women. Berkman and Syme (1979) noted that their social network index was associated with coronary heart disease deaths as a separate category.

In the Honolulu Heart Study, a prospective study of cardiovascular disease in a cohort of 8006 men of Japanese ancestry, Reed and his colleagues (1983) found that the prevalence of coronary heart disease was inversely associated with both factor-derived and conceptual scores describing social network size and complexity. However, there was no association between social network scores and the incidence of coronary disease during a seven-year follow-up period. This difference illustrates several weaknesses of cross-sectional or prevalence data. First, the occurrence of angina or a nonfatal myocardial infarction could reduce a person's ability or desire to maintain social interactions. Second, socially isolated people may be more sensitive to early signs of illness, such as anginal pain. Finally, prevalence data are incomplete because they do not include fatal cases that occurred before the survey.

Another study of Japanese American men (Josephs, unpublished report) also found that poor social support was correlated with the prevalence of coronary heart disease, but incidence data were not available. Rubberman and his associates (1984) studied 2320 participants 2–3 months after an acute myocardial infarction. They found that relatively high levels of life stress and social isolation made significant and independent contributions to the risk of death over a period of three years. Marital status was related to both in-hospital fatality rates and long-term survival in a sample of 1401 myocardial infarction patients, controlling for the severity of disease (Chandra *et al.*, 1983). An analysis of Finnish hospital discharge records (Koskenvuo *et al.*, 1981) demonstrated a lower incidence of coronary disease among married persons. Finally, evidence from a single study (Seeman and Syme, 1987) suggests that functional aspects of social support, such as instrumental assistance and "feeling loved", are more strongly associated with angiographically documented coronary athero-sclerosis than the structural measures used by most other investigators.

By comparison, few studies have looked at the relationship between social support and cancer survival (Vernon and Jackson, 1989). Psycholo-gists have long been interested in the role of personality factors and stress in the etiology of cancer (Fox, 1983), but have only recently considered social support as a possible determinant. Weisman and Worden (1975) used data from the Massachusetts Tumor Registry to calculate a standard-ized survival quotient, representing the difference between observed and expected survival for 35 patients with terminal lymphoma or cancer of the breast, cervix, colon, lung, or stomach. Extensive psychosocial infor-mation was submitted to factor analysis; a factor describing poor social relationships was negatively correlated with this survival quotient.

More recent studies of social support and cancer prognosis have pro-vided conflicting or equivocal results. No association was found between the availability of social support (defined as the number of persons to whom the respondent could turn in response to a personal problem) and the prevalence of significant breast abnormalities in 1052 women referred for mammography (Edwards *et al.*, 1990). Funch and Marshall (1983) determined the survival of 352 white women consecutively diagnosed with localized or regional breast cancer in the period 1958–1960. While both a subjective stress score and a stressful life events index were nega-tively related to survival, two out of three social support items (marital status, number of family and friends) were independent of survival. Only organizational involvement predicted survival in both bivariate and multivariate models. The best known negative study is that of Cassileth and her colleagues (1985, 1988), who found no association between social support and time to relapse in 158 patients with melanoma or stage II breast cancer. They employed several measures of social support: Berkman and Syme's (1979) Social Network Index, marital status, frequency of telephone contact with friends or relatives, and reported adequacy of one's friendship network. In a separate analysis of survival in 204 patients with advanced cancer (Cassileth *et al.*, 1988), those with the least social ties actually had *less* risk of death (relative risk 0.70 [0.51, 0.95]) than those with more ties. This result was apparently driven by a small number of patients with colorectal cancer.

When marital status was used as the sole measure of social support in two larger studies of cancer survival (Goodwin *et al.*, 1987; Neale *et al.*, 1986), it did emerge as a significant predictor. In the former study 2779 cases of staged epithelial cancers from the New Mexico tumor registry data were analyzed. The authors found that unmarried persons were more likely to be diagnosed at a regional or distant stage (odds ratio (OR) 1.19 [1.12, 1.25]) than married persons and, controlling for stage, were more likely to receive no treatment (OR 1.43 [1.33, 1.55]) or no definitive treatment (OR 1.35 [1.24, 1.47]). Proportional hazards regression models stratified by stage at diagnosis and treatment revealed a persistent but small deleterious effect of being unmarried (relative risk 1.18 [1.12, 1.23]). In the latter study, Neale and his associates (1986) found a similar effect for marital status (married versus widowed) on 10-year survival after controlling for age, socioeconomic status, delay and stage at diagnosis in 1261 women with breast cancer. The magnitude of the association in these studies suggests that Cassileth and Funch may not have had sufficient statistical power to detect a true effect.

Several recent studies on social support and cancer have tested 10 or more psychosocial variables and found just a few to be statistically significant. These studies must be regarded with caution, since chance alone could account for some of the reported results. For example, Stavraky and associates (1988) developed eight separate subscales: four measured the need for different dimensions of social support (overall support, care and sympathy, esteem and membership in a helping group), while the other four measured the supply of each. They dichotomized each subscale "in a way that best discriminated between ... outcomes", but found that only the perceived need for sympathy support was related to one-year survival in 224 patients newly diagnosed with lung cancer. None of the four measures indicating the actual supply or availability of social support was related to this outcome. Similarly, Hislop *et al.* (1987) examined 16 psychosocial factors and concluded that only three were significant independent prognostic factors for disease-free survival in 133 women under 55 years of age with recently diagnosed breast cancer. These three factors included the relative frequency of "expressive activities" away from home (e.g. club or church meetings, outside entertainment, visiting friends) and the frequency of such activities at home (e.g. entertaining, hobbies, playing games); however, the former was not associated with overall survival.

The most provocative study linking cancer survival with social support was a recently reported randomized trial of group therapy in 86 patients with metastatic breast cancer (Spiegel *et al.*, 1989a). Of the 50 women randomized to the intervention group 36 participated in weekly 90-min sessions for one year, in which participants expressed their feelings about their illness, discussed coping mechanisms and learned self-hypnosis. Mean survival from study entry to death was 36.6 months in the intervention group but only 18.9 months in the control group. This difference persisted after controlling for initial staging, socioeconomic status (Spiegel *et al.*, 1989b) and several treatment variables. Despite the strength of the randomized design in this trial, it remains unclear whether group therapy was effective because it provided social support or for other reasons.

In summary, there is mixed evidence that reduced social connections are related to mortality from cancer, and better evidence of a relationship with cardiovascular disease. Research on coronary heart disease has consistently found a threshold effect, whereby only those in the lowest quintiles of a social connection index have a substantially increased risk of mortality (Berkman and Syme, 1979; House *et al.*, 1982). There may be little improvement in health outcomes for levels of support above this threshold (Cohen and Wills, 1985). The studies looking at social ties, connectedness and cancer or heart disease suggest that many cardiac and cancer patients may have less adequate social resources than their healthy counterparts (Broadhead *et al.*, 1983; Syme and Seeman, 1983). Because the database is very limited, it is not possible to prove a causal relationship between social support and physical illness. However, the fact that many cancer or heart disease patients may not have enough social support when they need it most has important policy implications. The association between social support and physical illness therefore cannot be ignored.

Social support and psychological outcomes

The most frequently assessed mental health outcome is depression. Several prospective studies using mental health outcome measures have shown a positive relationship between social support and mental health (Cohen and Wills, 1985). Social isolation and social disruption are major contributors to the etiology of depression as well as physical illness. Numerous studies show that married persons are less subject to psychiatric problems than are non-married persons (Gove *et al.*, 1983; Hughes and Gove, 1981; Pearlin and Johnson, 1977). Social support and stressful life events have been directly related to depressive symptoms (Bell *et al.*, 1982). The size and homogeneity of social networks have been associated with symptoms of depression, with smaller networks being more common among the severely depressed (Goldberg *et al.*, 1985).

Sufficient evidence exists to suggest an association between social support and mental health which can affect the quality of one's life. For example, Larson (1978) showed that people who lived alone and had fewer social interactions had lower levels of satisfaction, contentment and morale.

EXPLANATIONS OF THE RELATIONSHIP

While the link between social support and various health outcomes is now undeniable, the mechanism for this relationship remains mysterious. Three basic mechanisms have been proposed: (1) a direct effect on stress, such that poor social support induces a stress response in the organism (Payne and Jones, 1987); (2) a "buffering" effect which posits that support "buffers" persons from the potentially pathogenic influence of stressful events (Cohen and Wills, 1985); and (3) a direct or "main" effect on health which is not dependent on the presence of stress. As Thoits (1983) cogently argued, the first two proposed mechanisms may be difficult to distinguish empirically, particularly with psychological outcomes such as distress. This problem arises because individuals who experience desirable events, such as marriage or childbirth, tend to have high life event scores, strong social support and excellent psychological or physical health. Conversely, individuals who experience undesirable events tend to have high life event scores, weak social support and poor psychological or physical health. It may therefore appear that social support has a particularly beneficial effect in persons under stress because of covariation between the cause of the stress and their health status. Despite this theoretical argument, Payne and Jones (1987) have argued after reviewing the literature that the relationship between social support and life events is surprisingly weak. Direct effects of social support on stress do not adequately explain the association between social support and health (Cohen and Wills, 1985). We will now discuss the other two hypothesized mechanisms in greater detail.

Social support and the buffering hypothesis

The indirect association between social support and health was first suggested in seminal articles by Cassel (1976) and Cobb (1976). They theorized that social relationships might promote health in several ways, but emphasized their role in moderating or buffering the potentially deleterious health effects of psychosocial stress. This hypothesis views social support as something that maintains or sustains the organism by promoting adaptive behavior or favorable neuroendocrine responses in the face of stresses or other health hazards (House, 1981).

Support may play a role at two different points in the causal chain linking stress to illness (Cohen and McKay, 1984; Gore, 1981; House,

1981). First, support may intervene between the stressful event (or expectation of that event) and a stress reaction by attenuating or preventing a stress appraisal response. This primary appraisal of the situation will affect whether the individual defines the situation as threatening (Lazarus, 1982). Knowledge of the success of treatment for breast cancer, for example, may determine whether the individual will define the diagnosis as life threatening. In the Peters-Golden (1982) study, women diagnosed as having cancer interpreted the diagnosis as less threatening than did the group of healthy women. The perception that others can, and will, provide necessary resources may redefine the potential for harm posed by a situation and/or bolster one's perceived ability to cope with imposed demands, and hence prevent a particular situation from being appraised as highly stressful. Other coping resources include being married, having a confidant or having an active orientation toward problem solving (Gore, 1981). Second, adequate support may intervene between the experience of stress and the onset of the pathological outcome by reducing or eliminating the stress reaction or by directly influencing physiological processes. Support may alleviate the impact of stress appraisal by providing a solution to the problem, by reducing the perceived importance of the problem, by tranquilizing the neuroendocrine system so that people are less reactive to perceived stress, or by facilitating healthful responses (House, 1981).

A survey of 139 women who were treated by mastectomy for early breast cancer provides evidence that the relationship between social supports and adjustment to mastectomy is mediated by coping (Bloom, 1982b). These cross-sectional data indicate that social support has direct effects on coping and indirect effects on three measures of adjustment to cancer – mood, self-esteem, and sense of efficacy. Thus, social support improved coping and coping was directly related to adjustment to cancer. A longitudinal study of 401 women (Bloom, 1986), 133 of whom were treated by mastectomy for breast cancer, provides further evidence of a buffering relationship between social support and coping. Emotional support and socioeconomic status have direct effects on coping style, whether appraised by Byrne's measure of Sensitization Repression (Byrne *et al.*, 1963), Spielberger's measure of trait anxiety (Spielberger *et al.*, 1970), the Locus of Control Scale (Levenson, 1974), or a factor-derived measure. Coping style is directly related to several measures of psychological well-being. These relationships held for each of four time periods after surgery: 0–3 months; 3–6 months; 6–9 months; 9–12 months (Bloom, 1986).

Cassel (1976) described a pathway by which social support could decrease susceptibility to physical health problems in stressed individuals. According to Cassel's hypothesis, psychosocial factors such as stress influence physiological reactions by acting as signs and symbols of danger.

The organisms responds to these signs and symbols by altering neuro-endocrine secretion, thereby changing the balance of hormonal effects and increasing susceptibility to disease agents. Laboratory experiments have shown that stressful social circumstances alter neural, hormonal and immunological control systems in ways that may lead to disease in suscep-tible animals (Ader *et al.*, 1963). These control systems include central neurotransmitters which affect cardiovascular function (Weiss *et al.*, 1975), endogenous opiates which modify pain responses and specialized lym-phocytes (natural killer cells) which are capable of destroying tumor cells (Shavit *et al.*, 1984; Kiecolt *et al.*, 1986). Although the evidence linking social networks to specific disease-producing physiological responses is not conclusive, plausible pathways via a range of physiological responses seem to exist.

While the mediating role of social support has been extensively sug-gested, the research evidence for such an interaction has been modest. In most of the studies where the mediating role of social support was examined, only selected values of the variables were involved. For example, Gore (1978) focused on the unemployed, a high life event group. Her results were meaningful but partial since their generalization to the entire range of values for the stress variable is unknown (Lin *et al.*, 1979). After an exhaustive literature review, Cohen and Wills (1985) concluded that previous studies only supported the buffering hypothesis when the social support instrument measured *perceived* types of support, as opposed to structural characteristics of the social network. The implication of this observation is that the perception of support, but not necessarily its pre-sumptive availability, buffers the impact of stressful events. A more recent review of several longitudinal studies on this topic found that "evidence for the buffering hypothesis is weak, and probably not greater than would be expected by chance" (Payne and Jones, 1987, p. 195).

Social support and the "main effect" hypothesis

This model proposes that social resources have a beneficial effect irrespec-tive of whether persons are under stress (Cohen and Wills, 1985). The evi-dence for this model derives from the demonstration of a statistical main effect of support with no interaction between stress and support. There are a variety of plausible mechanisms by which social support may reduce the incidence of cancer or prolong survival among patients already diagnosed with cancer. Some of these mechanisms have been evaluated as part of previous epidemiological studies of the link between social networks and overall mortality (Berkman and Syme, 1979; Schoenbach, 1986). However, none of the studies focusing specifically on cancer mortality have had the statistical power or quality of data to permit testing hypotheses about *how* social support exerts its beneficial effect. Elucidation of this question will require larger studies with more reliable, prospectively gathered data.

Several pathways by which poor social support may exert a deleterious main effect on health outcomes have been proposed. The first pathway is through high-risk health behaviors, such as smoking and alcohol abuse. The second pathway is through use of the health care system. In the specific case of cancer, such use might include screening tests which permit early detection of presymptomatic malignancies, prompt presentation for medical evaluation when symptoms arise and adherence to recommended therapies. The third and final pathway is through immunological or neuroendocrine mechanisms, similar to those postulated to mediate the relationship between stress and health outcomes.

Lifestyle factors

Smoking is the clearest example of a lifestyle factor which may mediate a relationship between poor social support and elevated cancer mortality. The 1987 National Health Interview Survey (US Department of Health and Human Services, 1989) contrasted the responses to four questions about social activities among never, former, and current smokers. Regardless of gender, persons who never smoked reported a greater likelihood of having participated in religious activities during the preceding year than former smokers (75.1% compared with 68.0% overall), who in turn reported greater participation than current smokers (55.5%). A parallel trend was noted for involvement in other group activities (67.4%, 64.1% and 53.8% among never, former, and current smokers, respectively). The smoking status categories did not differ so remarkably in the proportion of respondents who could call upon at least one relative or friend for help. The difference between current smokers and never smokers in the availability of friends was greater among men (87.0% compared with 82.5%) than among women (86.7% versus 87.0%).

In the absence of more detailed information, marital status is often used as a surrogate for social support. Indeed, the prevalence of smoking is considerably higher among separated or divorced persons than among those currently married or widowed. A multivariate analysis of data from the 1985 National Health Interview Survey (Novotny *et al.*, 1988) revealed that this association persisted after controlling for race, gender, poverty status, education and employment status. Using similar methods with data from the 1985 Current Population Survey, Waldron and Lye (1989) demonstrated that divorced or separated adults were more likely to be current smokers or never smokers and less likely to have quit than married adults, even after adjusting for age and educational level and stratifying by race and gender. While white respondents who had never married were less likely to smoke than those currently married, the quit rate was higher in the latter group and the difference in smoking behavior appeared to have originated during adolescence.

A recent study by our group (Romano *et al.*, 1991) examined stress and lack of social support as risk factors for smoking in a community-based sample of 1137 African American adults in two northern Californian cities. Social network size, as measured by Berkman and Syme's (1979) Social Network Index, was inversely related to current smoking only among women: in fact, men who reported that they turn to friends or family for help with personal problems were *more* likely to smoke than men who lacked such support. Functional measures of support were not associated with smoking among women. The contradiction between this finding and the favorable effect of emotional support noted in the National Health Interview Survey suggests that peer group interactions among African American men may promote smoking.

The observed relationship between smoking and poor social support may reflect the difficulty that socially withdrawn individuals experience in attempting to quit. Coppotelli and Orleans (1985) showed that female smokers who successfully quit had higher levels of perceived support from their partners than those who relapsed. The availability of someone to talk to about one's problems predicted cessation in another recent study (Mermelstein *et al.*, 1986). By contrast, participants in a worksite smoking cessation program did not appear to benefit from expected support for quitting from partners and friends (Curry *et al.*, 1989). These negative results may be due to inadequate measurement of the appropriate dimensions of social support.

Obesity is also believed to be a risk factor for some cancers (Lew and Garfinkel, 1979; Albanes, 1987), although it is clearly not as significant as tobacco. Social support from peers may augment the success of behavioral weight reduction programs (Perri *et al.*, 1987; Raeburn and Atkinson, 1986). Involving spouses in the treatment process has been shown to be effective in some studies (Brownell and Stunkard, 1981), but not in others (Dubbert and Wilson, 1984). Hence, social support may reduce the risk of cancer in certain high-risk individuals by facilitating long-term weight loss.

Finally, alcohol abuse is another risk factor for cancer which may be associated with poor social support. Excessive alcohol consumption has been linked to cancer of the mouth and pharynx (Rothman and Keller, 1972) and esophageal cancer (Pottern *et al.*, 1981; Tuyns *et al.*, 1979), although it remains unclear whether alcohol is a direct carcinogen or simply enhances the effects of other environmental carcinogens. Two recent reviews (Katz, 1981; Spiegel, 1980) have presented considerable empirical evidence for the effectiveness of alcohol treatment programs predicated upon mutual support. Alcoholics Anonymous is the best known example of a program which provides a supportive network to participants who may have lost their social networks as a result of prolonged alcohol abuse.

The importance of adequate social support for individuals attempting to modify these high-risk behaviors suggests that any effect of social support on cancer mortality may be partially mediated by such personal health habits as tobacco, alcohol and caloric consumption. The primitive state of current research on social support and cancer mortality precludes empirical validation of this hypothesis, yet Berkman and Syme (1979) explicitly controlled for these behaviors and still found an association between their Social Network Index and all-cause mortality. Schoenbach (1986) did not control for alcohol consumption but did show a persistent effect of social network size after adjusting for measured blood pressure and serum cholesterol. Other explanations must therefore be sought for the apparent relationship between social support and general health outcomes. Given the substantial contribution of cancer as a cause of mortality in the USA, we might expect cancer outcomes to follow the same pattern.

Seeking care for symptoms

It has long been recognized that many common types of cancer, most notably breast and colon cancer, have relatively favorable prognoses when diagnosed at an early stage. Indeed, the American Cancer Society has estimated that one-quarter of the individuals who die of cancer each year might have survived if their cancer had been detected earlier (American Cancer Society, 1977). The remediable causes of late diagnosis include delays in obtaining medical care by persons with symptoms of cancer, delays in the medical evaluation of such symptoms and failure to utilize diagnostic tests which can identify early malignancies in asymptomatic hosts. Social support may be hypothesized to operate on any or all of these levels, thereby promoting timely diagnosis of treatable cancers. Unfortunately, there is little empirical evidence to elucidate these relationships.

A multistage model of patient delay was originally proposed by Safer (Safer *et al.*, 1979) and revised by Cacioppo and his colleagues (1986). Safer's original model divided the total duration of delay into *appraisal*, which begins when the patient first notices a symptom and ends when he or she concludes that something is wrong; *illness delay*, which lasts from the recognition of illness to the decision to seek professional care; and *utilization delay*, which ends with the patient's first medical appointment. Cacioppo recognized that the last stage could be further divided into *behavioral* delay and *scheduling* delay, based upon whether the patient has acted on his or her decision to seek care by scheduling an appointment.

A brief review of the supportive functions of social relationships (Schaefer *et al.*, 1981; House *et al.*, 1982) will illuminate the pathways by which social support may minimize total patient delay. *Informational support* is the process of giving information or advice to facilitate problem solving. This type of support may shorten appraisal or illness delay by affirming the significance of new symptoms, and may also shorten utilization delay when it includes advice about when or where to seek care. *Instrumental support* represents tangible assistance with necessary tasks. By helping symptomatic individuals to locate a physician, schedule an appointment or get to a physician's office, such support may shorten utilization delay. *Emotional support,* which has been further characterized by different investigators as *appraisal* support (House *et al.*, 1982), *esteem* support (Cohen and Wills, 1985) and *confidant* support (Broadhead *et al.*, 1988), may help people overcome their initial fears and hence reduce illness delay. Fear is often cited as the major reason for delay in persons with symptoms of cancer (Smith and Anderson, 1985). Social networks may also enhance one's *motivation* to solve a worsening health problem in order to prevent suffering by friends and family (Cohen and Wills, 1985).

Several investigators have examined social factors related to delay among patients with cancer symptoms, but most have been unable to distinguish effects on the four stages of delay. The factors often found to be important include the patient's socioeconomic status and education, his or her knowledge concerning cancer, and the ready availability of medical care (Antonovsky and Hartman, 1974). Social support might be expected to reduce delay, since patients often report that advice from friends or family instigated their decision to seek care. Researchers who have tested this hypothesis have obtained conflicting results.

Samet and his colleagues (1988) interviewed 800 elderly New Mexicans newly diagnosed with any of nine cancers amenable to early, effective treatment. The site of cancer, the patient's ethnicity and a history of regular checkups were the only factors which significantly predicted delay. Berkman and Syme's (1979) structural measure of social support was independent of delay. In 125 consecutive patients with Hodgkin's disease, malignant melanoma or cancer of the breast, lung, or colon, Weisman and Worden (1975) found that marital status was not related to delay; however, a history of rejection or isolation in childhood and social introversion on the Minnesota Multiphasic Personality Inventory *were* so correlated. These findings are difficult to interpret due to the large but unspecified number of associations that the authors considered. Finally Berkanovic (1982) interviewed 1210 randomly selected individuals every six weeks for approximately one year, inquiring about any new symptoms and about whether a medical evaluation had been obtained. A panel of cancer specialists identified 35 cancer-relevant symptoms, which were reported on 345 occasions by 270 respondents. In a multiple regression model controlling for age, ethnicity, gender, income, and socioeconomic status, *symptom-specific* social network characteristics (e.g. the number of people contacted about the symptom) were strongly associated with visiting a physician. This positive finding suggests that social networks may only be effective in terminating delay if they are actively utilized by a person experiencing symptoms.

Utilization of cancer screening tests

There is mixed evidence from cross-sectional studies that social network characteristics may be associated with utilization of cancer screening tests. Factors relating to the practice of breast self-examination (BSE) have been the best studied. Rutledge (1987) reported that the frequency of BSE among 93 upper-middle-class women recruited at meetings of voluntary women's organizations was not related to scores on the Norbeck Social Support Questionnaire, which measures both structural features of the social network and its perceived quality. In a sample of 106 low-income Mexican American women attending a health clinic, Gonzales (1990) found no association between the perceived quality of social support and the frequency of BSE. By contrast, Norman and Tudiver (1986) developed a measure of social support specific to BSE (e.g. the proportion of female friends and family members who practice BSE, husband/partner's attitude toward BSE, and physician's attitude) which was highly correlated with the frequency of the procedure.

Preliminary evidence from our own work with a sample of 670 African American women (Kang, 1991) suggests that Berkman and Syme's (1979) Social Network Index is associated with having ever received routine mammography. Almost 30% of women with the largest social networks have had a routine mammogram, compared with just 10.7% of women with the smallest networks. This relationship does not appear to hold for routine Papanicolau screening or BSE, nor are functional measures of the social support network (instrumental support and emotional support (Seeman and Syme, 1987)) related to utilization of screening tests.

The implication of these analyses, which have yet to be confirmed in a prospective study controlling for all relevant confounders, is that malignancies may be diagnosed at earlier stages in persons with strong social support. Some evidence to the contrary has been presented by Broadhead *et al.* (1989), who found that persons with low confidant support visited an outpatient family practice clinic more often than those with optimal support. However, their social support indexes were *not* correlated with the number of laboratory tests ordered, suggesting the additional visits may have been inappropriate or psychosocial in nature. If the hypothesis that social support augments appropriate utilization is true, then medical and surgical therapy should be more effective in cancer patients who enjoy strong support.

Adherence to therapy

There is considerable evidence from studies of hypertension (Stanton, 1987), renal hemodialysis (O'Brien, 1990) and diabetes (Nagasawa *et al.*, 1989) that social support may enhance adherence to complex medical regimens. This effect is especially apparent in studies which have used *condition-specific* measures of support, centering around support for dietary or other lifestyle changes (Wilson *et al.*, 1986). If this relationship also holds for cancer therapy, then better adherence to effective therapies may lead to longer survival.

Immunological or other psychological mechanisms

Social support could be related to physical health outcomes directly through emotionally induced effects on neuroendocrine or immune system functioning (Jemmott and Locke, 1984). A recent study by Levy and her associates (1990) found that natural killer cell activity in 61 stage I and II breast cancer patients was associated with a perception of high quality emotional support from a spouse or partner and social support from a physician, even after controlling for estrogen receptor status, age, functional status and surgical history. This finding suggests a mechanism by which social support could improve cancer outcomes without buffering the effect of stress.

SOCIAL SUPPORT AND THE CANCER EXPERIENCE

The beneficial effects of social support

Several characteristics of social support are particularly beneficial to an individual at the time cancer or another health problem is diagnosed. *Emotional support*, defined as perception of being cared for and loved or having a confidant or intimate friend, has been related to lower levels of distress and depression (Gore, 1978; Holahan and Moos, 1981). A few studies have examined the relationship between emotional support and psychosocial adjustment following cancer. In one study, Bloom (1986) assessed 139 women with breast cancer on two occasions, two months apart. Emotional support as an explanation for adjustment was tested using multiple regression analysis in which variables were forced into the equation in three steps. The first step included measures of stress (illness-related measures and life events); secondly, social background factors were forced in; and in the final step the measure of emotional support was added. Emotional support made a significant contribution to each of three outcomes – psychological distress, self-esteem and sense of control.

Two different approaches to providing *informational and emotional support* for people undergoing stressful life experiences are described in the literature – individual counseling and support groups. Results of several studies indicate that these interventions are perceived as enjoyable, increase knowledge about cancer and its treatment, reduce the severity of cancer symptoms such as pain, reduce dysphoria, improve self-esteem and sense of efficacy, and may even lengthen survival in cancer patients (Jacobs *et al.*, 1983; Spiegel *et al.*, 1981, 1989a; Spiegel and Bloom, 1983; Ferlic *et al.*, 1979; Heinrich and Schag, 1985; Telch, unpublished report). However, none of these studies provides guidance as to whether the intervention produces these beneficial effects by changing the individual's support system. It is also unclear whether the intervention is more effective with individuals who are socially isolated than with ones who perceive that they are receiving less support than they want. For instance, Falk and Taylor's (1983) survey of support group members suggests that cancer patients turn to support groups because they perceive their needs as being inadequately met by their support system rather than because they are lacking in supportive ties.

While the evidence is quite sparse at present, it suggests that interventions can be effective in changing the individual's support system. When this occurs, both physical and mental health outcomes may improve. To date most intervention studies have either not been concerned about the support system *per se* or have assumed, but not measured, deficiences in the support system as an indication of the need for intervention. A study by Raphael (1977) is an exception. In this study, the support systems of recent widows were assessed. Most respondents who perceived their support systems to be inadequate (86%) reported poor health while only 22% of those reporting adequate support systems complained of poor health. When supportive counseling was offered to widows with inadequate support systems, the percentage reporting poor health decreased significantly. Of course, it would be instructive to know if the group of widows perceived their support systems to have improved as a function of intervention.

Tangible support may also be beneficial to patients with cancer. Finlayson (1976) reported that patients with the most favorable post myocardial infarction outcomes were those whose spouses received more assistance initially and over the course of the illness. A favorable outcome consisted of the patient's return to work and the wife's validation that the husband had recovered. Assistance consisted of visits by family members and their provision of services such as transport. Funch and Mettlin (1982) found that financial support was related to recovery from breast cancer surgery. In this study recovery was measured by an index composed of both physical and perceptual measures.

Erosion of support

It is generally accepted and fairly well substantiated that supportive relationships are a resource for an individual facing stressful life circumstances. The social support available to an individual is also becoming recognized as critical to maintaining or restoring one's health. Support from family and friends seems to facilitate one's ability to cope with the stressful and often nonmodifiable circumstances in one's life. Yet, for many, supportive relationships are not available at the time they are most needed. Oncology patients frequently report that their friends disappeared after their cancer was diagnosed.

Two plausible explanations of change in social support following cancer diagnosis are found in the literature: (1) the stigma associated with cancer; and (2) illness-imposed restrictions in one's activities.

Cancer as a stigmatized disease

The first explanation was provided by Cobb and his associate (Cobb, 1976; Cobb and Erbe, 1978). They argue that people feel uncomfortable in the presence of someone with cancer due to its stigma. Stigma is defined as negative evaluations attached to characteristics of a person which place the person outside some socially acceptable standard for human attributes and performance (Goffman, 1963). Even with recent advances in cancer treatment, 63% of an African American sample still believed in 1986 that cancer is a death sentence (Bloom *et al.*, 1987). Being in the presence of a cancer patient is the same as being in the presence of death. About the same proportion of this sample (62.5%) believed cancer to be contagious (Bloom *et al.*, 1987). People with a contagious disease or who remind one of one's own mortality are people to avoid.

Spending time with a cancer patient creates ambiguity in the normal course of social interaction. Individuals report that they don't know what to say, how to interact or when to help. This ambiguity is an additional source of discomfort or tension (Albrecht *et al.*, 1982). Seeking to reduce the tension, some will drop the patient completely as soon as they discover the cancer diagnosis. Others will withdraw more slowly by making visits shorter and intervals between visits longer. When physical withdrawal is not possible, social distancing will occur through psychological withdrawal. As Wiley and Sillman (1990) point out, this withdrawal may be mutual, i.e. the cancer patient may not actively seek social interaction. If the disease cannot easily be explained by the person's lifestyle (e.g. smoking), others become uncomfortable. The illness reminds them of their own vulnerability and their powerlessness in the face of this vulnerability; this is especially true for individuals perceiving themselves as similar in age or gender to the cancer patient. To avoid the threat, members of an individual's social network distance themselves either physically or by psychological means – e.g. "he brought it on himself".

The social activity hypothesis

Decreases in the perception of emotional support have also been explained in terms of role change and decreased activity. Serious illnesses such as cancer prevent individuals from carrying out their usual roles and responsibilities. As Gorsky and Calloway (1983) have noted, individuals who have reduced energy will initially continue to carry out obligatory activities, giving up discretionary activities – in other words, a cancer patient may continue to go to work, an obligatory activity, but due to low energy levels may do very little at home.

During cancer treatment, work may not be possible and family roles may change if illness-related disability occurs. Each social role carries with it a set of expected relationships and obligations to others. The individual comes to socially define himself or herself in terms of these roles. The assumption of these roles carries with it a set of expectations for one's behavior as well as a set of identities, a sense of permanence and coherence for the individual (Antonovsky, 1979). As Thoits (1983) and others have noted, "If one knows who one is (in the social sense), then one knows how to behave".

Role change may involve the loss of valued identities. Existential meaning and behavioral guidance provided by one's social identities become strained. This strain in identities contributes to feelings of being socially and emotionally isolated and may result in increased psychological distress. Some evidence indicates that emotional support by family and friends may partially prevent this outcome (Bloom, 1982a; Thoits, 1983).

One's social network is composed of people with whom one comes into contact through work, social, religious and recreational activities. The people in a social network provide social and emotional support in times of crisis. As the social activities which bring one into contact with others are given up, a gradual constriction of social network occurs. Constriction of social network decreases the ability to receive social support, whether it be emotional support, information or other instrumental (tangible) resources.

Several studies provide confirming evidence for the social activity hypothesis. In the first, Seeman and Syme (1987), in their study of coronary artery disease, found that social network size was related to emotional support, but not to instrumental support. Schaefer and her colleagues (1981) also found moderate correlations between emotional and informational support and social network size. This finding is consistent with that of Bloom and her colleagues (1991) for Hodgkin's disease survivors. They found significant correlations between both emotional and family support and social network index. Network size was strongly related to emotional support and moderately related to informational support, even after controlling for demographic and illness-related factors.

Longitudinal studies of cancer patients provide stronger support of the social activity hypothesis. Bloom and Kessler (1990) analyzed four panels of data on women during the year following mastectomy for breast cancer, cholecystectomy for gallbladder disease, biopsy for benign breast disease and a comparison group of women who did not have surgery, to assess whether reported emotional support was a result of the stigma of cancer or was due to illness-induced changes in the individual's social network. Contrary to the stigma hypothesis, they found that cancer patients reported receiving more emotional support during the three months following surgery than women experiencing other types of surgery. In other analyses of these data, women who had adjuvant therapy reported the highest levels of support during this time (Penman *et al.*, 1986). However, as time post surgery increased, the perceived support of this group decreased despite no significant change in the frequency of social contacts. By six months post surgery, their level of perceived support was equivalent to that of other groups. The frequency and number of social contacts was a significant predictor of emotional support during the year. Change in social contacts had no additional effect. Improvements in role functioning and in daily activities and decreased social isolation were also related to increases in perceived emotional support. Neither the measures of health prior to the diagnosis of cancer (concurrent conditions) nor following cancer treatment (health ratings) were related to emotional support, suggesting that most of the changes in emotional support are socially and psychologically based rather than physically based (Bloom and Kessler, 1990).

Two other studies of advanced cancer provide additional evidence of the importance of physical aspects of cancer on change in social support. In a study of 86 women with metastatic breast cancer, the women's activity level and perception of family support was related to their social functioning (Bloom and Spiegel, 1984). Thus, women who were able to visit and be visited, carry out simple errands and go shopping had opportunities to interact with others and receive social support. In the second study (Wiley and Sillman, 1990), a cross-sectional sample of 707 men and women newly diagnosed as having lung, breast or colorectal cancer was interviewed. Using multiple regression analysis it was found that the respondent's physical condition was related to lower levels of social activity, their measure of social support. This was true even though they controlled for the individual's background, living arrangements and the number of children who lived close enough to visit.

SUMMARY AND CONCLUSIONS

In this chapter we have attempted to integrate two disparate bodies of literature on the role of social support as a personal resource. The work of social epidemiologists has demonstrated the importance of social support in disease outcomes. Most clear is the relationship of social connectedness and social ties to mortality. There is also strong evidence that social connectedness is related to coronary heart disease. The evidence for such a relationship with cancer is less clear. These relationships hold for white, male populations. The subgroup analyses that are available do not provide as strong evidence of this relationship for women or for ethnic minorities. With the above caveats, we conclude that social support, defined as one's social ties to family, friends, and community, is related to both physical and mental health outcomes.

What is it about one's social relationships and interaction patterns that promotes health? In other words, what is transmitted over this network of interactions? We argue that individuals receive information that they are valued and cared for, that is *emotional support, information* about health matters, and *instrumental* supports such as assistance with transport, household chores and finances. Both informational and instrumental support communicate a sense of caring to the recipient, which reaffirms the individual's own sense of worth as well as having instrumental benefits such as giving them information about cancer prevention, getting them to cancer screening and providing assistance when they are already ill. Evidence for our argument comes from several provocative studies which demonstrate that illness-associated constrictions to one's social network are accompanied by decreases in the perception of emotional support. In the case of advanced disease, these constrictions may be physically based. However, they are more generally psychologically and socially based.

We have discussed several plausible pathways by which social supports transmitted within one's social network affect cancer outcomes. The most plausible and perhaps least understood are psychoneuroimmunological pathways, which are discussed in depth in Chapter 1. Second, there is good evidence that emotional support acts to improve the recipient's ability to cope, discussed in depth in Chapter 8. Third, there is evidence that social support influences lifestyle factors associated with the development of cancer, utilization of cancer screening tests, delays in presentation with cancer symptoms, and adherence to cancer therapy. The stresses associated with the cancer diagnosis are discussed more thoroughly in Chapter 7.

What are the implications of our findings? We believe that they suggest that research in the 1990s should include the study of support system interventions. If this research is to advance our understanding of social support as a resource for the individual undergoing a stressful life experience, then it must be concerned not only with outcomes, but also must assess whether changes in the support system actually took place. First, it will be important to develop reliable and valid methods of assessing the adequacy of support systems for people undergoing stressful life experiences. Second, it will be important to learn more about the outcomes of specific types of intervention (either individual or group). Third, it will be important to learn more about the mechanisms through which the interventions work, i.e. by changing host resistance, by changing immunological functioning, or perhaps by increasing the size and adequacy of the support system itself.

In conclusion, we encourage our colleagues to use our outline as a guide to research in the 1990s.

REFERENCES

Ader, R., Kreutner, A. and Jacobs, H.L. (1963) Social environment, emotionality and alloxan diabetes in the rat. *Psychosom. Med.*, **25**, 60–68.

Albanes, D. (1987) Caloric intake, body weight, and cancer: a review. *Nutrit. Cancer*, **9**, 199–217.

Albrecht, G.L., Walker, V.G. and Levy, J.A. (1982) Distance from the stigmatized: a test of two theories. *Sci. Med.*, **16**, 1319–1327.

Antonovsky, A. (1979) *Health, Stress and Coping.* Jossey-Bass, San Francisco.

Antonovsky, A. and Hartman, H. (1974) Delay in the detection of cancer: a review of the literature. *Health Education Monographs*, **2**(2), 98–127.

Bell, R.A., Leroy, J.B. and Stephenson, J.J. (1982) Evaluating the mediating effects of social support upon life events and depressive symptoms. *J. Commun. Psychol.*, **10**, 325–340.

Berkanovic, E. (1982) Seeking care for cancer relevant symptoms, *J. Chron. Dis.*, **35**, 727–734.

Berkman, L.F. and Syme, S.L. (1979) Social networks, host resistance, and mortality: a nine year follow-up study of Alameda County residents. *Am. J. Epidemiol.*, **109**, 186–204.

Berkson, J. (1962) Mortality and marital status – reflections on the derivation of etiology from statistics. *Am. J. Pub. Health*, **52**, 1318–1329.

Blazer, D.G. (1982) Social support and mortality in an elderly community population. *Am. J. Epidemiol.*, **115**, 684–694.

Bloom, J.R. (1982a) Social support systems and cancer: a conceptual view. In Cohen, J., Cullen, J. and Martin, R. (eds) *Research Issues in the Psychosocial Aspects of Cancer*. Raven Press, New York, pp. 129–149.

Bloom, J.R. (1982b) Social support, accommodation to stress and adaptation to breast cancer. *Soc. Sci. Med.*, **16**, 1329–1338.

Bloom, J.R. (1986) Social support and adjustment to breast cancer. In Anderson, B. (ed.) *Women and Cancer*. Springer-Verlag, New York, pp. 204–229.

Bloom. J.R. and Kessler, L. (1990) The continuity of social support following cancer: further evidence for the social activity hypothesis. *XV. International Congress on Cancer*, Hamburg, Germany.

Bloom, J.R. and, Spiegel, D. (1984) The relationship of two dimensions of social support to the psychological well-being and social functioning of women with advanced breast cancer, **19**(8), 831–837.

Bloom, J.R., Hayes, W.A., Saunders, F. and Flatt, S. (1987) Cancer awareness and secondary prevention practices in Black Americans: implications for intervention. *Family and Community Health*, **10**, 19–30.

Bloom, J.R., Fobair, P., Spiegal, D., Cox, R., Varghese, A. and Hoppe, R. (1991) Social supports and the social well-being of cancer survivors. In Albrecht, G. (ed.) *Advances in Medical Sociology*, Vol. 2, pp. 95–114.

Broadhead, W.E., Kaplan, B. and James, S. (1983) The epidemiological evidence for a relationship between social support and health. *Am. J. Epidemiol.*, **117**, 521–537.

Broadhead, W.E., Gehlbach, S.H., de Gruy, F.V. and Kaplan, B.H. (1988) The Duke-UNC functional social support questionnaire: measurement of social support in family medicine patients. *Medical Care*, **26**(7), 709–721.

Broadhead, W.E., Gehlbach, S.H., de Gruy, F.V. and Kaplan, B.H. (1989) Functional versus structural social support and health care utilization in a family medicine outpatient practice. *Medical Care*, **27**(3), 221–233.

Brown, D.R. and Gary, L.E. (1987) Stressful life events, social support networks, and the physical and mental health of urban black adults. *J. Human Stress*, **13**(4), 165–174.

Brownell, K.D. and Stunkard, A.J. (1981) Couple training, pharmacotherapy and behavior therapy in the treatment of obesity. *Arch. Gen. Psych.*, **38**, 1224–1229.

Byrne, D., Berry, J. and Nelson, D. (1963) Relationship of the revised repression-sensitization scale to measures of self-description. *Psycholog. Rep.*, **13**, 323–334.

Cacioppo, J.T., Andersen, B.L., Turnquist, D.C. and Tassinary, L.G. (1986) Psychophysiological comparison theory: on the experience, description and assessment of signs and symptoms. *Patient Education and Counseling*, **13**, 257–270.

Cassel, J. (1976) The contribution of the social environment to host resistance. *Am. J. Epidemiol.*, **104**(2), 107–123.

Cassileth, B.R., Lusk, E.J., Miller, D.S., Brown, L.L. and Miller, C. (1985) Psychosocial correlates of survival in advanced malignant disease. *New Engl. J. Med.*, **312**(24), 1551–1573.

Cassileth, B.R., Walsh, W.P. and Lusk, E.J. (1988) Psychosocial correlates of cancer survival: a subsequent report 3 to 8 years after cancer diagnosis. *J. Clin. Oncol.*, **6**(11), 1753–1759.

Chandra, V., Szklo, M., Goldberg, R. and Tonascia, J. (1983) The impact of marital status on survival after an acute myocardial infarction: a population-based study. *Am. J. Epidemiol.*, **117**, 320–325.

Cobb, S. (1976) Social support as a moderator of life stress. *Psychosom. Med.*, **38**(5), 300–314.

Cobb, S. and Erbe, C. (1978) Social support for the cancer patient. *Forum Med.*, 1(8), 24–29.

Cohen, S. and McKay, G. (1984) Social support, stress and the buffering hypothesis: a theoretical analysis. In Baum, A., Singer, J.E. and Taylor, S.E. (eds) *Handbook of Psychology and Health*, Vol. 4. Erlbaum, Hillsdale, pp. 253–267.

Cohen, S. and Syme, L.S. (eds) (1985) *Social Support and Health*. Academic Press, New York.

Cohen, S. and Wills, T.A. (1985) Stress, social support, and the buffering hypothesis. *Psycholog. Bull.*, 98(2), 310–357.

Coppotelli, H.C. and Orleans, C.T. (1985) Partner support and other determinants of smoking cessation maintenance among women. *J. Consult. Clin. Psychol.*, 53(4), 455–460.

Cox, P.R. and Ford, J.R. (1964) The mortality of widows shortly after widowhood. *Lancet*, i, 163–164.

Curry, S., Thompson, B., Sexton, M. and Omenn, G.S. (1989) Psychosocial predictors of outcome in a worksite smoking cessation program. *Am. J. Prevent. Med.*, 5(1), 3–7.

Dubbert, P.M. and Wilson, G.T. (1984) Goal setting and spouse involvement in the treatment of obesity. *Behav. Res. Ther.*, 22, 227–242.

Durkheim, E. and Simpson, G. (eds) (1951) *Suicide: A Study in Sociology*. The Free Press, Glencoe.

Edwards, J.R., Cooper, G.L., Pearl, S.G., de Paredes, E.S., O'Leary, T. and Wilhelm, M.C. (1990) The relationship between psychosocial factors and breast cancer: some unexpected results. *Behav. Med.*, 16(1), 5–14.

Ellis, J.M. (1958) Socio-economic differentials in mortality from chronic diseases. In Jaco, E.G. (ed.) *Patients, Physicians and Illness*. Free Press, Glencoe.

Falk, R.L. and Taylor, S.E. (1983) Support groups for cancer patients. *UCLA Cancer Bull.*, 10, 13–15.

Ferlic, M., Goldman, A. and Kennedy, J.J. (1979) Group counseling in adult patients. *Cancer*, 43, 760–766.

Finlayson, A. (1976) Social networks as coping networks, *Soc. Sci. Med.*, 10, 97–104.

Fox, B.H. (1983) Current theory of psychogenic effects on cancer incidence and prognosis. *J. Psychosoc. Oncol.*, 1(1), 17–31.

Funch, D.P. and Marshall, J.R. (1983) The role of stress, social support and age in survival from breast cancer. *J. Psychosom. Res.*, 27, 77–83.

Funch, D.P. and Mettlin, C. (1982) The role of support in relation to recovery from breast surgery. *Soc. Sci. Med.*, 16, 91–98.

Goffman, E. (1963) *Stigma*. Prentice-Hall, Englewood Cliffs.

Goldberg, E.L., Van Nata, P. and Comstock, G.W. (1985) Depressive symptoms, social networks and social support of elderly women, *Am. J. Epidemiol.*, 121, 448–456.

Gonzales, J.T. (1990) Factors relating to frequency of breast self-examination among low-income Mexican American women. *Cancer Nursing*, 13(3), 134–142.

Goodwin, J.S., Hunt, W.C., Key, C.R. and Samet, J.M. (1987) The effect of marital status on stage, treatment, and survival of cancer patients. *JAMA*, 258, 3125–3130.

Gore, S. (1978) The effect of social support in moderating the health consequences of unemployment, *J. Health Soc. Behav.*, 19, 157–165.

Gore, S. (1981) Stress-buffering functions of social supports: an appraisal and clarification of research models. In Dohrenwend, B.S. and Dohrenwend, B.P. (eds) *Stressful Life Events and Their Contexts*. Prodist, New York.

Gorsky, R. and Calloway, D. (1983) Activity pattern changes with decreases in food energy intake. *Human Biol.*, **55**, 577–586.

Gove, W.R., Hughes, M. and Style, C.B. (1983) Does marriage have positive effects on the psychological well-being of the individual, *J. Health Soc. Behav.*, **24**, 122–131.

Hanson, B.S., Isacsson, S.V., Janzon, L. and Lindell, S.E. (1989) Social network and social support influence mortality in elderly men: the prospective population study of men born in 1914, Malmo, Sweden. *Am. J. Epidemiol.*, **130**, 100–111.

Heinrich, R.L. and Schag, C.C. (1985) Stress and activity management: group treatment for cancer patients and spouses. *J. Consult. Clin. Psychol.*, **53**, 439–446.

Helsing, K.J. (1981) Factors associated with mortality after widowhood. *Am. J. Pub. Health*, **71**, 802–809.

Hislop, G.T., Waxler, N.E., Coldman, A.J., Elmwood, J.M. and Kan, L. (1987) The prognostic significance of psychosocial factors in women with breast cancer. *J. Chron. Dis.*, **40**(7), 729–735.

Holahan, C.J. and Moos, R. (1981) Social support and psychological distress: longitudinal analysis. *J. Ab. Psychol.*, **90**, 365–370.

House, J.S. (1981) *Work Stress and Social Support*. Addison-Wesley, Reading.

House, J.S., Robbins, C. and Metzner, H. (1982) The association of social relationships and activities with mortality: prospective evidence from the Tecumseh community health study. *Am. J. Epidemiol.*, **116**, 123–140.

House, J.S., Landis, K.R. and Umberson, D. (1988) Social relationships and health. *Science*, **241**, 540–545.

Hughes, M. and Gove, W.R. (1981) Living alone, social integration and mental health. *Am. J. Sociol.*, **87**, 48–74.

Jacobs, C., Ross, R.D., Walker, I.M. and Stockdale, F.E. (1983) Behavior of cancer patients: a randomized study of the effects of education and peer support groups. *Am. J. Clin. Oncol.*, **6**, 347–350.

Jemmott, J.B. III and Locke, S.E. (1984) Psychosocial factors, immunologic mediation, and human susceptibility to infectious diseases: how much do we know? *Psycholog. Bull.*, **95**, 78–108.

Jenkins, C. (1971) Psychologic and social precursors of coronary disease. *New Engl. J. Med.*, **284**, 244–255.

Jenkins, C. (1976) Recent evidence supporting psychologic and social risk factors for coronary disease. *New Engl. J. Med.*, **294**, 987–994.

Kang, S.H. (1991) Social support and the use of preventive services among African Americans. Doctoral Dissertation, University of California, Berkeley.

Kaplan, G.A. (1988) Social connections and mortality from all causes and from cardiovascular disease: prospective evidence from eastern Finland. *Am. J. Epidemiol.*, **128**, 370–380.

Katz, A.H. (1981) Self-help and mutual aid: an emerging social movement. *Ann. Rev. Sociol.*, **7**, 129–155.

Kiecolt, J., Glazer, R. and Strain, E. (1986) Modulation of cellular immunity in medical students. *J. Behav. Med.*, **46**, 15–23.

Koskenvuo, M., Kaprio, J., Romo, M. and Langinvainao, H. (1981) Incidence and prognosis of ischemic heart disease with respect to marital status and social class: a national record linkage study. *J. Epidemiol. Comm. Health*, **35**, 192–196.

Larson, R. (1978) Thirty years of research on the subjective well-being of older Americans. *J. Gerontol.*, **33**(1), 109–125.

Lazarus, R. (1982) Stress and coping as factors in health and illness. In Cohen, J., Cullen, J. and Martin, R.M. (eds) *Psychosocial Aspects of Cancer*. Raven Press, New York, pp. 163–190.

Levenson, H. (1974) Activism and powerful others: distinctions within the concept of internal-external control. *J. Person. Assess.*, **38**, 377–381.

Levy, S.M., Herberman, R.B., Maluish, A.M., Schlien, B. and Lippman, M. (1985) Prognostic risk assessment in primary breast cancer by behavioral and immunological parameters. *Health Psychol.*, **4**(2), 99–113.

Levy, S.M., Haberman, R.B., Whiteside, T., Sanzo, K., Lee, J. and Kirkwood, J. (1990) Perceived social support and tumor estrogen/progesterone receptor status as predictors of natural killer cell activity in breast cancer patients. *Psychosom. Med.*, **52**, 73–85.

Lew, E.A. and Garfinkel, L. (1979) Variations in mortality by weight among 750,000 men and women. *J. Chron. Dis.*, **32**, 563–576.

Lin, H., Simeone, R.S., Ensel, W. and Kuo, W. (1979) Social support, stressful life events, and illness: a model and an empirical test. *J. Health Soc. Behav.*, **20**, 108–119.

Mermelstein, R., Cohen, S., Lichtenstein, R., Baer, J.S. and Kamarck, T. (1986) Social support and smoking cessation and maintenance. *J. Consult. Clin. Psychol.*, **54**(4), 447–453.

Moore, M., Stunkard, A. and Srole, L. (1962) Obesity, social class and mental illness. *JAMA*, **181**, 962–966.

Nagasawa, M., Smith, M.C., Barnes, J.H. Jr. and Fincham, J.E. (1989) Meta-analysis of correlates of diabetes patients' compliance with prescribed medications. *The Diabetes Educator*, **16**(3), 192–200.

National Center for Health Statistics, (1963) *Family Income in Relation to Selected Health Characteristics*, Series 10, No. 2, US Government Printing Office, Washington.

Neale, A.V., Tidley, B.C. and Vernon, S.W. (1986) Marital status: delay in seeking treatment and survival from breast cancer. *Soc. Sci. Med.*, **23**, 305–312.

Norman, R.M.G. and Tudiver, F. (1986) Predictors of breast self-examination among family practice patients. *J. Family Pract.*, **22**(2), 149–153.

Novotny, T.E., Warner, K.E., Kendrick, J.S. and Remington, P.L. (1988) Smoking by Blacks and Whites: socioeconomic and demographic differences. *Am. J. Pub. Health*, **78**(9), 1187–1189.

Nuckolls, C.G., Cassel, J. and Kaplan, B.H. (1972) Psychosocial assets, life crisis, and the prognosis of pregnancy. *Am. J. Epidemiol.*, **95**, 431–441.

O'Brien, M.E. (1990) Compliance behavior and long-term maintenance dialysis. *Am. J. Kidney Dis.*, **15**(3), 209–214.

Parkes, C.M. (1972) *Bereavement: Studies of Grief in Adult Life*. International Universities Press, New York.

Payne, R.L. and Jones, J.G. (1987) Measurement and methodological issues in social support. In Kasl, S.V. and Cooper, C.L. (eds) *Stress and Health: Issues in Research Methodology*, John Wiley, Chichester, pp. 167–205.

Pearlin, L.I. and Johnson, J.S. (1977) Marital status, life-strains and depression. *Am. Sociolog. Rev.*, **42**, 704–715.

Penman, D., Bloom, J.R., Fotopolis, S., Cook, M., Murowski, B., Gates, C., Holland, J., Ross, R. and Flaerm, D.P. (1986) The impact of mastectomy on self-concept and social function: a combined cross-sectional and longitudinal study with comparison groups. *Women and Health*, 2(3–4). (Reprinted in Stellman, S. (ed.) *Women and Health*, Sage Press.)

Perri, M.G., McAdoo, W.G., McAllister, D.A. *et al.* (1987) Effects of peer support and therapist contact on long-term weight loss. *J. Consult. Clin. Pyschol.*, **55**, 615–617.

Peters-Golden, H. (1982) Breast cancer: varied perceptions of social support in the illness experience. *Soc. Sci. Med.*, **16**, 483–491.

Pottern, L.M., Ziegler, R.G. *et al.* (1981) Esophageal cancer among black men in Washington, DC: alcohol, tobacco and other risk factors. *J. Nat. Cancer Inst.*, **67**, 777–783.

Raeburn, J.M. and Atkinson, J.M. (1986) A low-cost community approach to weight control: initial results from an evaluated trial. *Prevent. Med.*, **15**, 391–402.

Raphael, B. (1977) Preventative intervention with the recently bereaved. *Arch. Gen. Psych.*, **34**, 1450–1454.

Reed, D., McGee, D., Yano, K. and Feinleib, M. (1983) Social networks and coronary heart disease among Japanese men in Hawaii. *Am. J. Epidemiol.*, **117**, 384–396.

Romano, P.S., Bloom, J.R. and Syme, S.L. (1991) Smoking, social support, and hassles in an urban African American community. *Am J. Public Health* (in press).

Rothman, K. and Keller, A. (1972) The effect of joining exposure to alcohol and tobacco on the risk of cancer of the mouth and pharynx. *J. Chron. Dis.*, **25**, 711–716.

Rubberman, W., Weinblatt, E. and Goldberg, J.D. (1984) Psychosocial influences on mortality after myocardial infarction. *New Engl. J. Med.*, **311**, 552–559.

Rutledge, D.N. (1987) Factors related to women's practice of breast self-examination. *Nursing Res.*, **36**(2), 117–121.

Safer, M.A., Tharps, Q.J., Jackson, T.C. and Leventhal, H. (1979) Determinants of three stages of delay in seeking care at a medical clinic. *Medical Care*, **17**(1), 11–29.

Samet, J.M., Hunt, W.C., Lerchen, M.L. and Goodwin, J.S. (1988) Delay in seeking care for cancer symptoms: a population-based study of elderly New Mexicans. *J. Nat. Cancer Inst.*, **80**(6), 432–438.

Schaefer, C., Coyne, J. and Lazarus, R. (1981) The health related functions of social support. *J. Behav. Med.*, **4**, 381–406.

Schoenbach, V.J. (1986) Social ties and mortality in Evans county Georgia. *Am. J. Epidemiol.*, **123**(4), 577–591.

Seeman, T.E. and Syme, S.L. (1987) Social networks and coronary artery disease: a comparison of the structure and function of social relations as predictors of disease. *Psychosom. Med.*, **49**, 341–354.

Seeman, T.E., Kaplan, G.A., Knudsen, L., Cohen, R. and Guralnik, J. (1987) Social network ties and mortality among the elderly in the Alameda County study. *Am. J. Epidemiol.*, **126**, 714–723.

Shavit, Y., Lewis, J. and Terman, G. (1984) Opioid peptides medicate the suppressive effect of stress in natural killer cell cytotoxicity. *Science*, **223**, 188–190.

Smith, E.M. and Anderson, B. (1985) The effects of symptoms and delay in seeking diagnosis on stage of disease at diagnosis among women with cancers of the ovary. *Cancer*, **56**, 2727–2732.

Spiegel, D. (1980) The recent literature: self-help and mutual support groups. *Commun. Mental Health Rev.*, **5**, 15–22.

Spiegel, D. and Bloom, J.R. (1983) Group therapy and hypnosis reduce metastatic breast carcinoma pain. *Psychosom. Med.*, **45**, 333–339.

Spiegel, D., Bloom, J.R. and Yalom, I. (1981) Group support for metastatic cancer patients: a randomized prospective outcome study. *Arch. Psych.*, **38**, 1117–1126.

Spiegel, D., Bloom, J.R., Kraemer, H.C. and Gottheil, E. (1989a) Effect of psychosocial treatment on survival of patients with metastatic breast cancer. *Lancet*, **2**, 888–891.

Spiegel, D., Bloom, J.R., Kraemer, H. and Gotheil, E. (1989b) Psychological support for cancer patients. *Lancet*, **ii**, 1447.

Spielberger, C.D., Gorsuch, R.L. and Lushene, R.E. (1970) *Manual for the State-Trait Anxiety Inventory*. Consulting Psychologists Press, Palo Alto.

Stanton, A.L. (1987) Determinants of adherence to medical regimens by hypertensive patients. *J. Behav. Med.*, **10**(4), 377–394.

Stavraky, K.M., Donner, A.P., Kincade, J.E. and Stewart, M.A. (1988) The effect of psychosocial factors on lung cancer mortality at one year. *J. Clin. Epidemiol.*, **41**(1), 75–82.

Syme, L. and Seeman, T. (1983) In Herd, A. and Weiss, S. (eds) *Sociocultural Risk Factors in Coronary Heart Disease, In Behavior and Arteriosclerosis*. Plenum Press, New York, pp. 55–71.

Thoits, P. (1983) Conceptual, methodological and theoretical problems in studying social support as a buffer against life stress. *J. Health Soc. Behav.*, **23**, 145–159.

Turner, R.J. and Noh, S. (1983) Class and psychological vulnerability among women: the significance of social support and personal control. *J. Health Soc. Behav.*, **24**, 2–15.

Tuyns, A.J., Pequignot, G. and Abbatucci, J.S. (1979) Esophageal cancer and alcohol consumption: importance of type of beverage. *Intern. Med. J. Cancer*, **23**, 443–447.

Vernon, S.W. and Jackson, G.L. (1989) Social support, prognosis and adjustment to breast cancer. In Markides, K.S. and Cooper, C.L. (eds) *Aging, Stress and Health*. John Wiley, New York, pp. 165–198.

Vital and Health Statistics (1989) *Smoking and other tobacco use: United States, 1987*. DHHS #89-1597, US Government Printing Office, Hyattsville.

Waldron, I. and Lye, D. (1989) Family roles and smoking. *Am. J. Prevent. Med.*, **5**(3), 136–140.

Ward, A.W.M. (1976) Mortality of bereavement. *Br. Med. J.*, **1**, 700–702.

Warheit, G.J. (1979) Life events, coping, stress, and depressive symptomatology. *Am. J. Psych.*, **136**, 502–507.

Weiss, J., Glazer, H. and Pohorecky, L. (1975) Effects of chronic exposure to stressors on avoidance-escape behavior and on brain norephinephrine. *Psychosom. Med.*, **37**, 522–534.

Weisman, A. and Worden, W. (1975) Psychosocial analysis of cancer deaths. *Omega*, **6**(1), 61–79.

Welin, L., Tibblin, G., Svandsudd, K., Tibblin, B., Ander-Peciva, S., Larsson, B. and Wilhelmsen, L. (1985) Prospective study of social influences on mortality. *Lancet*, **i**, 915–918.

Wiley, C. and Sillman, R.A. (1990) The impact of disease on the social support experiences of cancer patients. *Psychosoc. Oncol.*, **8**(1), 79–96.

Wills, T.A. (1983) Social comparison in coping and help-seeking. In DePaulo, B.M., Nadler, A. and Fisher, J.D. (eds) *New Directions in Helping*, Vol. 2. Academic Press, New York, pp. 109–141.

Wortman, C. (1983) Social support and the cancer patient: conceptual and methodological issues. *Cancer*, **53**, 2339–2360 (Supplement).

6

Studies of Psychological Factors and Cancer in China

ZHANG ZONG-WEI and GUO YAN-RONG
Beijing Institute for Cancer Research, Beijing, China

During recent years in China, a series of epidemiological studies have shown that there are positive correlations between cancer and psychological factors, which have been considered a very important cause of disease by the traditional theory of Chinese medicine. Qi-gong is the Oriental Psychotherapy and traditional treatment for cancer patients.

CANCER EPIDEMIOLOGY IN CHINA

Cancer has become a common disease and a serious public health problem in China. The national average annual age-adjusted cancer mortality rate for males was 80.17 per 100 000 and 54.27 per 100 000 for females. The proportionate mortality rate from cancer was 11.31% for males and 8.85% for females (see Table 1).

During the period 1973–1975, cancer was the second leading cause of death for males, following respiratory diseases, and the third for females, following respiratory and heart diseases. These mortality rates vary with age: among males aged 0–14 years, cancer was the cause of 0.88% of all deaths and ranked the ninth cause; among males aged 15–34 years, cancer comprises 8.27% of all deaths, and was the second leading cause of deaths; in the 35–54 and 55–74 year age groups, cancer accounted for 23.05% and 17.58% respectively, and was the leading cause of death for both groups. Females showed similar trends, indicating that not only was cancer a very important cause of death for the total population but also

Cancer and Stress: Psychological, Biological and Coping Studies
Edited by C. L. Cooper and M. Watson. © 1991 John Wiley & Sons Ltd

Psychosocial and Personality Factors

Table 1. The national average annual age-adjusted cancer mortality rate (per 100 000)

	Males	Females
Age-adjusted cancer mortality rate	80.17	54.27
Proportionate mortality rate from cancer (%)	11.31	8.85

that it severely affected the young and working population (The Editorial Committee, 1979).

Cancers of the digestive system are very common in China. In males, stomach cancer is the most frequent cause of cancer death. The national average mortality rate is 20.93 per 100 000, comprising 26.11% of all cancers. Next in frequency are oesophageal, liver, lung, colon and rectal cancers. In females, death due to stomach cancer continues to rank first, followed by cervical, oesophageal, liver and lung cancer. In recent years, the incidence of breast cancer has increased remarkably, especially in large cities (Wang, Qi-jun and Zhu, 1989).

Cancer mortality has ranked very highly as a cause of death in recent years. According to data for 1984, deaths due to cancer were the leading cause of mortality in Shanghai, with 26.7% of all deaths due to malignant disease (see Table 2). Deaths from cancer have also risen to third place in Beijing and Tianjin, with mortality rates of 18.95% and 19.35%, respectively (Beijing Health Bureau, 1984).

STUDIES OF PSYCHOLOGICAL FACTORS AND CANCER IN CHINA

Retrospective and prospective biobehavioral cancer studies in western countries have revealed that psychosocial stressors may play a pivotal role in the initiation and progression of malignant neoplasia. A well known medical model has been transformed from a simple biomedical model to a biopsychosocial medical model and there is increasing interest in multifactorial models of cancer aetiology. More and more scientists in China are beginning to think that psychosocial factors appear to play a greater role in cancer genesis than other risk factors. The application of this model appears to be of importance for further research, as well as for the detection of high risk individuals; also in regard to therapy, rehabilitation, early detection of, and possibly also prevention of, malignant disease.

Since 1984, a series of epidemiological studies have been conducted in Beijing, relating cancer to psychosocial factors. The aim of these studies was to explore the possible association of cancer with personality and negative life events. Death due to stomach cancer is most frequent in

Table 2. Constitution of causes of death in Beijing, Tianjin and Shanghai

Order	Beijing		Tianjin		Shanghai	
	Disease	%	Disease	%	Disease	%
1	Heart disease	24.88	Heart disease	28.46	Malignant tumour	26.70
2	Cerebrovascular	24.18	Cerebrovascular	25.93	Cerebrovascular	17.29
3	Malignant tumour	18.95	Malignant tumour	19.35	Heart disease	15.79
4	Respiratory disease	6.50	Respiratory disease	4.80	Respiratory disease	11.53
5	Digestive disease	4.12	Digestive disease	4.14	Infectious disease	5.96
6	Injury	3.08	Urinary disease	2.19	Digestive disease	4.02
7	Poisoning	2.25	Injury	1.96	Injury	3.55
8	Urinary disease	2.00	Poisoning	1.86	Nervous disease	1.92
9	Nervous disease	1.26	Tuberculosis	1.62	Urinary disease	1.67
10	Tuberculosis	1.19	Newborn disease	1.30	Endocrine disease	1.46
Total		88.41		91.61		89.89

males, and breast cancer is now the leading cancer in females. The studies focused on the relationship between psychological factors and the occurrence of cancer and used a self-administered questionnaire compiled by our research group.

Materials and methods

The data reported here are part of an epidemiological study of psychosocial factors and cancer, supported by the National Natural Science Foundation of China. All cases for the study were selected from the Beijing Cancer Registry. The patients with stomach cancer were diagnosed during January–December, 1984 and female patients with breast cancer were diagnosed during the period July 1986–February 1988. Subjects who were under 70 years old and residing in the Beijing urban area, were considered eligible for inclusion.

The method adopted was that of a case control study (Mausner and Bahn, 1985), with two controls matched to each case on sex, age within five years and educational level. One was a cancer-free control: the other was an "other cancers" control, that is cancer of any site except stomach or breast. All subjects and controls were invited to participate by personal letter. They were requested to complete a self-report questionnaire mailed beforehand, covering three areas. Information was obtained for both cases and controls, and covered the following.

General information

Age, educational level, family income, body mass index, marital status, reproduction and family history.

Personality traits

Depressive mood (D), Manifest Anxiety Scale (MAS), Social Control Ability (SC), Social Introversion (SI), Type A personality (TH4) and Lie Scale.

Life events

Interpersonal problems, work and study problems, marital and family problems, accidents and childhood experiences.

We also considered that one's personality may be changed after the diagnosis of cancer, so two different periods were covered in the questionnaire, with an assessment of concurrent psychological responses and a retrospective assessment covering the preceding three-year period. This was designed to try to overcome the shortcomings of using only a retrospective approach.

Results

By the end of 1984, we had obtained information from 132 subjects: 50 cases of stomach cancer, 43 cancer-free controls and 39 "other cancers" controls; 39 pairs on a 1:2 basis have been completed. The results of the present study, with respect to psychological factors, are summarized in Table 3.

Table 3 shows that when the stomach cancer and cancer-free groups were compared the risk of stomach cancer is seen to be significantly related to some personality styles, such as depressive mood and inflexibility. However, when the stomach cancer group and the "other cancers" group were compared this association was not found. Social introversion, depressive mood and inflexibility all showed significant associations between the "other cancers" group and the cancer-free group.

Recently another case control study of psychological factors and cancer has been carried out in the Beijing urban area. First, we examined possible change of one's personality before and after diagnosis of cancer. There were some statistically significant differences between the two periods only in the cancer group, not in the cancer-free group; these are shown in Table 4.

Thus it can be seen that the cognitive and behavioural responses may be changed when the patient receives a diagnosis of cancer. This study focused on personality *before* diagnosed cancer. Eighty-three cases of current breast cancer were selected for this study. They responded well, with low Lie scale scores ($P < 0.05$). Age distribution was 25–69 years;

Table 3. χ^2 test and U test of the psychological factors

	χ^2	U test		
		C and A	C and B	B and A
Social introversion (SI)	7.73	1.29	0.83	2.06[*]
Depression mood (D)	14.14[**]	3.87[*]	0.06	3.57[*]
Inflexibility (FX)	11.99[*]	1.67[*]	0.40	1.93[*]
Lie (L)	2.14	0.26	1.17	0.87
Life events	4.40	0.19	0.48	0.28

[*] $P < 0.05$; [**] $P < 0.01$; one-tailed test
C, cases of stomach cancer; A, cancer-free control; B, "other cancers" control.

Table 4. Personality changes between three years ago and at present (U test)

	Breast cancer group ($n = 83$)	"Other cancer" group ($n = 58$)	Cancer-free group ($n = 83$)
L	0.5206	0.9797	1.2686
D	5.2227**	3.2667**	1.3291
MAS	2.7403**	1.7866*	0.8906
SC	0.7320	0.4323	0.3757
SI	0.0152	0.5847	0.0289
TH4	0.8838	0.6514	0.2776
	$U = 1.64$; $P = 0.05$	$U = 2.39$; $P = 0.01$	

*$P < 0.05$; **$P < 0.01$.

93.99% were between the ages of 35 and 59 years, and 84.34% of educational level of junior middle school and above. The study also included 83 cancer-free controls and 58 "other cancers" controls.

Differences in personality traits between cancer group (including breast and other) and cancer-free group were first examined using Mantel–Haenszel Tests. Results are presented in Table 5.

Multiple Logistic Regression was used in this analysis; a total of 83 pairs of breast cancer and 58 pairs of other cancers were analysed. The results were similar to those indicated above: there was a positive correlation between depressed mood and breast cancer. The level of depression and the ability to control one's social situation are significantly related to other cancers. Depressive mood appears to be a high risk factor for both breast and other cancers.

Seven categories of life events were included in the questionnaire: relationships between individuals (interpersonal relations), problems in

Table 5. χ^2 Test of personality styles between cancer and cancer-free group

	Breast cancer cases matched with cancer-free controls		Other cancer cases matched with cancer-free controls	
	χ^2	RR	χ^2	RR
D	4.055*	1.081	7.595**	1.123
MAS	2.752	1.076	0.844	1.045
SC	0.080	1.016	4.782*	0.868
SI	0.068	1.008	2.519	0.943
TH4	0.283	0.979	0.101	1.017

*$P < 0.05$; **$P < 0.01$.

Table 6. χ^2 Test of life events scale between other cancers and cancer-free group

	χ^2	RR
Interpersonal relationships	10.332*	1.267
Life problems	1.204	1.051
Working or studying problems	4.023*	1.082
Accident	7.407**	1.187
Marital and family problems	12.354**	1.163
Childhood experience	3.124	1.100
Total scale	11.836**	1.045

* $P < 0.05$; ** $P < 0.01$.

life, problems in working or studying, marital and family problems, accident and childhood experiences. Each category consists of many items; a total of 48 items of negative life events were designed for our study.

We found no significant associations for breast cancer with life events scale in this study. However, there were statistically significant associations between four of the seven life events categories and the development of other cancers. The results are shown in Table 6.

More recently, we have expanded the sample size, and a total of 111 pairs of stomach cancer and 139 pairs of breast cancer were analysed. Each patient with stomach or breast cancer was matched to two controls individually, one cancer-free and the other an "other cancers" control. The results of this analysis are shown in Table 7.

This study indicated that life events may be more important than personality in the genesis of cancers at all sites.

Table 7. χ^2 Test of the psychological factors and cancer

	Stomach cancer (111 pairs)			Breast cancer (139 pairs)		
	Cs and As	Bs and As	Cs and Bs	C and A	B and A	C and B
D	0.203	4.277*	4.146	3.750	4.700*	0.236
MAS	0.184	2.132	4.551*	0.032	0.333	0.666
SC	0.107	1.187	1.596	0.287	3.811	1.616
SI	0.419	0.021	0.535	0.000	1.723	1.541
TH4	2.118	7.400**	1.679	0.553	0.983	0.047
Life events (total)	6.519**	12.034**	0.894	5.430*	20.360**	4.674*

* $P < 0.05$; ** $P < 0.01$
Cs, stomach cancer; As, cancer-free controls; Bs, "other cancers" controls; C, breast cancer; A, cancer-free controls; B, "other cancers" controls.

Discussion

The notion that cancer might be related in some way to stress or emotional factors is probably as old as the history of recorded medicine. Galen's treatise on tumors, *De Tumoribus*, noted that melancholy women who had too much black bile were more susceptible to cancer than other women. In 1701, the English physician Gendron emphasized the effect of "disasters of life as occasions for much trouble and grief" in the causation of cancer, and 80 years later Burrows attributed the disease to "the uneasy passions of the mind with which the patient is strongly affected for a long time". In the early 19th century, authors such as Nunn emphasized that emotional factors appeared to influence the growth of breast tumors, and Stern noted that cancer of the cervix appeared to be more common in sensitive and frustrated married women. Toward the end of the 19th century another English physician, Snow, reviewed more than 250 patients at the London Cancer Hospital and concluded that "the loss of a near relative was an important factor in the development of cancer of the breast" (Rosch, 1987).

It is now well known that psychosocial stress factors are conducive to a number of illnesses, ranging from mental disturbances to classic psychosomatic disorders and to "organic" disease. As to cancer, we have to ask which factors are especially important for the development and progression of malignant processes and whether there exists a certain risk profile for this disease (Baltrusch and Zhang, 1989).

In the area of cardiovascular disease behavioral medicine has been quite successful in discerning a Type A or coronary-prone pattern concept in large-scale epidemiologic studies in many countries. As an important moderating factor in the stress–disease nexus, this behavior pattern probably influences the cognitive processing of environmental stressors and the individual's emotional reactions to them. The psychological components underlying this particular behavior pattern are not completely understood, but hostility is seen as one important component, as well as a need for control. Type As respond to stressors with physiological hyper-reactivity. In a longitudinal study of coronary patients, the Type A pattern was found also to be associated with a psychological hyper-responsiveness at the cognitive and affective levels, particularly in respect to elevated anxiety (Baltrusch and Waltz, 1987).

More recently, behavioral oncologists have attempted to conceptualize and operationalize a Type C or cancer-prone pattern (Greer and Watson, 1987; Temoshok, 1987; Temoshok and Heller, 1984; Baltrusch *et al.*, 1987, 1988, 1989; Grassi, 1987). These researchers have noted suppression and repression of negative emotions and/or the inability to express emotions, in particular anger. Other marked traits are the avoidance of conflicts, so-called "harmonizing behavior", exaggerated social desirability and conformity, compliance, unassertiveness and overpatience, often camouflaged behind a façade of outer calmness and pleasantness. A recent Dutch study adds to these dimensions rationality, antiemotionality and elevated control of emotions as core factors in the psychosocial risk profile of cancer patients (van der Ploeg *et al.*, 1989).

Using the epidemiology method of a case-control study, we examined the possibility that psychological factors are related to occurrence of cancer, focusing on stomach cancer and breast cancer, which are leading cancers in China. We found that some dispositions, such as depressed mood and inflexibility, are associated with the development and outcome of stomach cancer (Zhang and Wang, 1988). We also found, in a subsequent investigation, a positive correlation between depressed mood and breast cancer. Other findings show that depression, the ability to control one's social situation and some negative life events are significantly related to other cancers. More recently, when the sample size was expanded, we found that life events may be a more important factor in cancer genesis than personality style: moreover, a suppression of negative emotions or the inability to express emotions has been noted in our investigations, particularly depression. It is generally believed that psychosocial factors are very important factors of high risk for cancer and seem to play a greater role than other risk factors, such as nutrition or pollution, in the genesis of cancer.

We consider that psychological factors may be a *promoter*. Personality styles may be internal causes, life events may be external causes, external causes become operative through internal causes in the development and outcome of cancer. Biobehavioral research in oncology has focused on stress as a dispositional factor associated with the development and clinical progression of malignant neoplasia. New insights into the transduction of environmental influences by the brain and neurotransmitters to the endocrine and immune systems have recently markedly increased the salience of this approach.

Our study represents initial work in this field in China. Many of these studies are limited by methodological problems, such as retrospective study design, lack of adjustment for confounding factors and small number of cases. Nevertheless, we firmly believe that research work in this field will be developed and become very useful in prevention, treatment and rehabilitation of cancer in the future.

TRADITIONAL CHINESE MEDICINE

The basic theories of traditional Chinese medicine consist of three parts:

- Yin–yang and five elements
- Zang-fu (internal organs)
- Channels and collaterals

Yin–yang and five elements

The theories of yin–yang and five elements were two kinds of outlook on nature in ancient China. They involved a naive concept of materialism and dialectics and actively promoted natural science. Physicians applied these two theories in their field, which have greatly influenced the formation and development of the theoretical system of traditional Chinese medicine and have guided clinical work up to the present.

Yin–yang: The theory of yin–yang holds that every object or phenomenon in the universe consists of two opposite aspects, *yin* and *yang*, which are at once in conflict and in interdependence: further, that this relation between yin and yang is the universal law of the material world, the principle and source of the existence of myriads of things, and the root cause for the flourishing and perishing of things.

The theory of yin–yang mainly expounds the opposition, interdependence, interconsuming-supporting and intertransforming relation of yin–yang. These relationships are extensively used in traditional Chinese medicine to explain the physiology and pathology of the human body and to serve as a guide to diagnosis and treatment in clinical work.

Five elements: The theory of five elements holds that wood, fire, earth, metal and water are the five basic materials constituting the material world. There is among them an interdepending and interrestraining relation which puts them in a state of constant motion and change.

The theory of five elements mainly explains the interpromoting, interacting, overacting and counteracting relation among the five elements. In traditional Chinese medicine it is used to classify natural phenomena together with the tissues and organs of the human body and the human emotional activities into different categories, and to interpret the relation between the physiology and pathology of the human body and natural environment with the law of interpromoting, interacting, overacting and counteracting of the five elements. It is used as a guide to medical practice.

Attribution of things to the five elements

Humans live in nature. The natural environment, weather changes and geographical conditions, exerts important influences on our physiological activities. This is manifested by the dependence of people on the environment on the one hand, and their adaptability to the environment on the other; it is known as *correspondency* between humans and nature. Proceeding from this recognition, traditional Chinese medicine comprehensively connects the physiology and pathology of the zang-fu organs and

Table 8. The five categories of things classified according to the five elements

Five elements	Human body					Nature					
	Zang	Fu	Five sense organs	Five tissues	Emotions	Season	Environmental factors	Growth and development	Colours	Tastes	Orientations
Wood	Liver	Gall bladder	Eye	Tendon	Anger	Spring	Wind	Germination	Green	Sour	East
Fire	Heart	Small intestine	Tongue	Vessel	Joy	Summer	Heat	Growth	Red	Bitter	South
Earth	Spleen	Stomach	Mouth	Muscle	Meditation	Late summer	Dampness	Transformation	Yellow	Sweet	Middle
Metal	Lung	Large intestine	Nose	Skin and hair	Grief and melancholy	Autumn	Dryness	Reaping	White	Pungent	West
Water	Kidney	Urinary bladder	Ear	Bone	Fright and fear	Winter	Cold	Storing	Black	Salty	North

tissues with many important factors of the natural environment. They are classified into different categories of the five elements, using similes and allegories to explain the complicated connections between physiology and pathology as well as the correlation between humans and their environment. Table 8 shows the five categories of things classified according to the five elements.

The interpromoting, interacting, overacting and counteracting relation of the five elements

Promoting implies promoting growth. The order of promoting is that wood promotes fire, fire promotes earth, earth promotes metal, metal promotes water and water, in its turn, promotes wood. In this interpromoting relation each element has the relations of "being promoted" and "promoting", the one which promotes being the "mother", and the one being promoted the "son". Hence this relation is known as the mother-and-son relation. Take wood as an example: the element by which wood is promoted is water, water is the "mother" of wood: wood promotes fire, fire is the "son" of wood.

Interacting connotes bringing under control or restraint. In the interacting relation, wood acts on earth, earth acts on water, water acts on fire, fire acts on metal and metal, in its turn, acts on wood. In this relationship, each of the five elements has the relations of "being acted on" and "acting on". Take wood as an example: the one acting on it is metal and the one being acted on by it is earth.

Overacting connotes launching an attack when the other element is weak. Clinically, it is conventionally also called interacting. The order of overacting is the same as that of interacting, only it is not a normal interacting relation but a harmful one occurring under certain conditions. *Counteracting* implies preying upon others. The order is opposite to that of interacting. The relations of the five elements are shown in Figure 1.

The theory of five elements is applied to the medical field by using the interpromoting, interacting, overacting and counteracting relation of the five elements to expound the interdepending and interrestraining relation among the zang-fu organs, sense organs and tissues and also the correlation between humans and nature. Above all it is used to explain the changes, aetiology and mechanism of disease. For example, the relations between emotional activities and zang-fu organs are: anger injures liver; meditation (overthinking) injures spleen and stomach; grief and melancholy injures lung.

Psychological factors have been considered a very important cause of diseases. Traditional theory of Chinese medical science even says that

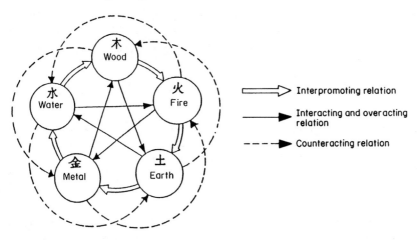

Figure 1. Interpromoting, interacting and overacting, and counteracting relations between the five elements: wood, fire, earth, metal and water

emotions are the cause for all disease. The Seven Human Emotions, Joy, Anger, Melancholy, Brooding, Sorrow, Fear and Shock are considered the internal factors causing diseases. This is an important component part of Chinese medical science.

Zang-fu (internal organs)

The term *zang-fu* in traditional Chinese medicine refers to the gross anatomical entities of the internal organs. At the same time, it is also a generalization of the physiological functions of the human body. The heart, liver, spleen, lung, kidney and pericardium grouped together are known as the six zang organs. Their main physiological functions are manufacturing and storing essential substances including vital essence, qi (vital energy), blood and body fluid. The small intestine, gallbladder, stomach, large intestine, urinary bladder and sanjiao are known collectively as the six fu organs. Their main functions are to receive and digest food, absorb nutrient substances and transmit and excrete wastes. There are in addition extraordinary fu organs including the brain and the uterus.

The zang organs are different in function from the fu, but the difference is only relative. In physiological activities, structural and functional connection and coordination exists not only among the zang and the fu organs separately, but also among the zang and fu organs collectively, and even among the zang-fu organs and the five sense organs and five tissues. The theory of zang-fu taking the five zang organs (six including the pericardium) as core explains the peculiarity of traditional Chinese medicine, i.e. the concept of regarding the body as an integral whole physiologically and pathologically.

Channels and collaterals

The channels and collaterals are distributed all over the human body, linking the interior zang-fu organs with the various tissues and organs of the superficial portion of the body to make the body an organic integrity. In the network of the channels and collaterals, the *channels* are the main trunks which pertain to the respective zang-fu organs, while the *collaterals* are their minor branches distributed over the entire body.

The system of channels and collaterals mainly consists of the twelve regular channels, the eight extra channels and the fifteen collaterals. The twelve regular channels, together with the Ren channel and the Du Channel of the eight extra channels, form the fourteen channels, along each of which are points for applying acupuncture and moxibustion.

The complete name of each of the twelve regular channels is composed of three parts: (1) hand or foot; (2) yin or yang (yin is further divided

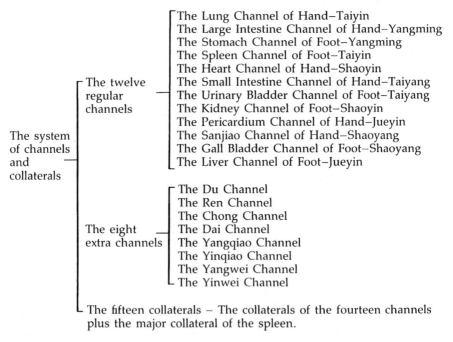

The system of channels and collaterals

The twelve regular channels
- The Lung Channel of Hand–Taiyin
- The Large Intestine Channel of Hand–Yangming
- The Stomach Channel of Foot–Yangming
- The Spleen Channel of Foot–Taiyin
- The Heart Channel of Hand–Shaoyin
- The Small Intestine Channel of Hand–Taiyang
- The Urinary Bladder Channel of Foot–Taiyang
- The Kidney Channel of Foot–Shaoyin
- The Pericardium Channel of Hand–Jueyin
- The Sanjiao Channel of Hand–Shaoyang
- The Gall Bladder Channel of Foot–Shaoyang
- The Liver Channel of Foot–Jueyin

The eight extra channels
- The Du Channel
- The Ren Channel
- The Chong Channel
- The Dai Channel
- The Yangqiao Channel
- The Yinqiao Channel
- The Yangwei Channel
- The Yinwei Channel

The fifteen collaterals – The collaterals of the fourteen channels plus the major collateral of the spleen.

Figure 2. Classification of channels and collaterals

into Taiyin, Shaoyin and Jueyin, and yang into Taiyang, Yangming and Shaoyang); and (3) a zang or a fu organ. The hand or foot in the name of a channel depends on whether the channel starts or terminates at the hand or the foot, while yin or yang and a zang or a fu organ are determined by whether it takes its course along the medial or the lateral aspects of the limb, and to which zang or fu organ it pertains. For instance, the channel which terminates at the hand, runs along the medial aspect of the upper limb and pertains to the lung is named the Lung Channel of Hand-Taiyin. Figure 2 shows the classification of channels and collaterals.

The theory of channels and collaterals is extensively used as a guide to treatment of diseases in the various clinical specialties, especially acupuncture and moxibustion. In acupuncture and moxibustion therapy, the affected channels or zang-fu organs are first detected. Points are then selected from adjacent areas or from the corresponding channels in distant areas. Therapeutic results may be obtained through regulating the circulation of qi and blood of the channels and collaterals.

Guo Lin Qi-gong system – the Chinese traditional treatment for cancer patients

The word Qi-gong consists of two independent Chinese characters.

What is qi?

Qi is the energy of life, qi is one of the fundamental concepts of Chinese thought. The manifestation of any invisible force in the body, forces which enable a person to move, to breathe, to digest food, to think, is called qi. Qi is involved in various aspects in physiology, pathology and clinical treatment. Generally speaking, the word qi connotes both substance and function. For instance, clean qi, waste qi and qi from essence of food are material qi; the qi of the heart, liver, spleen, kidney and stomach and the qi of channels and collaterals are functional qi.

What is gong?

Gong means Chinese Gongfu, and performing exercises assiduously.

The Guo Lin Qi-gong system was a new therapy developed by Guo Lin, a famous Qi-gong master in China, Guo Lin, alias Lin Guanming or Meishu, was born in Zhongshan county of Guangdong province in April, 1909. Doing Qi-gong (breathing exercises) since childhood, Guo was well versed in this exercise in its ancient form. In the late 1940s, she underwent six operations for cancer, but the tumor remained in her. To remove this threat to human lives she began to improve ancient qi-gong. She studied intensively both Chinese and Western medicines, sought the advice of two qi-gong masters to whom she had access, and practised the reformed exercise for 20 years. The result; a new system of qi-gong therapy which cured her of the lingering cancer.

Guo Lin died of cerebral haemorrhage on December 14, 1984 at the age of 75. Since her death her achievements have been carried further by the Guo Lin Qi-gong Research Society, beneficiaries of her system and qi-gong enthusiasts. Doctor Guo Lin will be remembered by the people for her contribution to the development of Chinese qi-gong exercises.

The Guo Lin Qi-gong system is also known as the New Qi-gong therapy (New Qi-gong for short), Self control therapy, Self bioelectric therapy, New Qi-gong five animal exercise, common saying Xixihu (means inhale, inhale and exhale).

The system has been accepted as one of the important therapies for cancer patients especially for cancer rehabilitation, and is the most outstanding example of preventing and treating cancer since its initiation in 1971. The system has also proved effective for other chronic diseases and difficult and complicated cases such as cardiovascular disorders.

The Guo Lin Qi-gong system consists of four phases of exercise: the preliminary, intermediate, advanced and special qi-gong exercises. For treatment of disease, there is a subsystem for cancer and another for chronic, difficult and complicated disorders. The system is an integral therapy that puts emphasis on motivating internal qi or energy through meditation, body movement, breathing, vocal utterance and a combination of these. Diagnosis uses a dialectical analysis of an illness. Treatment combines movement and stillness, such as concentrating one's mind on an object to achieve consciousness of our natural being, and breathing in wholesome air to trigger unconscious movement of the hands and feet, leading through three steps of breathing, meditation and movement. The exercises are easy to perform and produce few undesirable side-effects.

The exercises of the Guo Lin Qi-gong system include natural exercise, fixed step exercise, toe step exercise, fast exercise, hands lifting–lowering–extending–closing exercise, vocal exercise, slow step exercise, hand roller exercise, yongquan massage exercise, head massage exercise, feet roller exercise, eight-section exercise, back relaxing exercise, tri-circle exercise, five-animal exercise, standing exercise, sitting exercise and lying-down exercise. Patients and qi-gong enthusiasts can choose any of these that best serve their needs.

Clinical observations have shown that the Guo Lin Qi-gong system has remarkable curative effects and vitalizes the exerciser's energy. It can be learned by any one strong enough to walk unaided and anyone who does it as prescribed will soon find that their appetite has improved, they sleep

Table 9. Therapeutic effects of Guo Lin Qi-gong (percentages of patients treated)

Curative effect	Disease		
	Cancer	Heart disease	Hypertension
Highly effective	5	10	25
Remarkably effective	20	30	30
Effective	70	55	42
Non-effective	5	5	3

better, their blood becomes healthier, and their pain has eased, signs that help to build up confidence in fighting illness. If they continue the exercises, their health will be improved, their immune system strengthened, they stand a better chance of being cured of disease, thus lengthening their lifespan.

The Guo Lin Qi-gong does not exclude other means of medical treatment. In fact, it is believed that combined with Chinese and Western medicines, the therapy will be even more effective.

Incomplete statistics show that there are over one million patients who have practised the Guo Lin Qi-gong system; cases of 36 different kinds of cancer (including cancer of the lungs, liver, colon, stomach, breasts, uterus, kidney, lymphoma and leukaemia), and those suffering from 24 chronic diseases such as heart disease, hypertension, hepatitis, nephritis, diabetes, hard skin disease and lupus erythematosus. Most cases showed satisfactory therapeutic effects. The results are shown in Table 9.

Case histories

When Gao Wenbin, a naval officer, was found to be suffering from lung cancer in 1976, it was too late for surgery. He started practising the Guo Lin Qi-gong system. In two years he had recovered and was strong enough to work again; he has been in good health ever since. Doctors called his recovery a miracle.

Li Yiming, a factory worker, fell victim of liver cancer in 1984. After surgery he started practising the Guo Lin Qi-gong system. His liver now functions normally, so do the gallbladder, pancreas and spleen. He is now an active qi-gong coach and practitioner at the qi-gong coaching center.

Yu Dayuan of the General Political Department of the army developed cancer of the colon in 1978. The tumor metastasized after surgery. After a year of exercise in qi-gong, the focus disappeared. Now, he is physically capable of working more than eight hours a day.

Gu Pingdan of the China Art Research Institute was found to have stomach cancer in 1981. He was too weak after surgery for chemotherapy. Five years of qi-gong exercises enabled him to work again.

A middle-school teacher in Chengdu, Wan Niwen, developed breast cancer in 1975. After surgery the tumor metastasized to the lungs. After two years of practising the Guo Lin Qi-gong system, the tumor was gone. She is now a qi-gong activist.

Han Quisheng of the Beijing Railway Bureau suffered from chronic disease for many years. As he did not respond to any medicine, he turned to the Guo Lin Qi-gong system. The exercises were more effective on him than he expected. Since then he has fallen in love with qi-gong, teaching the exercises and working to develop a theory of the therapy.

A Beijing factory worker, Zhang Mingwu, developed coronary heart disease and angina pectoris in 1974. After the medical treatment he received failed to cure him, he began to practise the Guo Lin Qi-gong system in 1975. It took him only nine months to rid himself of the illness. He is now back to work and is a qi-gong enthusiast.

Another Beijing factory worker Shan Changli contracted protracted hepatitis in 1973. He was cured after a year of exercise prescribed in the Guo Lin Qi-gong system. He now works at the Shengli Oilfield as a qi-gong coach.

The magical effect of qi-gong for cancer patients has been recognized by more and more scientists in China. They think that the Chinese traditional Qi-gong system is a special psychotherapy and that it is necessary to make a thorough investigation and study this oriental medicine scientifically.

To sum up, a whole set of rehabilitation medicine for cancer patients has been set up in China, and the Chinese Cancer Rehabilitation Society (CCRS) was established in 1990. Chinese Cancer Rehabilitation Medicine involves western psychotherapy, the New Qi-gong system, Chinese herbal medicines and dietetic treatment. Chinese herbal medicines are considered to possess an ability to increase the immunity of the body against the tumor – this is far beyond what many chemosynthetic medicines do. The CCRS thereby uses comprehensive rehabilitation treatment in order to increase survival rate, extend survival time and improve the quality of survival.

REFERENCES

Baltrusch, H.J. and Waltz, M.E. (1987) Stress and cancer: A sociobiological approach to aging, neuroimmunomodulation and the host–tumor relationship. *Human Stress: Current Selected Research*, **2**, 153–200.
Baltrusch, H.J.F. and Zhang, Z.W. (1989) The role of psychosocial stressors, per-

sonality and coping in the multifactorial origin, initiation and clinical course of neoplastic disease in host-defense. *Chin. J. Cancer Res.*, **1**(4), 65–75.

Baltrusch, H.J.F., Stangel, W. and Waltz, M.E. (1988) Cancer from the bio-behavioral perspective: the Type C pattern. *Act. Nerv. Super. Praha*, **30**, 18–21.

Beijing Health Bureau (1984) *Annual Statistical Data.*

The Editorial Committee for the Atlas of Cancer Mortality in the People's Republic of China (1979) *Atlas of Cancer Mortality in the People's Republic of China.* China Map Press, Beijing.

Greer, S. and Watson, M. (1985) Towards a psychobiological model of cancer: psychological considerations. *Soc. Sci. Med.*, **20**, 773–777.

Mausner, J.S. and Bahn, A.K.A. (1985) *Epidemiology – An Introductory Text*, 2nd Edition. W.B. Saunders Company, Philadelphia.

Rosch, P.J. (1987) *Stress and Cancer.*

Temoshok, L. (1987) Personality, coping style, emotion and cancer: towards an integrative model. *Cancer Surveys*, **6**, 545–567.

Temoshok, L. and Heller, B.W. (1984) On comparing apples, oranges and fruit salad: a methodological overview of medical outcome studies in psychosocial oncology. In Cooper, C.L. (ed.) *Psychosocial Stress and Cancer.* John Wiley, Chichester, pp. 231–260.

van der Ploeg, H. M., Kleijn, W.Chr., Mook, J., van Donge, M., Pieters, A.M.J. and Leer, J.-W.H. (1989) Rationality and antiemotionality as a risk factor for cancer: concept differentiation. *J. Psychosom. Res.*, **33**, 217–225.

Wang, Qi-jun and Zhu, W.X. (1989) Analysis of the cancer mortality and incidence in Beijing urban area. *J. Prac. Oncol.*, **2**, 1–4.

Zhang, Z.W. and Wang, T.G. (1988) Use of psychological personality inventory method in cancer epidemiological survey. *Chin. J. Epidemiol.*, **4**(9), 230–232.

Section III
COPING AND PSYCHOSOCIAL INTERVENTIONS

7

The Stress of Cancer: Psychological Responses to Diagnosis and Treatment

PAUL B. JACOBSEN and JIMMIE C. HOLLAND

Psychiatry Service, Memorial Sloan-Kettering Cancer Center, New York, USA

Other chapters in this book consider the effects of stress on the development of cancer and its subsequent clinical course. The aim of this chapter is to analyze the diagnosis and treatment of cancer in terms of its stressful properties and to review the literature on this topic.

One of the difficulties in reviewing research on stress is the imprecise use of the term. As Endler and Edwards (1982) point out, stress has been defined as a stimulus, a response, and an intervening state of the individual. In this chapter, the term *stressors* will be used to describe external events or conditions (i.e. stimuli) that impinge on individuals. The term *stress response* will be used to refer to the reactions of the individual to stressors.

A PSYCHOLOGICAL MODEL OF STRESS

The definitions offered above are very broad and, as applied to cancer, would include all research into both the physical and the psychological effects of neoplastic diseases and their treatments. To narrow the scope, we will limit our review to *psychogenic stressors* associated with cancer and its treatment.

What defines a psychogenic stressor? In answer to this question we present a model of stress that incorporates ideas put forth by Hamilton

Cancer and Stress: Psychological, Biological and Coping Studies
Edited by C. L. Cooper and M. Watson. © 1991 John Wiley & Sons Ltd

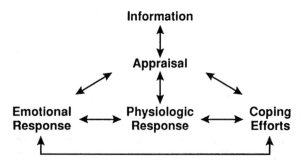

Figure 1. A psychological model of stress

(1980, 1982) and Lazarus (Lazarus and Folkman, 1984) (see Figure 1). According to this model, an event or an anticipated event is a psychogenic stressor if it provides information that is appraised as having unfavorable implications or potentially unfavorable outcomes. Lazarus and Folkman (1984) have described the three types of appraisals that characterize stressful encounters: harm/loss, threat, and challenge. *Harm/loss* refers to an appraisal of the extent of damage that is perceived to have already occurred. *Threat* refers to an appraisal that harm or loss can be anticipated. *Challenge* refers to an appraisal that there is a potential for gain or mastery in a situation that also has the potential for harm. Our definition of psychogenic stressors emphasizes the role that cognitive processes play in determining whether or not an event is stressful. It is not the *event* itself that is necessarily stressful, rather the individual's *interpretation* of the event. Thus, the same event may have very different meaning for two individuals based on their individual appraisals of the situation. This definition stands in contrast with "objective" views (e.g. Holmes and Rahe, 1967), which hold that certain life events (such as being diagnosed with cancer) are inherently stressful for all individuals.

The other part of the model involves the multidimensional nature of the stress response. As conceptualized here, there are three major components. The first component is the *emotional response*. The experience of psychogenic stressors (i.e. the appraisal that a situation is harmful or threatening) is usually associated with the subjective experience of negative emotional states such as anxiety and dysphoria. The second component is the *physiologic response*. Physiologic changes (e.g. autonomic nervous system activation) may be concomitants of the emotional response and of efforts to respond to harm, threat, and challenge. The third component of the stress response is *coping efforts*. As Holroyd and Lazarus (1982) have pointed out, "stressful circumstances do not take their toll from a passive individual ... but from an individual who is imbuing stressful circumstances with personal meaning and is struggling to control and master these circumstances". Any discussion of stress must consider the individual's ongoing cognitive and behavioral efforts to cope with internal and external demands.

A key feature of the model depicted in Figure 1 is the possibility for interaction among the components. Three examples illustrate this principle. The first involves the possible bidirectional relationship between appraisal and information. Appraisal is viewed as an ongoing process which can influence the subsequent search for information. Based on the appraisal, an individual may or may not seek additional information or may seek only information which confirms the initial appraisal (i.e. that a threat exists or that there is no threat). A second example involves the reciprocal relationship between emotional responses and coping. A powerful emotional response to a threatening situation may lead to a reliance on emotion-focused coping efforts (e.g. avoidance of thoughts related to the threat) which, in turn, serve to blunt the emotional response. The third example is that the nature of the stress response can shape subsequent appraisals; this is particularly true when the psychogenic stressor is chronic or occurs repeatedly. Based on previous experience, the degree of threat an individual associates with a particular situation may increase or decrease over time.

Using this model, we will organize our review of the stress of cancer and its treatments around situations in which individuals encounter information that may lead to appraisals of harm, threat, or challenge. The model suggests that the impact of cancer-related psychogenic stressors should also be examined in terms of the emotional responses, physiologic responses, and coping efforts to which they give rise. Although not explicit in the model, there are characteristics of the individual that are important to consider since they may contribute to differences in appraisal and in stress responses. For example, an individual who has strong beliefs about personal control over events may be more likely to view an event such as cancer diagnosis as a challenge and undertake problem-solving efforts. Situational factors may also affect appraisal and coping. Situations characterized by a high degree of uncertainty (such as awaiting biopsy results) create conditions likely to give rise to appraisals of threat.

The term cancer refers to a diverse group of over 100 different diseases. In order to provide an in-depth discussion, we limit this review to a critical analysis of the psychogenic stressors of breast cancer and its treatments. We have chosen to focus on breast cancer because it has been extensively researched from a psychological perspective. Moreover, the diagnosis and treatment of breast cancer involves a series of medical events and procedures (mammography, biopsy, surgery, chemotherapy, and radiation) with the potential to serve as psychogenic stressors. Our examination of the literature is not exhaustive. For more extensive reviews, the reader is referred to other sources (Andersen, 1986; Cooper, 1988; Rowland and Holland, 1989). We have chosen to review studies that allow us to characterize the stress of breast cancer and its treatments within the model we have described.

INITIAL STRESSORS

One might assume that the stress of breast cancer only begins with the discovery of a breast lump. However, according to the model we have outlined even the *threat* of detecting a breast abnormality can serve as a psychogenic stressor. Any situation which leads to the appraisal that harm could occur has the potential to cause a stress response. By this reasoning, all routine screening procedures (breast examination, thermography, mammography) may function as psychogenic stressors since they can detect abnormalities requiring further evaluation to rule out the presence of cancer. Unfortunately, there has been relatively little research on the stressful effects of breast screening procedures. In one of the few studies of this topic, Bartolucci and colleagues (1989) used a self-report measure of emotional distress (Kellner, 1987) to measure stress responses before and after thermography and mammography. Among patients undergoing thermography, emotional distress decreased over time regardless of whether the procedure yielded normal or abnormal results. There was a similar, although less sizable, decrease in distress over time in women who received negative mammography results (women who had abnormal mammograms were not studied). Results of this research provide initial support of the view that these routine screening procedures can serve as psychogenic stressors and should encourage additional study.

The first tangible stressor that most women encounter is a sign or symptom of breast disease. The abnormality may first be noted by the patient herself (e.g. the sensation of a painless lump) or may be found by her physician during a routine physical examination. In terms of the model outlined earlier, the detection of a breast abnormality is likely to lead to an appraisal of harm or threat ("there is something wrong with my breast") which could evoke a stress response.

In the few studies which have examined stress responses to undiagnosed symptoms of breast disease, women have typically been assessed during outpatient clinic visits. For example, Romsaas *et al.* (1986) studied women who were either self- or physician-referred to an outpatient "breast problem clinic". Stress response was assessed using a self-report measure of psychological distress (McNair *et al.*, 1971), which was administered just before the physician's examination. Contrary to expectations that distress would be high, scores on the self-report measure were significantly lower than norms for psychiatric outpatients. While distress was not at the level associated with psychiatric disorder, it remains unclear from this study if women with breast problems are more distressed than women without breast problems.

Morris and Greer (1982) also measured stress responses in women self- and physician-referred to a breast clinic. This sample included women with breast problems as well as asymptomatic women undergoing screening. Patients completed self-report measures of sociability, emotional lability, and dissimulation (Eysenck and Eysenck, 1975), and trait and state anxiety (Spielberger *et al.*, 1970) just prior to physical examination. Results are provided only for patients found to have benign breast disease or no breast pathology (normal). While these two groups scored similarly on most measures, women later found to have benign disease exhibited higher state anxiety and a greater tendency to dissimulate. The observed difference is attributed by Morris and Greer to the higher prevalence of physical symptoms among the benign disease patients. This finding suggests that the presence of physical symptoms provides additional information that could lead to the appraisal that breast disease (and possibly cancer) is present.

Hughes *et al.* (1986) assessed women with clinical signs of disease who were physician-referred to a breast clinic. Stress response was assessed with self-report measures of current anxiety and depression (Zigmond and Snaith, 1983) and by an interview-based measure of depressive symptomatology (Hughes *et al.*, 1986). These measures were administered in the patient's home several days before the first appointment. On the self-report measures, current anxiety was characterized as "high" in 25% of patients later found to have benign disease and 42% of patients later found to have cancer; current depression was "high" in only 7% of the benign disease patients and none of the cancer patients. These findings suggest that anxiety may be a more common emotional response to undiagnosed breast problems than depression. Interview data indicated that major and "minor" depression had been present in 29% of patients with benign disease and 36% of patients with cancer during the past month. However, for many of these patients the onset of depressive symptoms predated their breast problems and were related to the occurrence of other stressors such as bereavement or marital discord.

Taken together, the results of these studies provide partial support for the view that undiagnosed symptoms of breast disease evoke a stress response. One possible explanation for the mixed findings is that patients may differ greatly in their appraisal of undiagnosed symptoms. For some patients the symptoms may not be appraised as threatening ("It's probably nothing"), while for others they may be quite threatening ("What if it's cancer?"). By including measures of appraisal in future research, it may be possible to explain individual differences in stress response to breast symptoms. Moreover, measurement of appraisal would help to establish that observed responses are related to breast symptoms and not to other concurrent or antecedent psychogenic stressors.

BIOPSY

The next event to occur in the diagnostic evaluation of breast disease is surgical biopsy. Biopsy has the potential to be a psychogenic stressor since results demonstrating that cancer is present are likely to be appraised as harmful and challenging. Anticipation of biopsy results can also serve as a psychogenic stressor given the uncertainty of the situation and the potential for harm (i.e. the diagnosis of cancer). The biopsy procedure itself may also be appraised as threatening or harmful, as it is an invasive procedure performed on a part of the body that may be invested with great emotional significance.

In most studies of biopsy, researchers have focused on the anticipatory period. For example, Scott (1983) assessed women in hospital just prior to biopsy using self-report measures of state anxiety (Spielberger *et al.*, 1970) and capacity for critical thinking (Watson and Glaser, 1964). Mean anxiety was reported to be high, comparable to that of patients hospitalized for acute anxiety reactions. A unique feature of the Scott study was that patients found to have benign disease were reassessed 6–8 weeks later. Consistent with predictions, these patients exhibited significant decreases in anxiety and improvements in critical thinking from their prebiopsy levels.

Greer and colleagues have published two studies in which stress responses were assessed on the day before biopsy. In the first study (Greer and Morris, 1975), stress response was measured using clinical ratings of depressive symptomatology (Hamilton, 1967). Results showed that only 7% of patients later found to have cancer and 5% of patients later found to have benign disease had symptoms of mild or greater intensity. These findings are consistent with research reviewed earlier (Hughes *et al.*, 1986) which suggested that depression is a relatively uncommon response to undiagnosed breast problems. In the second study (Morris *et al.*, 1981), stress response was assessed using self-report measures of state and trait anxiety (Spielberger *et al.*, 1970), and emotional lability (Eysenck and Eysenck, 1975). Among patients later found to have benign disease, levels of trait and state anxiety were significantly higher than published norms, suggesting that these patients were distressed in anticipation of biopsy. Among patients later found to have malignant disease, heightened anxiety was evident among older women (aged 50–69 years) but not younger women (40–49 years). Direct comparison of the positive and negative biopsy groups also indicated that patients with cancer scored lower on the measure of emotional lability. Thus, results suggest that cancer patients (especially younger patients) are likely to experience less emotional distress in anticipation of biopsy.

Several other studies have reported that the presence of malignancy is associated with lowered distress before biopsy. For example, Hughson *et al.* (1988) reported that, prior to biopsy, patients found to have cancer scored lower on interviewer ratings of depression and irritability (Maguire, 1976; Maguire *et al.*, 1978) than patients found to have benign disease. However, in this study younger cancer patients were noted to be more anxious than older ones. Schonfield (1975) also reported differences in emotional reactions prior to biopsy based on malignancy status. Participants in this study were Israeli women who completed self-report measures of emotional distress and personality functioning on the day before biopsy. Among younger women, denial (Hathaway and McKinley, 1951) and covert anxiety (Cattell and Scheir, 1963) were higher in patients with cancer than in patients with benign disease. In addition, among women of European and American ancestry, more denial was evident among patients with cancer. Finally, Wirsching and colleagues have conducted two studies in which emotional expression and personality functioning were measured on the day prior to biopsy. In the first study (Wirsching *et al.*, 1982), patients underwent a semistructured interview which assessed level of emotional distress and use of defense mechanisms. Consistent with predictions, patients found to have malignant disease were more likely than patients found to have benign disease to suppress anxiety and to express optimism and self-sufficiency. In the second study (Wirsching *et al.*, 1985), patients completed a self-report personality measure (Hehl and Wirsching, 1983) and underwent a semistructured interview similar to that used in the previous study. Results confirmed predictions that patients with malignant disease would be characterized by more optimistic and independent attitudes, a tendency towards rationalization, and an absence of expressed anxiety.

The results of these studies suggest that the presence or absence of malignancy is related to differences in patients' responses to psychogenic stressors. What remains unclear is the mechanism that may underlie a relationship between malignancy and stress responses prior to biopsy. Two explanations can be offered. One possibility is that women who develop breast cancer are more likely to suppress emotions and that, under the stress of impending biopsy, they will experience less emotional distress. Using retrospective data collected just before biopsy, Greer and colleagues (Greer and Morris, 1975; Morris *et al.*, 1981) reported that women found to have malignant disease are more likely to have engaged in a pattern of anger suppression throughout adult life. This link could reflect a causal relationship. It has been hypothesized that chronic abnormal release of emotions may play a biological role in the development of breast cancer via neuroendocrine or neuroimmune mechanisms (Pettingale *et al.*, 1977). A second explanation is that the results obtained reflect differences in appraisal. Patients found to have cancer may have formed accurate expectations that their breast lumps were malignant. These expectations could be based on information acquired before surgical consultation (i.e. patient's knowledge that family history placed her at increased risk for breast cancer) or information communicated by medical personnel involved in the diagnostic evaluation. In at least two of the studies reported above (Wirsching *et al.*, 1982, 1985) a percentage of patients had been informed about the anticipated results of their biopsies. However, even in studies where patients were believed to be "blind" to their diagnosis, appraisals based on beliefs and on previously acquired information could have influenced stress responses. These expectations could have served to reduce distress in patients with malignancy either by lowering the appraised uncertainty about the test results or by evoking emotion-focused coping efforts. This explanation could be tested by including measures of patients' appraisals and coping efforts in future studies of biopsy.

In the studies reviewed thus far, stress response has typically been defined in terms of observer-rated or self-reported levels of emotional distress. According to the model outlined, stress responses also have a physiological component. Relationships between psychological and physiological functioning have been examined in two studies of women awaiting biopsy. In a landmark study, Katz *et al.* (1970) conducted assessments of both psychological and endocrine functioning during the week before biopsy. Endocrine activity was measured by administering an intravenous dose of radiolabelled hydrocortisone and collecting urine output over the next 72 h for analysis. Psychological functioning was assessed via a semistructured interview (Wolff *et al.*, 1964) which was rated for the patient's level of affective distress, functional disruption (psychophysiologic symptomatology), and defensive reserve (i.e. ego strength). These three ratings were then combined to create an index labelled "defensive failing". The main findings were that greater defensive failing, affective distress, and functional disruption were each correlated with higher rates of hydrocortisone production. In their discussion, the researchers offer an interpretation of the findings consistent with a psychological model of stress: "It is not a 'stress' situation *per se* that evokes psychic distress and a concomitant adrenal corticosteroid outpouring, but rather that both depend upon how the stress is perceived, interpreted, and defended against". In other words, emotional and physiological reactions to the psychogenic stressor of biopsy appear to be mediated by the cognitive process of appraisal and the individual's ongoing coping efforts.

In the other biopsy study that included a physiological measure, Pettingale *et al.* (1977) concurrently assessed emotional expressiveness and levels of serum immunoglobulins (IgG, IgA, IgM and IgE). Assessments were performed prior to biopsy, and at three, 12 and 24 months post-operatively. Examining the prebiopsy data showed that serum IgA levels were significantly higher in women who showed extreme suppression of anger than in women who showed normal anger expression. This relationship was evident both in women found to have benign disease and in those with malignant disease. At subsequent assessments there continued to be relationships between suppression of anger and serum IgA levels in the malignant disease group, but not in the benign disease group. The results suggest that psychogenic stressors (i.e. impending biopsy at the first assessment and diagnosed cancer at subsequent assessments) may have selective physiological effects depending on the patient's style of emotional expression.

SURGICAL TREATMENT

There is an extensive research literature on psychological reactions to surgical treatment of breast cancer. We include only studies that fall within the model of stress outlined earlier. Our focus is on studies of breast surgery patients which have measured the process of appraisal as well as the emotional, physiological and coping responses to psychogenic stressors.

What are the psychogenic stressors associated with surgical treatment of breast cancer? There are at least two forms of information that can be appraised as stressful. First, there is the diagnostic and prognostic information yielded by surgery. As part of the process of surgery, patients may expect to receive or may have received information as to the seriousness of their disease (e.g. tumor size, extent of lymph node involvement) or their need for further treatment. Such information clearly would have the potential of conveying unfavorable implications and/or unfavorable outcomes for the patient. Secondly, there is the sensory and perceptual information associated with the surgery itself. Patients may anticipate or may be experiencing new physical sensations and visual cues that are appraised as threatening or harmful; for example, sensory information could serve as a psychogenic stressor by eliciting an appraisal that breast surgery will result, or has resulted, in physical unattractiveness.

MASTECTOMY

Although several surgical options now exist for treatment of breast cancer, most of the psychological literature has focused on mastectomy. In a large number of these studies, patients were first assessed weeks or even months following mastectomy. Relatively little is known about stress responses before mastectomy or during the immediate postoperative period. In one of the few studies conducted in the immediate postoperative period, Watson *et al.* (1984) examined the relationship between denial and the degree of emotional distress experienced during the week following mastectomy. Emotional distress was assessed using self-report measures of state anxiety (Spielberger *et al.*, 1970; McNair *et al.*, 1971) and denial/acceptance of cancer diagnosis was assessed using a semistructured interview. Consistent with predictions, patients who denied the implications of their cancer diagnosis reported less distress. While these results suggest that denial is an effective coping strategy, the researchers caution that the longer term implications of denial remain unknown. Moreover, the low rates of emotional distress reported by deniers could also reflect an unwillingness to admit psychological distress on a self-report instrument. Thus, it is possible that the same patients may have exhibited heightened stress responses if observer-rated or physiological measures of stress response had been administered.

Using a retrospective design, Jamison *et al.* (1978) assessed emotional adjustment to mastectomy in women who had been operated on an average of 22 months previously. When asked to describe the quality of their postoperative emotional adjustment, 83% of the sample rated it as good, very good, or excellent. Only 10% rated their adjustment as not very good, poor or very poor, suggesting that severe distress reactions were relatively uncommon following hospital discharge. Age differences emerged as an important predictor of adjustment. Younger women (those under 45 years of age) provided poorer ratings of their adjustment than older women and were more likely to have sought professional help for psychological problems related to mastectomy. One possible explanation for these age differences is that younger women may perceive that mastectomy has resulted in more serious harm in important areas of their lives. Along these lines, Jamison *et al.* reported that younger women were more likely to perceive that mastectomy had a negative influence on their sexual relationships.

A number of longitudinal studies have examined short- and long-term changes in stress response among women treated for breast cancer. Using a prospective design, Morris *et al.* (1977) assessed women just prior to biopsy and at three, 12, and 24 months following mastectomy. Stress response was measured using interview-based measures of perceived stress and psychological response to diagnosis. Three months following surgery 46% of the sample reported experiencing psychological stress related to surgery. Most patients attributed this stress to feelings of loss and disfigurement. The incidence of stress responses declined to 28% by one year and 25% by two years. Throughout the follow-up period, the most common reaction to diagnosis was a stoic acceptance (acknowledgement of the diagnosis not accompanied by excessive concern). The percentage of patients in whom stoic acceptance was evident increased from 53% to 71% over the period of the study. In contrast, there was a notable decline (from 16% to 2%) in the percentage of patients who responded with a "fighting spirit" (hopefulness combined with information seeking). The results of this study illustrate that coping is a dynamic process subject to changes over time (Folkman and Lazarus, 1985) and that stress responses are related to appraisals that harm or loss has occurred.

Maguire *et al.* (1978) also used a prospective design to study stress responses following mastectomy. Patients were first assessed at the time of initial referral for breast biopsy and reassessed one year following mastectomy. The responses of patients who underwent mastectomy were compared with those of patients who also underwent breast biopsy but were found to have benign disease. Stress response was measured using a semistructured interview rated for the frequency and extent of psychiatric symptomatology. One year after surgery, symptoms of anxiety and/or depression were moderate to severe in 25% of mastectomy patients but in only 10% of benign disease patients. While these differences are attributed to the impact of mastectomy, it should be noted that most of the breast cancer patients in this study also underwent radiotherapy. Since radiotherapy may also elicit stress responses (see pp. 159–160), it is not clear to what extent the observed reactions are specific to mastectomy.

The Psychological Aspects of Breast Cancer Study Group (1987) conducted a prospective study in which women who underwent modified radical mastectomy were compared with three other groups: women who had benign breast disease, women who underwent cholecystectomy, and women with medical disorders who had not undergone surgery in the past year. All participants were assessed four times over a one-year period, with the mastectomy group first assessed within three months of surgery. Responses to a battery of self-report and interview-based measures were subjected to principal components analysis which yield seven summary scores. Across time, mastectomy patients scored higher than the other groups on four of the summary measures: somatic distress; self-deprecation; irritability and physical complaints; and impairment in everyday social functioning. No differences were observed on the measures of psychopathology, negative attitude, or separation and death anxiety. As the researchers point out, the reported differences in physical complaints and somatic distress may reflect the effects of adjuvant chemotherapy administered to many of the mastectomy patients. Indeed, other research (see pp. 159–160) has shown that adjuvant chemotherapy often gives rise to psychological distress.

The results of these studies permit few conclusions to be drawn about stress responses to mastectomy. On the one hand, findings suggest that most patients do not experience significant emotional distress in the months following mastectomy (Jamison *et al.*, 1978; Psychological Aspects of Breast Cancer Study Group, 1987), but on the other, research suggests that approximately 25% of mastectomy patients are experiencing moderate to severe emotional distress one year after surgery (Morris *et al.*, 1977; Maguire *et al.*, 1978). Two explanations can be offered for this discrepancy. One possibility is that societal or cultural differences are responsible. In the research reviewed, the higher rates of distress were obtained in studies in the UK while the lower rates were obtained in studies in the USA. Differences in attitudes towards breast cancer and mastectomy and in the information provided to patients may have existed between the two countries. The second and more likely explanation is differences in research methodology. Each of the studies reviewed used different defini-tions of emotional distress and different assessment techniques. Until common research methodology is adopted, direct comparisons across medical centers or across countries cannot be made.

MASTECTOMY VERSUS LUMPECTOMY

Depending on such factors as the size and location of the the tumor, women may be offered alternatives to mastectomy. Surgical procedures which preserve the breast (e.g. lumpectomy), sometimes combined with radiotherapy, have been shown to yield similar disease-free intervals as mastectomy (Fisher *et al.*, 1985; Veronesi, *et al.*, 1981). A major reason for developing breast-conserving techniques has been to reduce the presumed psychological impact of mastectomy. To test whether breast conservation is less traumatic than mastectomy, a number of studies have directly com-pared psychological outcome following the two procedures. Although the focus has been on determining the benefits of breast conservation, this research paradigm also addresses issues related to the model of stress presented earlier. For example, are procedures which preserve the breast appraised as being less threatening or harmful than procedures in which the breast is removed? A second issue involves the effects of offering patients a choice of surgical procedures. Does the opportunity to choose, a situation which should enhance appraisal of personal control over events, reduce or increase stress responses to breast surgery?

In general, studies have found few differences in emotional distress in the months after surgery based on whether patients underwent mastec-tomy or lumpectomy (Fallowfield *et al.*, 1986; Steinberg *et al.*, 1985; Wolberg *et al.*, 1989; Schain *et al.*, 1983; Kemeny *et al.*, 1988). However, there are exceptions to this pattern. Kemeny *et al.* (1988) found that women who underwent mastectomy recalled the experience of first viewing the results of surgery as more traumatic than did women who underwent lumpectomy, suggesting that differences in appraisal and emotional distress between the procedures may be limited to the immediate postoperative period.

Another exception was reported by Levy *et al.* (1989), who found that, during the three months following surgery, patients who underwent lumpectomy scored higher on self-report measures of depression, confusion, and anger (McNair *et al.*, 1971) than patients who underwent mastectomy. These results are based on a sample in which all the lumpectomy patients and an unknown percentage of the mastectomy patients *chose* which procedure they would undergo. In a comparison sample of patients *randomized* to mastectomy or lumpectomy, Levy did not find differences in emotional distress. To further evaluate the role of choice, patients who chose lumpectomy over mastectomy were directly compared with patients who were randomly assigned to lumpectomy. Patients who chose the procedure were more emotionally distressed (on the fifth postoperative day) than patients who were randomized to the procedure. According to the researchers, "... one implication that could be drawn here is that to make a treatment choice within a risky context of perceived unknowns is threat-producing". Much of the information patients encounter in making this choice is highly technical and does not provide definitive conclusions about the superiority of one procedure over another. While few would argue that patients should not be offered a choice of breast treatment procedures, it appears that the uncertainty inherent in this situation may serve to increase appraisals of threat and heighten stress responses.

RADIATION THERAPY AND ADJUVANT CHEMOTHERAPY

Two forms of treatment have been developed to slow or prevent the recurrence of breast cancer following initial surgical treatment. Radiation therapy involves the administration of fractionated doses of radiation on a frequent basis (up to five times weekly) over several weeks. It is typically administered to breast cancer patients with small tumors and no evidence of regional or distant spread of disease. Adjuvant chemotherapy involves intravenous and oral administration of cytotoxic drugs on a weekly to monthly basis over periods extending up to one year. It is typically initiated with patients in whom there is evidence or suspicion of a regional disease spread (i.e. nodal involvement). These treatments present patients with several forms of information which may be appraised as stressful. First and foremost is the experience of aversive side-effects and the meaning attached to them by the patient. Depending on the specific treatment regimen symptoms may include nausea and vomiting, anorexia, hair loss, fatigue, mouth sores, diarrhea, tingling, or numbness. For some patients, the treatment administration itself has stressful properties. In the case of chemotherapy, research has shown that almost 60% of adjuvant patients experience conditioned nausea and anxiety in anticipation of treatment (Andrykowski *et al.*, 1988). In the case of radiotherapy, clinical reports indicate that physical isolation in the treatment room can be a potent elicitor of emotional distress in certain individuals (Holland, 1989).

In one of the few studies to examine stress responses to radiotherapy among breast cancer patients, Holland *et al.* (1979) conducted a prospective study of women who had recently undergone mastectomy. Stress responses were measured by performing a content analysis (Gottschalk and Gleser, 1969) on speech samples obtained prior to the first radiation treatment, during the second week of treatment, and near the end of treatment 2–4 weeks later. The level of anxiety was higher than published norms for both non-psychiatric and psychiatric comparison groups at the initial assessment and did not decrease over time. Moreover, levels of outward and inward hostility (i.e. depression) increased significantly during the course of radiation treatment. The researchers attribute the continued emotional distress to the cumulative effects of treatment in producing anorexia, fatigue, and a general lack of wellbeing.

A study by Hughson *et al.* (1986) directly compared the stress responses to radiotherapy and adjuvant chemotherapy. The impact of treatment was studied in patients who had been randomized to one of three regimens: three weeks of daily radiotherapy, one year of adjuvant chemotherapy administered twice monthly, and combined radiotherapy and adjuvant chemotherapy. Stress responses were assessed using both self-report and interview-based measures of general psychiatric disturbance, anxiety, and depression (Goldberg, 1979; Snaith *et al.*, 1976; Maguire *et al.*, 1978). Data collected at one, three, and six months following mastectomy showed no differences in stress response as a function of treatment assignment. However, by 13 months patients in the treatment arms that included chemotherapy evidenced higher rates of anxiety, depression, and general psychiatric disturbance than patients treated solely with radiotherapy. This pattern corresponds to differences among the treatments in their side-effect profiles. During the second six months of the study, patients treated with chemotherapy reported more physical side-effects (e.g. nausea, vomiting, and hair loss) and were more likely to have anticipatory nausea than patients treated with radiotherapy. Along the same lines, almost all patients who received combined therapy rated the side-effects of chemotherapy to be worse than those of radiotherapy.

The relationship between stress responses and the side-effects of adjuvant chemotherapy treatment was examined closely by Leventhal *et al.* (1986). Patients' emotional reactions to adjuvant chemotherapy were assessed over the first six cycles of treatment using self-report and interviewer ratings developed specifically for the study. Results indicated that a greater number of treatment side-effects was associated with higher emotional distress. The actual number of side-effects emerged as a better predictor of distress than the occurrence of any single side-effect. As part of the same study, the researchers also examined the impact of coping on chemotherapy-related distress. Women who perceived their coping efforts to be ineffective against side-effects experienced greater distress than women who believed they coped successfully. The researchers speculate that unsuccessful coping serves to increase distress by reducing the patient's sense of control and increasing the perceived unpredictability of treatment outcome. In future research, it will be useful to examine whether there are specific coping efforts (e.g. meditation, exercise) that are associated with lower reported distress. This could have important implications for the clinical management of stress reactions during chemotherapy.

CUMULATIVE EFFECTS OF TREATMENT

Thus far, the focus has been on stress responses to discrete events: discovering a breast lump, having it biopsied, undergoing surgical treatment, and receiving postoperative radiotherapy and/or chemotherapy to prevent recurrence. In addition to research on these discrete events, there are a number of studies which have examined the cumulative effects of the events comprising breast cancer diagnosis and treatment. While these studies can provide insight into the overall impact of breast cancer, there are drawbacks to this approach. A major disadvantage is that the relative contribution of individual psychogenic stressors to the aggregate cannot be measured; this problem is compounded when patients who have received different surgical treatments followed by different adjuvant regimens are grouped together. Under such circumstances, researchers may be overlooking important differences in the types of psychogenic stressors to which patients are responding. With these limitations in mind, the following studies were selected for review because of their innovative use of techniques for assessing appraisal and coping in breast cancer patients.

Taylor *et al.* (1984) assessed appraisals about cancer and their relationships to psychological adjustment. The sample studied was heterogeneous and included breast cancer patients who had undergone different surgical procedures and received different postoperative treatments. Moreover, patients were assessed at widely different time points following surgery (range 1–60 months). Two forms of appraisal were measured using a semistructured interview: attribution of the cause of cancer and beliefs about the control of cancer. The measure of psychological adjustment used in this study was derived from a factor analysis of 10 self-report and observational measures of psychosocial adjustment and emotional distress administered to each patient. Content analysis indicated that the most common attribution for the development of cancer was stress, which was cited by 42% of patients. Contrary to predictions, causal attributions were generally not related to adjustment. According to Taylor *et al.*, this suggests that, "... for a continuing threat such as cancer, finding the reasons for its occurrence may be less important than finding a way to modify its course now". This view is corroborated by results regarding the role of beliefs about control over cancer. Patients who believed they could control their cancer or that others (e.g. physicians) could control it evidenced better psychological adjustment than patients who did not hold these beliefs. The results of this study illustrate how the appraisal process can influence the emotional response to a psychogenic stressor. Findings further suggest that perceived control may be an important aspect of how patients appraise the potential stress of cancer treatment.

Vinokur *et al.* (1990) examined appraisals regarding breast cancer and their change over time. In this study, patients were administered a battery of self-report measures at four and 10 months following mastectomy. Among the many variables measured were the patient's appraisal of her ability to control the impact of cancer on her life and the degree of threat and uncertainty about the future evoked by breast cancer. Over the six-month period of the study, women generally perceived that breast cancer had become less threatening and was more controllable and predictable. These changes occurred in the context of improvements in physical functioning. As predicted, appraisal of threat was significantly related to the degree of emotional distress reported at both times of assessment. Indeed, the subjective appraisal of threat by the patient appeared to have more influence on distress than an objective measure of prognosis (stage of disease at diagnosis).

A study by Bloom (1982) focused on the role of social support and coping in adjustment to breast cancer. Patients who had undergone surgical treatment from one week to 2.5 years previously completed self-report measures of social support and coping designed for this study. Stress response was assessed using a standardized measure of emotional distress (McNair *et al.*, 1971). The main finding of the study was that the use of more "negative" behaviors to cope with stress (e.g. smoking, drinking, worrying) was strongly related to greater emotional distress. While this finding is hardly surprising, the results of this study indicate the type of coping responses that accompany emotional distress in breast cancer patients. An important goal for future research will be to identify whether there are "positive" coping behaviors associated with lowered distress. Additional analyses suggested that social support was indirectly related to distress through its effects on coping responses: patients who felt they received greater social support used fewer negative coping behaviors. The role of social support as a potential buffer for the effects of stressors has been the topic of much discussion and research (for reviews see Wortman, 1984; Cobb, 1976; Cohen and Wills, 1985). In terms of our model, social support can be viewed as a factor which influences both appraisal and coping. With regard to appraisal, social support in the form of information or advice from others can influence the degree to which a situation is appraised as threatening (Cohen and McKay, 1984). With regard to coping, results reported by Bloom (1982) and others suggest that the availability of emotional support may serve to influence the choice of coping responses. Along these lines, Thoits (1986) has pointed out that many forms of social support (such as offering advice) are techniques that can assist distressed individuals in their coping efforts. Given its central role in modulating responses to health-related psychogenic stressors, social support would appear to be an important variable to consider in future research on the stress of cancer and its treatment.

RECURRENCE OF DISEASE

After undergoing surgical treatment and postoperative radiotherapy and/or chemotherapy, many breast cancer patients will unfortunately experience a recurrence of their disease. Despite clinical reports that the diagnosis of recurrent disease often precipitates acute stress responses (Holland, 1989), there has been relatively little empirical research on this topic. In our review of the literature, we found only two published studies that had examined the psychological effects of disease recurrence in breast cancer patients.

Hughson *et al.* (1986) used data from their longitudinal study of radiotherapy and chemotherapy to measure the impact of recurrence. Among the radiotherapy patients, 31% had suffered a recurrence of disease by 18 months after mastectomy. Observer rating of psychiatric symptomatology (Maguire *et al.*, 1978) performed at 18 months indicated that all the patients who had recurred displayed clinical signs of anxiety and depression whereas none of the disease-free patients were classified as anxious or depressed.

Silberfarb *et al.* (1980) assessed the psychological impact of recurrence by comparing three groups with breast cancer: patients who had undergone mastectomy approximately four months previously, patients who had suffered a first recurrence of breast cancer within the last 12 weeks, and patients in the final stage of disease. Stress response was assessed using observer ratings of psychiatric symptomatology (Spitzer *et al.*, 1970). Results indicated that the recurrent group scored highest on an overall index of psychiatric disturbance as well as on subscales measuring depression, anxiety, suicidality, social isolation, and impairment in daily routine. The results of these two studies corroborate clinical reports that disease recurrence is a powerful psychogenic stressor. However, many psychological issues related to recurrence remain unexamined. A particularly important question yet to be addressed is whether patients differ in their stress responses to recurrence.

CONCLUSIONS

In this review we have applied a psychological model of stress to the study of breast cancer. The two main features of this model are that events become stressors depending on how they are cognitively appraised and that responses to stressors are characterized by an emotional response, a physiological response, and efforts to cope. By focusing on a series of discrete events related to breast cancer diagnosis and treatment we have examined the explanatory value of this model.

Several conclusions can be drawn. First, the literature confirms the view that situations in which individuals receive, or anticipate receiving, information about the threat or presence of cancer are psychogenic stressors. These include attending clinics for evaluation of undiagnosed breast symptoms, undergoing breast biopsy to establish/rule out cancer, and being informed about the recurrence of disease. Second, research supports the view that situations in which patients anticipate or experience sensory information perceived to be aversive function as psychogenic stressors. With regard to breast cancer, these situations include undergoing surgical treatment which alters physical appearance and receiving postoperative treatments (radiotherapy and chemotherapy) which produce aversive side-effects. The third conclusion supported by the literature is that the same situation may have very different stressful properties based on the individual's appraisal and her coping efforts. Studies reviewed show that appraisal and coping processes explain individual differences in stress responses to breast biopsy, mastectomy, and adjuvant chemotherapy, and the cumulative effects of cancer treatment.

The fourth and final conclusion we wish to consider is the direction for future research. Our review has revealed several gaps in knowledge about the stress of breast cancer and its treatments: one notable gap is the relative lack of data on how patients appraise and cope during encounters with potential stressors. While every study reviewed included measures of emotional distress or psychiatric symptomatology, few included any assessment of appraisal or coping. Moreover, when these processes were assessed, instruments of questionable reliability and validity were often used; this was particularly true in the case of coping. The number of coping processes assessed was typically quite limited, the specific forms of coping assessed were generally not specified, and the rationale for combining different forms of coping into a single summary index was seldom provided. One solution to this problem would be to use or to adapt existing measures of coping that have been used widely in other psychological studies of stress (for reviews see Moos and Billings, 1982; Lazarus and Folkman, 1984).

Another important gap is that relatively little is known about the physiological component of the stress response. With a few notable exceptions (Katz *et al.*, 1970; Pettingale *et al.*, 1977), biological measures have not been included in studies of the stress of breast cancer and its treatment. A growing body of laboratory and clinical research has shown that both endocrine and immune functions in humans are affected by emotional reactions to stressful conditions (for review see Chapter 1). An important goal for future research will be to systematically investigate physiological responses to the stress of cancer and its treatments. The significance of this research lies in the possibility that stressor-induced physiological changes may have important implications for responses to cancer treatment and subsequent disease course. Along these lines, the results of one recent study have suggested that an intervention which reduces emotional distress in breast cancer patients may also prolong survival (Spiegel *et al.*, 1989).

Much progress has been made in understanding the stress of cancer and its treatments. Instruments for measuring patient's emotional responses have been created or identified and have been used to measure reactions to most of the major diagnostic and treatment procedures. However, much remains to be learned. Future advances in the study of cancer-related stress will probably be achieved by using theoretical models to generate hypotheses and develop research methodology. In this chapter, we have examined the usefulness of a general psychological model of stress which emphasizes the roles of appraisal and coping processes. A consideration of these processes can further our understanding of why particular events in the diagnosis and treatment of cancer are stressful and why individuals differ in their responses to these events.

REFERENCES

Andersen, B.L. (1986) *Women with Cancer: Psychological Perspectives*. Springer, New York.
Andrykowski, M.A., Jacobsen, P.B., Marks, E., Gorfinkle, K., Hales, T.B., Kaufman, R.J., Currie, V.E., Holland, J.C. and Redd, W.H. (1988) Prevalence, predictors, and course of anticipatory nausea in women receiving adjuvant chemotherapy for breast cancer. *Cancer*, **62**, 2607–2613.

Bartolucci, G., Savron, G., Fava, G.A., Grandi, S., Trombini, G. and Orlandi, C. (1989) Psychological reactions to thermography and mammography. *Stress Med.*, 5, 195–199.

Bloom, J.R. (1982) Social support, accommodation to stress and adjustment to breast cancer. *Soc. Sci. Med.*, 16, 1329–1338.

Cattell, R.B. and Scheir, I.H. (1963) *Handbook for the IPAT Anxiety Scale* (Self Analysis Form). Institute for Personality and Ability Testing, Champaign.

Cobb, S. (1976) Social support as a moderator of life stress. *Psychosom. Med.*, 38, 300–313.

Cohen, S. and McKay, G. (1984) Interpersonal relationships as buffers of the impact of psychological stress on health. In Baum, A., Singer, J.E. and Taylor, S.E. (eds) *Handbook of Psychology and Health*. Erlbaum, Hillsdale, pp. 253–267.

Cohen, S. and Wills, T.A. (1985) Stress, social support, and the buffering hypothesis. *Psychol. Bull.*, 98, 310–357.

Cooper, C.L. (1988) *Stress and Breast Cancer*. John Wiley, Chichester.

Endler, N.S. and Edwards, J. (1982) Stress and personality. In Goldberger, L. and Breznitz, S. (eds) *Handbook of Stress*. Free Press, New York, pp. 36–48.

Eysenck, H.J. and Eysenck, S.B.G. (1975) *Manual of the Eysenck Personality Questionnaire*. Hodder and Stoughton, London.

Fallowfield, L.J., Baum, M. and Maguire, G.P. (1986) Effects of breast conservation on psychological morbidity associated with diagnosis and treatment of early breast cancer. *Br. Med. J.*, 293, 1331–1334.

Fisher, B., Bauer, M., Margolese, R., Poisson, R., Pilch, Y., Redmond, C., Fisher, E., Wolmark, N., Deutsch, M., Montague, E., Saffer, E., Wickerham, L., Lerner, H., Glass, A., Shibata, H., Deckers, P., Ketcham, A., Oishi, R. and Russell, I. (1985) Five-year results of a randomized clinical trial comparing total mastectomy and segmental mastectomy with or without radiation in the treatment of breast cancer. *New Engl. J. Med.*, 312, 665–673.

Folkman, S. and Lazarus, R.S. (1985) If it changes it must be a process: Study of emotion and coping during three stages of a college examination. *J. Person. Soc. Psychol.*, 48, 150–170.

Goldberg, D.P. (1979) *Manual of the General Health Questionnaire*. NFER Publishing Company, Windsor.

Gottschalk, L. and Gleser, G.C. (1969) *The Measurement of Psychological States Through the Content Analysis of Verbal Behavior*. University of California Press, Berkeley.

Greer, S. and Morris, T. (1975) Psychological attributes of women who develop breast cancer: A controlled study. *J. Psychosom. Res.*, 19, 147–153.

Hamilton, M. (1967) Development of a rating scale for primary depressive illness. *Br. J. Soc. Clin. Psychol.*, 6, 278–296.

Hamilton, V. (1980) An information processing analysis of environmental stress and life crises. In Sarason, I.G. and Spielberger, C.D. (eds) *Stress and Anxiety*, vol. 7. Hemisphere, Washington, pp. 13–30.

Hamilton, V. (1982) Cognition and stress. In Goldberger, L. and Breznitz, S. (eds) *Handbook of Stress*. Free Press, New York, pp. 105–120.

Hathaway, S.R. and McKinley J.C. (1951) *Minnesota Multiphasic Personality Inventory*. Psychological Corporation, New York.

Hehl, F.J. and Wirsching, M. (1983) *Psychosomatischer Einstellungsfragebogen (PEF)*. Hogrefe, Gottingen.

Holland, J.C. (1989) Radiotherapy. In Holland, J.C. and Rowland, J.H. (eds) *Handbook of Psychooncology*. Oxford University Press, New York, pp. 134–145.

Holland, J.C., Rowland, J., Lebovits, A. and Rusalem, R. (1979) Reactions to cancer treatment: Assessment of emotional response to adjuvant radiotherapy as a guide to planned intervention. *Psych. Clin. N. Am.*, **2**, 347–358.

Holmes, T.H. and Rahe, R.H. (1967) The Social Readjustment Rating Scale. *J. Psychosom. Res.*, **11**, 213–218.

Holroyd, K.A. and Lazarus, R.S. (1982) Stress, coping, and somatic adaptation. In Goldberger, L. and Breznitz, S. (eds) *Handbook of Stress*. Free Press, New York, pp. 21–35.

Hughes, J.E., Royle, G.T., Buchanan, R. and Taylor, I. (1986) Depression and social stress among patients with benign breast disease. *Br. J. Surg.*, **73**, 997–999.

Hughson, A.V.M., Cooper, A.F., McArdle, C.S. and Smith, D.C. (1986) Psychological impact of adjuvant chemotherapy in the first two years after mastectomy. *Br. Med. J.*, **293**, 1268–1271.

Hughson, A.V.M., Cooper, A.F., McArdle, C.S. and Smith, D.C. (1988) Psychosocial morbidity in patients awaiting breast biopsy. *J. Psychosom. Res.*, **32**, 173–180.

Jamison, K.R., Wellisch, D.K. and Pasnau, R.O. (1978) Psychosocial aspects of mastectomy: I. The woman's perspective. *Am. J. Psych.*, **135**, 432–436.

Katz, J.L., Weiner, H., Gallagher, T.F. and Hellman, L. (1970) Stress, distress, and ego defenses. *Arch. Gen. Psych.*, **23**, 131–142.

Kellner, R.A. (1987) A symptom questionnaire. *J. Clin. Psych.*, **48**, 268–274.

Kemeny, M.M., Wellisch, D.K. and Schain, W.S. (1988) Psychosocial outcome in a randomized surgical trial for treatment of primary breast cancer. *Cancer*, **62**, 1231–1237.

Lazarus, R.S. and Folkman, S. (1984) *Stress, Appraisal, and Coping*. Springer, New York.

Leventhal, H., Easterling, F., Coons, H.L., Luchterhand, C.M. and Love, R.R. (1986) Adaptation to chemotherapy treatments. In Andersen, B.L. (ed.) *Women with Cancer: Psychological Perspectives*. Springer, New York, pp. 172–203.

Levy, S.M., Herberman, R.B., Lee, J.K., Lippman, M.E. and d'Angelo, T. (1989) Breast conservation versus mastectomy: Distress sequelae as a function of choice. *J. Clin. Oncol.*, **7**, 367–375.

Maguire, G.P., Lee, E.G., Bevington, D.J., Kuchemann, C.S., Crabtree, R.J. and Cornell, C.E. (1978) Psychiatric problems in the first year after mastectomy. *Br. Med. J.*, **1**, 963–965.

Maguire, P. (1976) The psychological and social sequelae of mastectomy. In Howells, J.G. (ed.) *Modern Perspectives in the Psychiatric Aspects of Surgery*. Bruner Mazel, New York, pp. 390–421.

McNair, D.M., Lorr, M. and Droppleman, L.F. (1971) *Manual for the Profile of Mood States*. Educational and Industrial Testing Service, San Diego.

Moos, R.H. and Billings, A.G. (1982) Conceptualizing and measuring coping resources and processes. In Goldberger, L. and Breznitz, S. (eds) *Handbook of Stress*. Free Press, New York, pp. 212–230.

Morris, T. and Greer, S. (1982) Psychological characteristics of women electing to attend a breast screening clinic. *Clin. Oncol.*, **8**, 113–119.

Morris, T., Greer, H.S. and White, P. (1977) Psychological and social adjustment to mastectomy. *Cancer*, **40**, 2381–2387.

Morris, T., Greer, S., Pettingale, K.W. and Watson, M. (1981) Patterns of expression of anger and their psychological correlates in women with breast cancer. *J. Psychosom. Res.*, **25**, 111–117.

168   *Coping and Psychosocial Interventions*

Pettingale, K.W., Greer, S. and Tee, D.E.H. (1977) Serum IgA and emotional expression in breast cancer patients. *J. Psychosom. Res.*, **21**, 395–399.

Psychological Aspects of Breast Cancer Study Group (1987) Psychological response to mastectomy. *Cancer*, **59**, 189–196.

Romsaas, E.P., Malec, J.F., Javenkoski, B.R., Trump, D.L. and Wolberg, W.H. (1986) Psychological distress among women with breast problems. *Cancer*, **57**, 890–895.

Rowland, J.R. and Holland, J.C. (1989) Breast cancer. In Holland, J.C. and Rowland, J.H. (eds) *Handbook of Psychooncology*. Oxford University Press, New York, pp. 188–207.

Schain, W., Edwards, B.K., Gorrell, C.R., de Moss, E.V., Lippmann, M.E., Gerber, L.H. and Lichter, A.S. (1983) Psychosocial and physical outcomes of primary breast cancer therapy: mastectomy vs excisional biopsy and irradiation. *Breast Cancer Res. Tr.*, **3**, 377–382.

Schonfield, J. (1975) Psychological and life-experience differences between Israeli women with benign and cancerous breast lesions. *J. Psychosom. Res.*, **19**, 229–234.

Scott, D.W. (1983) Anxiety, critical thinking and information processing during and after breast biopsy. *Nursing Research*, **32**, 24–28.

Silberfarb, P.M., Maurer, L.H. and Crouthamel, C.S. (1980) Psychosocial aspects of neoplastic disease: I. Functional status of breast cancer patients during different treatment regimens. *Am. J. Psych.*, **137**, 450–455.

Snaith, R.P., Bridge, G.W. and Hamilton, M. (1976) The Leeds scales for the self assessment of anxiety and depression. *Br. J. Psych.*, **128**, 156–165.

Spiegel, D., Bloom, J.R., Kraemer, H.C. and Gottheil, E. (1989) Effect of psychosocial treatment on survival of patients with metastatic breast cancer. *Lancet*, **ii**, 888–891.

Spielberger, C.D., Gorsuch, R.L. and Lushene, R.E. (1970) *STAI Manual*. Consulting Psychologists Press, Palo Alto.

Spitzer, R.L., Endicott, J., Fleiss, J.L. and Cohen, J. (1970) The Psychiatric Status Schedule. *Arch. Gen. Psychiat.*, **23**, 41–55.

Steinberg, M.D., Juliano, M.A. and Wise, L. (1985) Psychological outcome of lumpectomy versus mastectomy in the treatment of breast cancer. *Am. J. Psych.*, **142**, 34–39.

Taylor, S.E., Lichtman, R.R. and Wood, J.V. (1984) Attributions, beliefs about control, and adjustment to breast cancer. *J. Person. Soc. Psychol.*, **46**, 489–502.

Thoits, P.A. (1986) Social support as coping assistance. *J. Consult. Clin. Psychol.*, **54**, 416–423.

Veronesi, U., Saccozzi, R., Del Vecchio, M., Banfi, A., Clemente, C., DeLena, M., Gallus, G., Greco, M., Luini, A., Marubini, E., Muscolino, G., Rilke, F., Salvadori, B., Zecchini, A. and Zucali, R. (1981) Comparing radical mastectomy with quadrantectomy, axillary dissection, and radiotherapy in patients with small cancer of the breast. *New Engl. J. Med.*, **305**, 6–11.

Vinokur, A.D., Threatt, B.A., Vinokur-Kaplan, D. and Satariano, W.A. (1990) The process of recovery from breast cancer for younger and older patients. *Cancer*, **65**, 1242–1254.

Watson, G., and Glaser, E.M. (1964) *Manual for Forms YM and ZM: Watson–Glaser Critical Thinking Appraisal*. Harcourt, Brace and World, New York.

Watson, M., Greer, S., Blake, S. and Shrapnell, K. (1984) Reactions to a diagnosis of breast cancer. *Cancer*, **53**, 2008–2012.

Wirsching, M., Stierlin, H., Hoffmann, F., Weber, G. and Wirsching, B. (1982)

Psychological identification of breast cancer patients before biopsy. *J. Psychosom. Res.*, **26**, 1–10.

Wirsching, M., Hoffmann, F., Stierlin, H., Weber, G. and Wirsching, B. (1985) Prebioptic psychological characteristics of breast cancer patients. *Psychother. Psychosom.*, **43**, 69–76.

Wolberg, W.H., Romsaas, E.P., Tanner, M.A. and Malec, J.F. (1989) Psychosexual adaptation to breast cancer surgery. *Cancer*, **63**, 1645–1655.

Wolff, C.T., Friedman, S.B., Hofer, M.A. and Mason, J.W. (1964) Relationship between psychological defenses and mean urinary 17-OHCS excretion rates: I. A predictive study of parents of fatally ill children. *Psychosom. Med.*, **26**, 576–591.

Wortman, C.B. (1984) Social support and the cancer patient. *Cancer*, **53**, 2339–2362.

Zigmond, A.S. and Snaith, R.P. (1983) The hospital anxiety and depression scale. *Acta Psych. Scand.*, **67**, 361–370.

8

What Good is Psychotherapy when I am Ill? Psychosocial Problems and Interventions with Cancer Patients

CYNTHIA M. MATHIESON and HENDERIKUS J. STAM
Department of Psychology, University of Calgary, Calgary, Alberta, Canada

Stress, like many broad psychological terms, can be seen as a contested topic. It is viewed simultaneously as a stimulus (as in stressful events) and as a response (as in experienced stress). It is characterized simultaneously as destructive (the experience of incapacitating stress) and motivating (the stress required for action). The limitation implied in the phrase "stress and cancer" makes the task of specifying the subject under discussion no simpler. In effect, the diagnosis, treatment and course of cancer are almost universally viewed as extremely stressful. Nevertheless, determining precisely what it is that is stressful about the illness and when and how this is manifest is not at all obvious.

In this chapter we will focus on only two aspects of cancer as a stressor. First, assuming cancer to be a psychologically debilitating disease, how do we come to determine which patients suffer most and might benefit from psychotherapy? Second, having determined who needs therapy, when and what therapy ought to be provided? In the course of the discussion we will consider the assumptions embedded in various assessment techniques as well as questions about the nature of chronic illness and its

Cancer and Stress: Psychological, Biological and Coping Studies
Edited by C. L. Cooper and M. Watson. © 1991 John Wiley & Sons Ltd

treatment. When considering therapy we will also address the questions raised by recent research on the attempts to ameliorate the disease itself via psychotherapy.

ASSESSING PSYCHOSOCIAL PROBLEMS

The use of psychotherapeutic interventions by cancer patients is an important topic, if only because little is documented about why patients avail themselves of these services. It is also complex, since a great diversity of interventions claim to have similar objectives. Before we review these interventions, we will attempt to provide a framework to guide our understanding of the nature of referrals (that is, the manner and timing of assessment) and its implication for intervention. Providing psychosocial support to cancer patients is not a simple matter of dealing with post-diagnosis stress. When we ask how best to intervene in patients' lives, we commit ourselves to understanding how patients deal with the demands of a chronic illness, which inevitably implicate the individual in a broader social (and often medical) world.

The major prerequisite for providing effective psychosocial interventions for cancer patients is the accurate assessment of the patient's problems. Reported rates of psychosocial problems vary dramatically, as these are influenced by the manner of assessment, the timing of the assessment, the ability to differentiate psychosocial problems from physical ones. Studies which rely primarily on psychiatric diagnoses report much higher rates of distress than those using other criteria (Holland and Rowland, 1989). In a prototypical study carried out by Derogatis *et al.* (1983), cancer patients were interviewed using DMS-III criteria. Of the 215 patients interviewed, 47% exhibited symptomatology sufficient to warrant a diagnosis of psychiatric disorder. Not surprisingly, the most frequent disturbances were found in adjustment disorders (i.e. depression and/or anxiety). Diagnoses of depression predominate in psychiatric studies, estimating rates of depression close to 50% (Craig and Abeloff, 1974; Bukberg *et al.*, 1984; Massie and Holland, 1988; Razavi *et al.*, 1990). Within this psychiatric framework there is an assumption that depressive symptoms will frequently go untreated (Maguire, 1985; Rodin and Voshart, 1986; Mayou *et al.*, 1988) leading some researchers to suggest that we search for biological markers of depression in cancer patients (Evans *et al.*, 1986).

In contrast to the above approach, a variety of studies have employed standardized scales within the framework of semistructured interviews to assess negative affect and psychosocial problems. For example, the Profile of Mood State (POMS, McNair *et al.*, 1971) has been used to assess recent emotional state. The Center for Epidemiologic Depression Scale (CES-D,

Devins *et al.*, 1988; Radloff, 1977) has also been used to assess depressive symptoms in nonpsychiatric groups. In fact, it has become a preferred instrument for assessment because of its strong psychometric properties and ease of administration. Neither of these assessment tools assumes that the reference group to which patients should be compared is psychiatric patients.

For studies using the above approach, reported rates of depressive symptomatology fall in the 10–30% range (Weisman *et al.*, 1980; Wellisch *et al.*, 1983; Cassileth *et al.*, 1984, 1986c; Stam *et al.* 1986). In fact, several studies have confirmed that psychopathological symptoms were absent or within normal limits for oncology patients. Using scores from the Mental Health Index, Cassileth *et al.* (1984) found cancer patients to have *better* psychological status than patients under treatment for depression. Farber *et al.* (1984) found levels of psychological distress which were elevated in comparison to nonpatients, but which nonetheless fell within normal limits. Bloom *et al.* (1987) concluded that psychopathological symptoms over the year following surgery were conspicuously absent in 412 mastectomy patients. In five studies conducted by Stam and colleagues at the Tom Baker Cancer Centre in Calgary over a five-year period, the CES-D was used to measure depression. The scope of these studies included assessments of chronic pain in 75 adults undergoing radiotherapy (Stam *et al.*, 1985); delay to diagnosis in 80 newly diagnosed lung and gastrointestinal patients (Pullin and Stam, 1986); lag time to diagnosis in 103 newly diagnosed breast cancer patients (Pullin and Stam, 1990, unpublished report); anticipatory nausea and vomiting in 70 patients receiving chemotherapy (Challis and Stam, 1991), and quality of life for 57 laryngectomy patients (Stam *et al.*, 1991). In none of these studies were abnormally high levels of depressive symptomatology found. We would like to emphasize, however, that when patients scored above the traditional cutoff score of 16 on the CES-D, these scores were invariably correlated with measures of pain, stage of disease, number of chemotherapy/radiotherapy sessions and presence of other psychosocial problems.

House (1988) has also pointed out that preoccupation with screening for, and diagnosis of, depression has led to the tacit assumption that depression in the physically ill is synonymous with mood disorder, especially when employing psychiatric criteria. House then goes on to argue, quite rightly, that as a result, other important aspects of adjustment tend to be neglected. In recent studies which investigate anxiety levels in cancer patients, we can surmise that patients who were anxious due to cancer do not necessarily differ from normal control patients on measures of state anxiety (Robinson *et al.*, 1985; Cassileth *et al.*, 1986b). The exceptions to this occur in specific medical situations such as treatment protocols, points of recurrence, or palliative care (Andersen and Tewfik, 1985; Cassileth *et al*. 1986a, b; Schag and Heinrich, 1989).

Even more striking than the lower prevalence rates for depressive symptomatology found with nonpsychiatric criteria, are the findings in many studies that negative affect rarely occurs in isolation (Cassileth *et al*., 1986c; Fobair *et al*., 1986; Petersen *et al*., 1988; Vinokur *et al*., 1990). Stam *et al*. (1986), for example, assessed the range and type of psychosocial problems encountered by a referred population of cancer patients. The psychosocial problem category reported with the highest frequency was family/significant other concerns, including impairment in relationships with significant others, familial role difficulties, sexual dysfunction; bereavement issues and anticipatory grief. Personal concerns (i.e. denial, body image concerns, adjustment reaction, other mood disturbances) were reported with the next highest frequency. In their evaluation of the psychosocial problems of the homebound cancer patient, Wellisch *et al*. (1983) reported a similar constellation of problem categories. The most frequent problem categories were:

(a) somatic side-effects, of which pain accounted for almost half;
(b) mood disturbances;
(c) equipment problems;
(d) family/relationship impairment;
(e) cognitive impairment.

These findings are indicative of the multiple interrelated problems typical of this population. Houts *et al*.(1986) reported that patients felt that their unmet needs were a combination of emotional problems (including family difficulties), economic problems, medical information problems, and instrumental difficulties. Likewise, Petersen *et al*. (1988) found that, compared with controls, patients had elevated scores for depressed mood, loss of work and interests, agitation, general somatic symptoms, hypochondriasis and loss of weight. Taken together, these data are good indicators that the patient's emotional status is closely bound to other psychosocial events set in motion by the trajectory of the disease.

The illness trajectory

Logically, depressive symptoms might be expected to occur concomitantly with initial diagnosis, the onset of treatment or changes in prognosis. One well-documented phase of distress has been the "existential plight" which occurs for patients in approximately the first three months following diagnosis (Cassileth *et al*., 1984; De Haes and Van Knippenberg, 1985; Weisman *et al*., 1980). Events which occur rapidly within this phase include surgery and the beginning of treatment. It is precisely at these times that separating psychological state from physical symptoms which co-occur with the disease is most problematic. For example, the following statements from the CES-D lend themselves to interpretation strictly as side-effects of chemotherapy: "I did not feel like eating, my appetite was poor", "My sleep was restless", "I could not get going". Likewise, the following adjectives from the POMS checklist reflect the physical concerns of patients on treatment: "unable to concentrate, restless, worn-out, fatigued, exhausted, bushed". Given these constraints, it is not surprising that assessment at these points may lead to exaggerated levels of symptomatology, especially with psychiatric measures which were not designed for chronic illness populations.

The last point warrants further elaboration. *When* and *how* a patient is assessed are critical, but not only in reference to the course of the disease *per se*. Most of us have an understanding of the characteristic physical phases of illness on a physical level. For cancer, this usually means acute periods followed by periods of remission, although even in this regard cancer is unpredictable. We are, however, referring to understanding the illness trajectory, a term used by Strauss *et al.* (1985) to refer "... not only to the physiological unfolding of a patient's disease but to the total organization of work done over that course, plus the impact on those involved with that work and its organization. For different illnesses, the trajectory will involve different medical and nursing actions, different kinds of skills and other resources, a different parceling out of tasks among the workers (including, perhaps, kin and the patient), and involving quite different relationships – instrumental and expressive both – among the workers". For purposes of our discussion, the key point about the illness trajectory is that, while health care professionals have an understanding of what to expect as the illness trajectory unfolds, cancer patients usually do not. This means that patients, aside from a transformation in physical status, are thrust into a series of dynamic psychosocial changes and institutional events for which they are basically unprepared. Furthermore, because of the chronicity of the disease, the trajectory carries long-term as well as short-term ramifications past the point of diagnosis. The nature of this chronicity is not well assessed in studies using traditional measures of distress and psychopathology. Strauss *et al.* (1985) argue that, unlike acute illness, chronic illnesses are long-term, uncertain illnesses which may have acute *episodes*, require large efforts at palliation, are intrusive upon the lives of patients and their families, require a wide variety of ancillary services and often lead to conflicts of interpretation and authority among patients and healthcare workers. DSM criteria and other, one-time measures of distress may vary dramatically depending upon where in a patient's trajectory the assessment is conducted. We still do not have very good studies indicating what problems arise when in a cancer patient's illness trajectory. Obviously, this research is more difficult to carry out than the traditional single assessment study. Nevertheless, until we have such data, our knowledge of the true problem rates and stress points in cancer patients' illness will not be understood.

PSYCHOSOCIAL INTERVENTIONS WITH CANCER PATIENTS

As Feinstein (1983) documents, the systematic use of psychological approaches in the treatment of cancer and cancer-related problems is a relatively recent clinical development (also see Goldberg, 1981). Broadly conceived, these interventions include individual psychotherapy, supportive group therapy, broad-based behavioral therapies adapted for cancer populations and psychopharmacological interventions. A wide range of outcomes (e.g. changes in physical or emotional status, changed self-concept, increased survival time or time to recurrence, spontaneous remission) has been examined with these interventions. While some of these outcomes appear fairly straightforward, others, such as the use of psychological interventions to alter the course of the disease, remain controversial and need to be considered as a separate research issue.

Psychotherapy with cancer patients

Although lacking a unified framework, traditional psychotherapy with cancer patients has been generally oriented towards helping the patient manage the emotional trauma of the diagnosis and its implications for personal meaning (LeShan, 1977, 1989; Mahrer, 1980). In some cases this implies assisting the patient with the terminal phases of the illness. Here the goal of psychotherapy is to provide psychological support while encouraging the patient to cope realistically with the disease and impending death (Bahson, 1975; Hackett, 1976; Sampson and Whitfield, 1977; Spiegel and Glafkides, 1983; Spiegel and Yalom, 1978) and it may involve a family systems approach (Cantor, 1978; Cohen and Wellisch, 1978; Rait and Lederberg, 1989). Some psychotherapy has been offered individually to spouses of patients (Goldberg *et al.*, 1984; Goldberg and Wool, 1985).

Spiegel and Yalom (1978) have summarized the process that helps patients in group psychotherapy for terminal illness as

(a) modeling effective coping strategies of other patients;
(b) detoxifying dying;
(c) working through family problems;
(d) encouraging communication with health care professionals;
(e) living a full life in the face of dying.

In their paper on the effects of group confrontation with death and dying, Spiegel and Glafkides (1983) found that exposure to physically deteriorating cancer patients stimulated discussion of meaningful issues, but did not promote negative affect. The evidence to date suggests that group psychotherapy in particular is helpful in assisting patients and families to adjust to terminal illness.

Psychotherapeutic interventions have also been used to assist cancer patients in coping with the course of the disease. On a basic level, psychotherapy may be oriented towards helping the patient determine and achieve a realistic quality of life at different stages of illness (Luce and Dawson, 1975). More specifically, a study by Gordon *et al.* (1980) is indicative of multilevel counseling received by patients as part of a psychotherapeutic intervention. In this study, 157 patients (breast cancer, lung cancer and melanoma) were provided with educational support regarding the disease, counseling for monitoring thoughts and feelings, counseling for ventilating feelings; and health consultations and further referrals. When compared with appropriate controls, the patients receiving the intervention showed a decrease in negative affect on measures of anxiety, hostility, and depression, and a more realistic outlook on life. Additionally, a greater proportion of intervened patients returned to their previous employment.

Project Omega (Weisman *et al.*, 1980) was a seminal study which highlighted not only possible interventions with cancer patients, but also the changing psychosocial needs of the patient during the course of the disease. This study was important from a psychotherapeutic perspective in several respects. First, it suggested that between the initial cancer diagnosis (the existential plight) and terminality, there were other psychosocial phases with characteristic transitional problems. Second, the study found that patients who were good copers had characteristics which might suggest a future avenue for short-term interventions which encourage these attributes. Third, the study evaluated two different types of individual intervention. The first was a standard psychotherapeutic model. This consultation therapy was patient-centred, with the therapist's role as facilitator of identifying problems. The alternative intervention was a cognitive skills training intervention in which patients were taught to recognize, confront and solve commonly encountered cancer problems. In the second intervention patients were taught how to solve future tasks. In general, Project Omega found that patients receiving interventions exhibited lower emotional distress and reduced levels of denial than control patients. Both interventions were equally effective in reducing distress. The numbers and types of psychosocial problems reported by patients did not differ between the two intervention groups, or between the intervened and non-intervened groups. Intervention did made a difference in bringing about a better resolution of problems, though not a reduction in their number.

Because patients in the above study were assessed in a two-, four- and six-month follow-up, the data from Project Omega also suggest that newly diagnosed cancer patients can be given appropriate interventions to reduce psychological distress which may occur at some point in the future. Other studies have been less successful at establishing the longer term benefits of intervention for cancer patients. A study by Lonngvist *et al.* (1981), for example, found no significant differences between a control group and intervened patients who had received short-term group psychotherapy on a follow-up assessment at six months and one year. Their measures included a self-rating scale to chart attitudes towards cancer, self-concept evaluation, the Beck Depression Inventory and a Rorschach test. Nonsignificant results in this area of research should not be considered unusual, however, considering that (a) few empirical data are available regarding the impact of the cancer experience on long-term survivors of adult cancer (Loescher *et al.*, 1989, 1990; Welch-McCaffrey *et al.*, 1989) and (b) a framework for conceptualizing the disease impact and treatment outcomes is largely absent (see Ware, 1984).

Psychotherapy during specific medical protocols

Early studies on the psychosocial problems of cancer patients did not directly address the problems of emotional distress and adjustment induced by specific medical protocols (i.e. chemotherapy, radiotherapy). Likewise, there are few studies which report psychotherapeutic interventions with patients during these precise time periods (Nerenz *et al.*, 1982; Love *et al.*, 1989). The main reason for the lack of research in this area is that only in the last decade has there been a trend away from perceiving cancer patients as a homogeneous group. The emerging literature confirms that these tasks vary with medical variables, course of the disease, and the demands placed on the individual patient: for example, Holley (1983) found that a psychotherapeutic intervention was successful in motivating patients to learn to speak after laryngectomy – a task unique to the laryngectomee.

A study by Forester *et al.* (1985) is illustrative of interventions which can be carried out during medical protocols. The authors determined the effects on the symptoms of patients undergoing a six-week course of radiotherapy of ongoing weekly individual psychotherapy. The psychotherapy sessions consisted of weekly nonstructured sessions conducted by a physician in which patients were free to discuss whatever they chose, although the researchers classified their therapeutic sessions as combinations of supportive therapy with educational, interpretive and cathartic components. A statistically significant reduction was found on both emotional distress and physical symptoms, using the Schedule of Affective Disorders and Schizophrenia (SADS), in patients receiving psychotherapy when compared with the control group. This study highlights two important points. First, there is a need for more studies investigating factors contributing to emotional distress during scheduled treatment protocols, and the extent to which psychotherapy can reduce this distress. Perhaps more importantly, the basic question remains as to why psychotherapy was successful. As the researchers quite rightly point out, psychotherapy may have met a need for increased professional contact. On the other hand, very recent research in communicating with medical patients in general (see Stewart and Roter, 1989) and with oncology patients in particular (Degner *et al.*, 1989) implies that patient distress is related to many outcome variables, among them patient–practitioner communication. Health care professionals who provide psychotherapeutic interventions should be aware that they may in effect be improving emotional status as a result of their willingness to serve as information providers.

Group therapies

As with other chronic illnesses, group therapy remains a popular form of support for cancer patients. Galinsky (1985) proposed five objectives for group therapy for cancer patients:

- support
- sharing feelings
- developing coping skills
- gathering information and education
- considering existential issues.

Of course, it is also frequently the case that simply meeting others who have experienced cancer is itself supporting (Zimpfer, 1989). Probably the most well known cancer support groups are those patterned after Simonton (Simonton *et al.*, 1978) and Siegel (1986), where support is encouraged on both an individual and group level. According to this approach, group work can foster an optimistic attitude because it is believed that patients can help program their bodies towards greater health. This will be discussed in greater detail later.

Some of the real attractiveness of group work is that it remains flexible enough to include the patient's family in psychotherapy. Depending on its setting, it is also flexible enough to include patients who might not otherwise be referred for counseling. For example, Arnowitz *et al.* (1983) report on group therapy conducted with patients in the waiting room of an oncology clinic. Furthermore, although not considered therapy *per se*, group interactions involving patient–family–health care provider constellations may serve an important function in psychological preparation after diagnosis but before treatment protocols (Cassileth and Steinfeld, 1987). Why do patients join support groups? Taylor *et al.* (1986) report that although most patients claim high levels of support following diagnosis, some patients experience isolated instances of rejection or do not receive the type of support they would find helpful. This is one motive. Taylor *et al.* also found that support group attenders were more likely than nonattenders to be white, middle-class female, to report having more problems, and to access support services of all kinds. Negative experience with the medical community was a predictor of joining a group, suggesting that patients were using the group to vent feelings which were the result of difficulties experienced elsewhere in the medical system. Finally, among other findings, Taylor *et al.* found that attenders showed no greater psychological distress than nonattenders. At the very least, this research suggests that cancer patients willing to take part in group therapy are not necessarily better or worse off than other patients, but may be more likely to recognize the benefits of a support group.

Models of group therapy

In general, a variety of strategies for group therapy has been reported to reduce emotional distress and psychosocial problems of cancer patients (Schwartz, 1977; Wellisch *et al.*, 1978; Ferlic *et al.*, 1979; Capone *et al.*, 1980; Ringler *et al.*, 1981; Cain *et al.*, 1986; Telch and Telch, 1986; Phillips and Osborne, 1989). Supportive group therapy has perhaps been most widely utilized (see review by Telch and Telch, 1985). A recent study by Telch and Telch (1986) illustrates the supportive group therapy concept and compares it with an alternative group therapy, coping skills instruction, and a no treatment control group. Forty-one cancer patients were randomized to one of the above conditions. Supportive group sessions were nondirective and encouraged the sharing of mutual feelings. Group coping skills instruction presented the group members with different instructional modules intended to facilitate coping in common patient situations. Behavioral strategies included in coping instructions were:

● homework assignments
● goal setting
● self-monitoring
● behavioral rehearsal and role playing
● feedback and coaching.

Results indicated a consistent superiority of the coping skills intervention on a number of measures related to affect, satisfaction with lifestyle activities, cognitive distress, communication and coping with medical procedures. Patients in the supportive group therapy showed little improvement in psychological distress; control patients' psychological status appeared to have deteriorated.

A slightly different model for short-term counseling with high information and problem solving components was detailed by Cain *et al.* (1986). They call their model a structured thematic counseling model. The group sessions themes include:

(a) what is cancer?
(b) what are the causes of cancer?
(c) the impact of treatment on body image and sexuality
(d) relaxation
(e) diet and exercise
(f) relating to caregivers
(g) talking with family and friends
(h) goal setting.

In this study, the psychosocial status of 80 women with newly diagnosed gynecological cancer was assessed precounseling, immediately postcounseling and six months later. Compared with a control group, women who participated in counseling sessions were found to be less depressed and anxious, reported fewer sexual difficulties, had better relationships with caregivers, and seemed to have more factual knowledge of their illness.

Philips and Osborne (1989) used a "phenomenological method" to investigate the impact of a group therapy program called "forgiveness therapy". In general, therapy focused on the relief of negative feelings, leading to a change in perspective where the patient realizes she cannot condemn herself or others. Some therapy sessions began with mini-lectures on specific topics (e.g. holistic approach to mind–body, forgiveness), and all sessions included the sharing of experiences by group members. The researchers concluded that forgiveness is a process with stages, that patients can draw inspiration and courage from the therapeutic value of the forgiving experience, and that forgiveness therapy can promote catharsis and peace. What is unusual with this particular study, however, is the implicit assumption that patients experience guilt for their cancer.

The wide diversity of group therapies for cancer patients poses a major problem in interpreting the efficacy of group therapy in general. A review of both randomized and retrospective studies of group intervention for cancer patients indicates that the literature lacks a theoretical framework (see van den Borne *et al.*, 1986). When studies focus on patient contact in self-help groups, it is often unclear as to whether the results can be generalized to other types of group intervention. As in most psychotherapy research, the therapist's indirect contribution to the effect is often in question. Finally, outcome measures are incredibly varied among the research as a whole, with little evidence of replicability. Exceptions to this seem to be measures of depression, some of which will be discussed below, and outcomes related to self-esteem (Stecchi, 1979, unpublished report; Spiegel *et al.*, 1981; Jacobs *et al.*, 1983).

In a study by Farash (1978), 80 breast cancer patients were randomly assigned to one of three conditions: individual counseling given once a week for 12 weeks, once a week self-help group counseling for 12 weeks, or no treatment. The mastectomy group without intervention exhibited more body image disturbance than the intervened groups. Individual psychotherapy and self-help groups did not differ from each other or from controls on levels of depression measured with the Beck Depression Inventory. In another study of breast cancer patients by Spiegel *et al.* (1981), participants were randomly assigned to either a self-help group or no fellow-patient contact. Intervened patients met in small groups for 90 minutes per week. The structure of discussion groups was jointly determined by patients and volunteer counselors. Data gathered for a year included baseline measures, the Profile of Mood States (POMS), Health Locus of Control (HLOC), self-image, coping responses, phobias and denial measures. After one year of fellow-patient contact, women in the experimental group showed a significant decrease in negative feelings (anxiety, tension, fatigue, confusion), in inadequate coping responses and in experiencing phobias. There were no significant changes in self-image and locus of control. What is important about this study is not only its methodological soundness, but also the emphasis on continuing patient contact as an effector of change.

In a study by Vachon *et al.* (1982), 64 breast cancer patients in a self-help group were compared with 104 patients who received no such intervention. All women were receiving radiotherapy. The women in the "Coping with Cancer" group exhibited better improvement in their general health perception (using the General Health Questionnaire, Goldberg and Hillier, 1979) than patients in the control group. This study suggests that supportive group meetings contributed to decreases in level of distress.

While standardized measures of distress may give researchers some idea of a patient's negative affect at the time of interview, the study by Telch and Telch (1986) discussed earlier is to be highlighted for including broader measures of dynamic psychosocial changes in their attempt to understand the effect of therapy. The psychosocial oncology literature as a whole suggests that these variables include lifestyle changes, instrumental difficulties, communication with healthcare providers and relationship changes (including sexual functioning). Any long-term effects attributed to psychotherapy, either individual or group, should optimally be interpreted in light of these psychosocial constraints.

Behavior therapies and cognitive-behavior therapies

Behavior therapies and cognitive-behavior therapy form a group of interventions which have long been adapted for use with cancer patients. Some of these therapies attempt to treat specific symptoms. For example, the following have been reported to reduce nausea, vomiting, and emotional distress associated with chemotherapy episodes:

(a) systematic desensitization (Morrow and Morrell, 1982);
(b) progressive muscle relaxation plus guided imagery (Burish and Lyles, 1981; Lyles *et al.*, 1982);
(c) hypnosis and imagery.

The use of hypnosis for control of cancer pain and anticipatory nausea and vomiting (ANV) will be discussed briefly later. Stam and Bultz (1986) used somatic focusing and imagery to treat a cancer patient suffering from insomnia. Hopwood and Maguire (1988) used cognitive behavior therapy to enhance self-esteem of mastectomy patients, arguing that for patients with body image problems, negative thoughts and cognitive distortions must be challenged.

Behavior therapy with cancer patients has also been used to reduce negative affect, namely depression and anxiety (Tarrier *et al.*, 1983; Tarrier and Maguire, 1984; Moorey and Greer, 1989). Along these lines, Easterling and Leventhal (1989) have argued for the use of cognitive behavior therapy in controlling disease-worry elicited from neutral symptoms. Ultimately, the use of cognitive behavior therapy with this group of patients derives from the theorized role of cognitive factors in stress reduction (see Lazarus and Folkman, 1984; Leventhal, 1990).

Moorey and Greer (1989) have used the phrase Adjuvant Psychological Therapy (APT) to describe a behavior therapy which predicts that emotional distress experienced by patients is mediated by interpretations and evaluations that the patient assigns to her illness. The structure and content of therapy is derived from Beck's cognitive model. Therapy is problem-oriented, with regular homework assignments to facilitate restructuring maladaptive thoughts and developing new coping strategies. Its aims are to reduce anxiety and depression, to induce a fighting spirit, to promote patients' sense of autonomy and to develop effective coping strategies for cancer-related problems. Similarly, Bates *et al.* (1989) reported several case studies to describe how cognitive behavior therapy modified distorted thinking patterns of patients. These clinicians report treating guilt, anxiety, shame, and indecisiveness with this approach.

At the heart of cognitive behavior therapy is the therapist's intent to assist the patient in the cognitive restructuring of negative automatic thoughts and irrational concerns. Extensive use is made of prospective hypothesis testing and the explicit focus is on systematic distortions in information processing. It is conceivable however that this treatment strategy, devised for a general population, is inappropriate for a cancer population.

Cognitive therapy and pharmacology

Blackburn *et al.* (1981) argued that cognitive therapy is most effective when the depressed mood is first alleviated, followed by cognitive restructuring. The use of pharmacology to treat depression and anxiety is not unique to cancer patients, but a few studies have been published arguing for Blackburn's conclusions as an intervention for specific cancer problems. Tarrier and Maguire (1984), for example, showed with a group of breast cancer patients who failed to adjust to breast loss that short term cognitive behavior therapy used in conjunction with antidepressant medication was superior to antidepressant alone. Maguire *et al.* (1985) reported treating depression in breast cancer patients with antidepressant medication with or without cognitive therapy. Both treatments alleviated depression in the short term but improvement was sustained only in groups given combination treatments.

Hypnosis

The use of hypnotic interventions for cancer-related problems is typically aimed at the alleviation of symptoms of the disease or its treatment, such as the reduction of pain, nausea, emesis or anxiety (see Stam, 1989a for a review). The most common use of hypnosis in cancer appears to be related to symptom control, with the most frequently reported use in the control of pain. Stam (1989a) summarizes the pain literature by saying that while hypnosis may ameliorate pain in some individuals under some circumstances, few studies substantiate that hypnosis provides a unique analgesic. In the past decade symptom control has also included the use of hypnosis for ANV and postchemotherapy nausea (PCNV). Often, the use of hypnosis is coupled with other techniques, such as relaxation or imagery (Redd *et al.*, 1982; Kaufman *et al.*, 1989). The mechanism by which hypnotic procedures reduce nausea and emesis may in fact be those operating in relaxation-oriented procedures (Challis and Stam, 1991).

CAN PSYCHOTHERAPY ALTER THE ONSET OR COURSE OF CANCER?

The treatment of cancer by psychological means is neither recent nor surprising given the probabilistic nature of cancer treatment. Nevertheless, a popularized literature on treating cancer through psychological means emerged vigorously in the 1970s. This literature has steadily grown to include hypnosis, meditation, imagery and psychotherapy among its techniques. That these interventions may be useful in altering the onset or progression of cancer originates in the concept of the cancer-prone personality, which itself derives from psychosomatic medicine (for selective reviews see Stam and Steggles, 1987; Stam, 1989b). In the new, updated version of psychoneuroimmunology, it is claimed that person variables play an important role in tumorogenesis and in various other chronic disease states (see reviews by Eysenck, 1985, 1987a, b). Within this framework, the role of the behavior therapies and the cognitive behavior therapies is conceived as (a) altering relevant personality characteristics which will in turn prevent the occurrence of cancer in a predisposed group of individuals and (b) bolstering immune functioning.

Visualization techniques

The utility of imagery and visualization for treating cancer, sometimes used interchangeably with hypnotherapy, has achieved popular stature (see review by Krippner, 1985), largely based on the work of Simonton and his associates (Simonton *et al.*, 1978). Their work relies on relaxation techniques, the use of imagery to visualize cancer and the body's defenses, and a rhetoric of mobilizing immune functioning. From this framework, clinicians have argued that psychological factors such as denial of the disease, negative self-concept and perceived loss of control are related to disease status (Achterberg *et al.*, 1977a, b; Achterberg and Lawlis, 1979; Schneider *et al.*, 1983, unpublished report). In fact, Achterberg and Lawlis (1984) developed a diagnostic tool called the Imagery of Disease Test to rate how patients imagine tumors, white blood cells and current treatment. Achterberg and Lawlis found that, for some samples of cancer patients, the score on this test could predict patients' health status two months later. Lansky (1982), arguing that cancer is a result of psychosomatic replacement of a significant loss or suppressed anger, proposed a therapeutic strategy whereby the patient learns to "love his tumor". (Presumably this must be done under trance in order to contact those deep-seated pathologies which caused tumor growth in the first place.) There have also been reports of cases of regression of cancer based on special forms of meditation (Meares, 1982/83).

Sometimes these studies report not only the psychological state but also the immunological status of the patients. Gruber *et al.* (1988) report a study where patients systematically engaged in relaxation and guided imagery exercises over the course of a year. Several changes in measures of immune system function drawn from blood samples, and psychological measures from the MMPI (Minnesota Multiphasic Personality Inventory) and Rotter's Test for locus of control, were found to parallel the use of relaxation and imagery. The researchers concluded that relaxation and imagery can influence immune responsiveness.

The precise physiological mechanism which explains how these immune factors are affected by psychological variables is never delineated in any of the above studies. Rather, the key notions in this literature may be summarized by the following popularized ideas:

- cancer cells develop in most, if not all, individuals sometime during their life
- the immune system normally destroys these cells before they develop abnormally
- the immune system can be influenced by psychological variables
- these psychological variables can be mobilized to destroy cancer cells.

Survival studies

Several recent psychotherapy studies have attempted to delineate a causal role for stress and coping in promoting the survival of cancer patients. Higher rates of recurrence-free survival have been reported for patients exhibiting attitudes of "fighting spirit" (Greer *et al.*, 1990), active information seeking (Nelson *et al.*, 1988), positive expectations (Roud, 1986/87), joy (Levy *et al.*, 1988) and denial (Dean and Surtees, 1989; Greer *et al.*, 1990). From this framework the psychotherapy literature argues that psychological variables can be manipulated to alter the course of the disease, or that behavior therapy can be used prophylactically to reduce the risk of developing cancer (Eysenck, 1987b, 1988). Two studies are illustrative of this literature.

A study by Grossarth-Maticek *et al.* (1984) is frequently quoted to support these contentions. The researchers studied four groups of 25 patients each. Some received chemotherapy, some received behavior therapy, some received both behavior therapy and chemotherapy and some received neither. Grossarth-Maticek *et al.* used a type of behavior therapy called "creative novation therapy". This cognitive therapy, aimed at reducing depression and feelings of hopelessness, was a hybrid of Wolpe's (1958) desensitization, Beck's cognitive orientation, and Lazarus and Folkman's emphasis on teaching coping strategies. In summary, patients receiving no therapy did worst with a mean survival time of 11.3 months; the two-therapy group did best with a survival mean of 22.4 months. Patients receiving only one treatment had a mean survival time of 14.5 months, with the two types of therapy equally efficacious. This study concluded that the effects of the therapeutic combination was clearly synergistic; survival length was greater in combination than simple additive effects of each therapy alone.

In a reanalysis and follow-up of their original group therapy study,

Spiegel *et al.* (1989) examined the effect of psychosocial treatment on the survival rates of women with metastatic breast cancer. Eighty-six women participated in a prospective study for one year. The intervention consisted of weekly supportive group therapy with self hypnosis for pain. At a 10-year follow-up, patients randomized to weekly therapy lived significantly longer than controls, by an average of nearly 18 months. Although Spiegel *et al.* exercised caution in drawing the conclusion that group therapy had a direct effect on the physiology of the disease, they did suggest that the immune system may be a major link between emotional process and the progression of cancer.

In some respects, this research stands in striking contrast to the findings of Jamison *et al.* (1987) and Cassileth *et al.* (1988), both of whom failed to find consistent psychosocial factors associated with length of survival or remission. Contrary to certain claims in the literature, definitive studies have not been performed and long-term outcome studies are too few to be reliable indicators of the efficacy of psychotherapy as a treatment to prevent the onset or slow the course of cancer.

Quite apart from methodological considerations and the difficulties inherent in conducting the requisite research, this entire strategy is premised on the questionable assumption (long a stable element in western culture) of the relationship between psychological state and the onset of a major illness such as cancer. Not only must patients bear the consequences of their disease but they are frequently affronted by the notion that they bear a direct responsibility for their plight. Furthermore, should therapy fail, they will be responsible for its failure, having obviously succumbed to a death wish (albeit unconsciously) or having simply failed to cope appropriately.

There are two issues here that present themselves to the researcher. First, what relationship may exist between the immune system and central nervous system is an empirical question; whatever the outcome of such research as takes place in immunology laboratories, the results are already finding their way into the new biotherapeutics for treating cancer. It seems unlikely that research at the level of psychological treatment will have nearly the same impact. Second, there are serious moral questions invoked by a treatment strategy that implicitly assigns blame to the patient for the onset and outcome of a disease, *the biological origins of which are still not clearly known*. At the very least, a heavy dose of moderation is required to those who make claims of the sort discussed.

"WHAT GOOD IS PSYCHOTHERAPY WHEN I AM ILL?"

To put this diverse group of studies in perspective, we suggest that a major problem exists with the assumption that psychotherapy for cancer patients must be oriented towards intrapsychic events. This is not to say that patients do not experience themselves as genuinely depressed, nor that they are sometimes helped by traditional treatment methods – quite the opposite: the use of behavior therapy for ANV is a good example of the latter. But an exclusive intrapsychic focus leads either to claims that most patients must have psychological problems, as the DSM-III studies have done, or to the equally inaccurate claim that patient distress is due to the disease alone. The use of measures of depression to evaluate therapeutic efficacy reflects the same bias. As Weisman et al. (1980) have shown, most cancer patients do not need professional assistance to help them through their periods of psychological stress. For patients at risk for psychosocial distress, however, a focus on depressogenic cognitions is at best incomplete.

In a recent study (Mathieson and Stam, 1991, unpublished data), we interviewed over 70 patients in a semistructured interview; 34 were interviewed in a repeated measures design. Interviews lasted approximately 2 h. Open-ended responses were audio taped for content analysis. Structured psychosocial measures included standardized measures of psychological distress (i.e. Center for Epidemiologic Studies Depression Scale (CES-D; Radloff, 1977; Devins et al., 1988), the Profile of Mood States (POMS; McNair et al., 1971; Shacham, 1983; Malouff et al., 1985), Spielberger's State-Trait Inventory (STAI: Spielberger et al., 1970), and cancer-specific measures of quality of life: the Project Omega Screening Inventory (Weisman et al., 1980) and the Functional Living Index: Cancer (FLIC, Schipper et al., 1984)). Several common themes have emerged from the open-ended content analyses, many of which would be construed, according to a cognitive behavioral approach, as negative thinking. The most outstanding of these examples are: (a) fear of recurrence; (b) the extent to which patients feel stigmatized as the result of having cancer; (c) the manner in which this sense of stigma is almost always related to the patient's contacts with her larger social world (e.g. healthcare professionals, employers, friends, family); (d) the patient's difficult task of developing a voice with health care professionals in institutional medicine; and (e) the dramatic, and sometimes traumatic, changes a diagnosis of cancer makes to a patient's lifestyle, long-term as well as short-term. To interpret this constellation of psychosocial problems as a product of negative, automatic thinking or irrational beliefs fails to place the experience of chronic illness in the context of the social and historical referents of the patient as well as the demands arising from the institutional context of medicine. To date we are still in the process of determining the relationship of the above issues to standardized measures of distress and quality of life. However, we believe our research supports our contention that there are alternative ways to interpret episodes of negative affect expressed by cancer patients.

A more useful conceptualization of the role of psychotherapy might focus on the patient's need for continual readjustment of identity in the face of chronic illness (Stam, 1989b). A patient who lives with cancer finds themselves in a nexus of dynamic psychosocial events, including bodily changes, relationship stressors, time management constraints and institutional events. Placing the illness experience in the context of identity development simultaneously accounts for the individual's experience of chronic illness as well as the social organization of the patient's world and the medical arena. This approach is dramatically opposed to interpreting the trajectory of chronic illness as only a series of physiological processes which stress one's immune system (Kline Leidy, 1989) or as a problem to be solved through the adoption of appropriate coping techniques.

For patients who suffer from any chronic illness, it is imperative that they renegotiate their identity status with family, friends, co-workers and medical personnel. In our own studies, we have found that patients often report that they "feel like different persons" as a result of their cancer experience. We believe these reports reflect loss of productive function, financial strain, family stress, stigma and threats to former self-images. In effect, the patient's identity forcibly undergoes transformation. In this light, the experience of depression , so well documented in many cancer studies, may serve an important role in *communicating* the identity work undertaken by the patient. This social–psychological conception of negative affect in cancer patients calls for a move away from the psychiatric model of psychotherapy and the role of therapist as diagnostician. No therapist who really understands the illness trajectory of cancer would be willing to focus on mental events to the exclusion of the psychosocial processes set in motion by the illness itself.

Our final point is a simple one, and may throw some light on the recurring references to the role of social support in chronic illness. It is simply not possible to renegotiate one's identity alone. Rebuilding one's identity of necessity involves the larger social world. The experience of cancer introduces into the patient's world new constraints and contingencies which also impinge on those who care for them physically or emotionally. Ultimately, our interventions with cancer patients become effective only when we understand that we are engaging in psychotherapy not for the disease, but for the person.

REFERENCES

Achterberg, J. and Lawlis, G.F. (1979) A canonical analysis of blood chemistry variables related to psychological measures of cancer patients. *Multivar. Exp. Clin. Res.*, **4**, 1–10.

Achterberg, J. and Lawlis, G.F. (1984) *Imagery and disease: A diagnostic tool for behavioral medicine.* Institute for Personality and Ability Testing, Champaign.

Achterberg, J., Lawlis, G.F., Simonton, O.C. and Matthews-Simonton, S. (1977a) Psychological factors and blood chemistries as disease outcome predictors for cancer patients. *Multivar. Exp. Clin. Res.*, **3**, 107–122.

Achterberg, J., Matthews-Simonton, S. and Simonton, O.C. (1977b) Psychology of the exceptional cancer patient: A description of patients who outlived predicted life expectancies. *Psychotherapy Theory, Practice, and Research*, **4**, 426–436.

Andersen, B.L. and Tewfik, H.H. (1985) Psychological reactions to radiation therapy: Reconsideration of the adaptive aspects of anxiety. *J. Person. Soc. Psychol.*, **48**(4), 1024–1032.

Arnowitz, E., Brunswick, L. and Kaplan, B. (1983) Group therapy with patients in the waiting room of an oncology clinic. *Social Work*, September/October, 395–397.

Bahson, C.B. (1975) Psychologic and emotional issues in cancer: The psychotherapeutic care of the cancer patient. *Semi. Oncol.*, **3**, 293–309.

Bates, A., Burns, D. and Moorey, S. (1989) Medical illness and the acceptance of suffering. *Int. J. Psych. Med.*, **19**(3), 269–280.

Blackburn, J., Bishop, S., Glen, A., Walley, L. and Christie, J. (1981) The efficacy of cognitive therapy in depression: a treatment trial using cognitive therapy and pharmacotherapy, each alone and in combination. *Br. J. Psych.*, **139**, 181–189.

Bloom, J., Cook, M., Flamer, D., Gates, C., Holland, J.C., Muenz, L., Murawski, B., Penman, D. and Ross, R. (1987) Psychological response to mastectomy: A prospective comparison study. *Cancer*, **59**(1), 189–196.

Bukberg, J., Penman, D. and Holland, J.C. (1984) Depression in hospitalized cancer patients. *Psychosom. Med.*, **46**, 199–212.

Burish, T.G. and Lyles, J.N. (1981) Effectiveness of relaxation training in reducing adverse reactions to chemotherapy. *J. Behav. Med.*, **4**, 65–78.

Cain, E., Kohorn, E., Quinlan, D., Latimer, K. and Schwartz, P. (1986) Psychosocial benefits of a cancer support group. *Cancer*, **57**, 183–189.

Cantor, R.C. (1978) *And A Time to Live: Toward Emotional Well-being During the Crisis of Cancer*. Harper and Row, New York.

Capone, M.A., Westie, K.S. and Good, R.S. (1980) Sexual rehabilitation of the gynecologic cancer patients: An effective counseling model. *Front. Rad. Ther. Oncol.*, **14**, 123–129.

Cassileth, B. and Steinfeld, A. (1987) Psychological preparation of the patient and family. *Cancer*, **60**, 547–552.

Cassileth, B., Lusk, E., Strouse, T., Miller, D., Brown, L., Cross, P. and Tenaglia, A. (1984). Psychosocial status in chronic illness: A comparative analysis of six diagnostic groups. *New Engl. J. Med.*, **311**, 506–511.

Cassileth, B.R., Knuiman, M.W., Abeloff, M.D., Falkson, G., Ezdinli, E. and Mehta, C.R. (1986a) Anxiety levels in patients randomized to adjuvant therapy versus observation for early breast cancer. *J. Clin. Oncol.*, **4**(6), 972–974.

Cassileth, B., Lusk, E. and Walsh, W. (1986b) Anxiety levels in patients with malignant disease. *The Hospice Journal*, **2**(2), 57–69.

Cassileth, B., Lusk, E., Brown, L., Cross, P., Walsh, W. and Hurwitz, S. (1986c) Factors associated with psychological distress in cancer patients. *Med. Pediat. Oncol.*, **14**, 251–254.

Cassileth, B.R., Walsh, W.P. and Lusk, E.J. (1988) Psychosocial correlates of cancer survival: A subsequent report 3 to 8 years after cancer diagnosis. *J. Clin. Oncol.*, **6**(11), 1753–1759.

Challis, G.B. and Stam, H.J. (1991) A longitudinal study of the development of anticipatory nausea and vomiting in cancer chemotherapy patients. *Health Psychology* (in press).

Cohen, M. and Wellisch, D. (1978) Living in limbo: Psychosocial interventions in families with a cancer patient. *Am. J. Psychother.*, **32**, 561–571.

Craig, T.J. and Abeloff, M.D. (1974) Psychiatry symptomatology among hospitalized cancer patients. *Am. J. Psych.*, **13**, 1323–1327.

De Haes, J.C. and Van Knippenberg, F.C. (1985) The quality of life of cancer patients: A review of the literature. *Soc. Sci. Med.*, **20**, 809–817.

Dean, C. and Surtees, P.G. (1989) Do psychological factors predict survival in breast cancer? *J. Psychosom. Res.*, **33**(5), 561–569.

Degner, L., Farber, J. and Hack, T. (1989) *Communication between cancer patients and health care professionals: An annotated bibliography.* The Joint Medical Affairs Committee of the Canadian Cancer Society and The National Cancer Institute of Canada.

Derogatis, L.R., Morrow, G.R., Fetting, J., Penman, D., Piasetsky, S., Schmale, A.G., Henrichs, M. and Carnicke, C.L. Jr. (1983) The prevalence of psychiatric disorders among cancer patients. *JAMA*, **249**, 751–757.

Devins, G., Orme, C., Costello, C., Binik, Y., Frizzell, B., Stam, H. and Pullin, W. (1988) Measuring depressive symptoms in illness populations: Psychometric properties of the Center for Epidemiologic Studies Depression (CES-D) Scale. *Psychol. Health*, **2**, 139–156.

Easterling, D. and Leventhal, H. (1989) Contribution of concrete cognition to emotion: Neutral symptoms as elicitors of worry about cancer. *J. App. Psychol.*, **74**(5), 787–796.

Evans, D., McCartney, C., Nemeroff, C., Raft, D., Quade, D., Golden, R., Haggerty, J., Holmes, V., Simon, J., Droba, M., Mason, G. and Fowler, W. (1986) Depression in women treated for gynecological cancer: Clinical and neuroendocrine assessment. *Am. J. Psych.*, **143**(4), 447–452.

Eysenck, H.J. (1985) Personality, cancer, and cardiovascular disease: A causal analysis. *Person. Indiv. Diff.*, **6**(5), 535–556.

Eysenck, H.J. (1987a) Anxiety, learned helplessness, and cancer: A causal theory. *J. Anx. Dis.*, **1**, 87–104.

Eysenck, H.J. (1987b) Personality as a predictor of cancer and cardiovascular disease, and the application of behavior therapy in prophylaxis. *Eur. J. Psych.*, **1**(1), 29–41.

Eysenck, H.J. (1988) Behavior therapy as an aid in the prevention of cancer and coronary heart disease. *Scand. J. Behav. Ther.*, **17**(314), 171–188.

Farash, J.L. (1978) Effects of counselling on resolution of loss and body image disturbance following mastectomy. *Diss. Abs. Int.*, **39**, 8B:4027.

Farber, J.H., Weinerman, B.H. and Kuypers, J.A. (1984) Psychosocial distress in oncology outpatients. *J. Psychosoc. Oncol.*, **2**(314), 109–118.

Feinstein, A.D. (1983) Psychological interventions in the treatment of cancer. *Clin. Psychol. Rev.*, **3**, 1–14.

Ferlic, M., Goldman, A. and Kennedy, B.J. (1979) Group counseling in adult patients with advanced cancer. *Cancer*, **43**, 760–766.

Fobair, P., Hoppe, R., Bloom, J., Cox, R., Varghese, A. and Spiegel, D. (1986) Psychosocial problems among survivors of Hodgkin's disease. *J. Clin. Oncol.*, **4**(5), 805–814.

Forester, B., Kornfeld, D. and Fleiss, J. (1985) Psychotherapy during radiotherapy: Effects on emotional and physical distress. *Am. J. Psych.*, **142**(1), 22–27.

Galinsky, M.J. (1985) Groups for cancer patients and their families: Purposes and group conditions. In Sundel, M., Glasser, P., Sarri, R. and Venter, R. (eds) *Individual Change Through Small Groups*, 2nd ed. Free Press, New York, pp. 27–42.

Goldberg, D. and Hillier, V. (1979) A scaled version of the General Health Questionnaire. *Psycholog. Med.*, **9**, 139–146.

Goldberg, J.G. (ed.) (1981) *Psychotherapeutic Treatment of Cancer Patients*. Macmillan, Riverside, New Jersey.

Goldberg, R. and Wool, M. (1985) Psychotherapy for the spouse of lung cancer patients: Assessment of an intervention. *Psychother. Psychosom.*, **43**, 141–150.

Goldberg, R., Wool, M., Tull, R. and Boor, M. (1984) Teaching brief psychotherapy for spouses of cancer patients: Use of a codable supervision format. *Psychother. Psychosom.*, **41**, 12–19.

Gordon, W.A., Friedenbergs, I., Diller, L., Hibbard, M., Wolf, C., Levine, L., Lipkins, R., Ezrachi, O. and Lucido, D. (1980) Efficacy of psychosocial intervention with cancer patients. *J. Consult. Clin. Psychol.*, **48**, 743–759.

Greer, S., Morris, T., Pettingale, K. and Haybittle, J. (1990) Psychological response to breast cancer and 15-year outcome. *Lancet*, **335**(8680), 49–50.

Grossarth-Maticek, R., Schmidt, P., Vetter, N. and Arndt, S. (1984) Psychotherapy research in oncology. In Steptoe, A. and Mathews, S. (eds). *Health Care and Human Behavior*. Academic Press, London, pp. 325–342.

Gruber, B., Hall, N., Hersh, S. and Dubois, P. (1988) Immune system and psychological changes in metastatic cancer patients using relaxation and guided imagery: A pilot study. *Scand. J. Behav. Ther.*, **17**(1), 25–46.

Hackett, T.P. (1976) Psychological assistance for the dying patient and his family. *Ann. Rev. Med.*, **27**, 371–378.

Holland, J.C. and Rowland, J.H. (eds) (1989) *Handbook of Psychooncology*. Oxford University Press, New York.

Holley, B. (1983) Counseling the head and neck cancer patient: Laryngectomy. *Prog. Clin. Biol. Res.*, **121**, 215–225.

Hopwood, P. and Maguire, G.P. (1988) Body image problems in cancer patients. *Br. J. Psych.*, **153** (suppl. 2), 47–50.

House, A. (1988) Invited review: Mood disorders in the physically ill – Problems of definition and measurement. *J. Psychosom. Res.*, **33**(415), 345–353.

Houts, P., Yasko, J., Kahn, B., Schelzel, G. and Marconi, K. (1986) Unmet psychological, social, and economic needs of persons with cancer in Pennsylvania. *Cancer*, **55**(10), 2355–2361.

Jacobs, C., Ross, R.D., Walker, I.M. and Stockdale, F.S. (1983) Behavior of cancer patients: A randomized study of the effects of education and peer support groups. *Am. J. Clin. Oncol.*, **6**, 347–350.

Jamison, R.N., Burish, T.G. and Wallston, K.A. (1987) Psychogenic factors in predicting survival of breast cancer patients. *J. Clin. Oncol.*, **5**, 772–786.

Kaufman, K.L., Tarnowski, K.J. and Olson, R. (1989) Self-regulation treatment to reduce the aversiveness of cancer chemotherapy. *J. Adolesc. Health Care*, **10**, 323–327.

Kline Leidy, N. (1989) A physiological analysis of stress and chronic illness. *J. Adv. Nursing*, **14**, 868–876.

Krippner, S. (1985) The role of imagery in health and healing: A review. *Saybrook Review*, **5**(1), 32–41.

Lansky, P. (1982) Possibility of hypnosis as an aid in cancer therapy. *Perspect. Biol. Med.*, **25**(3), 147–148.

Lazarus, R.S. and Folkman, S. (1984) *Stress, Appraisal and Coping*. Springer, New York.

Le Shan, L.L. (1977) *You can Fight for Your Life*. Jove, New York.

Le Shan, L.L. (1989) *Cancer as a Turning Point*. Plume, New York.

Leventhal, H. (1990) Emotional and behavioral processes. In Johnston, M. and Wallace, L. (eds) *Stress and Medical Procedures*. Oxford University Press, Oxford, pp. 25–57.

Levy, S., Lee, J., Bagley, C. and Lippman, M. (1988) Survival hazards analysis in first recurrent breast cancer patients: Seven-year follow-up. *Psychosom. Med.*, **50**, 520–528.

Loescher, L.J., Welch-McCaffrey, P.W., Leigh, S., Hoffman, B. and Meyskens, F. (1989) Surviving adult cancers (part I): Physiological effects. *Ann. Intern. Med.*, **111**(5), 411–432.

Loescher, L., Clark, L., Atwood, J., Leigh, L. and Lamb, G. (1990) The impact of the cancer experience on long-term survivors. *Oncology Nursing Forum*, **17**(2), 223–229.

Lonngvist, J., Achte, K., Gohn, P., Korhonen, P., Lehvonen, R., Mustonan, U. and Sevila, A. (1981) Adaptation to cancer. *Psych. Fennica Suppl.*, 179–188.

Love, R., Leventhal, H., Easterling, D. and Nerenz, D. (1989) Side effects and emotional distress during cancer chemotherapy. *Cancer*, **63**, 604–612.

Luce, J.K. and Dawson, J.J. (1975) Quality of life. *Sem. Oncol.*, **2**, 323–327.

Lyles, J.N., Burish, T.G., Krozley, M.G. and Oldhan, R.K. (1982) Efficacy of relaxation training and guided imagery in reducing the aversiveness of cancer chemotherapy. *J. Consult. Clin. Psychol.*, **50**, 509–524.

Maguire, P. (1985) Improving the detection of psychiatric problems in cancer patients. *Soc. Sci. Med.*, **20**(8), 819–823.

Maguire, P., Hopwood, P., Tarrier, N. and Howell, T. (1985) Treatment of depression in cancer patients. *Acta Psych. Scand.*, **72** (suppl. 320), 81–84.

Mahrer, A.R. (1980) The treatment of cancer through experiential psychotherapy. *Pyschother. Theor. Res. Pract.*, **17**, 335–342.

Malouff, J.H., Schutte, N.S. and Ramerth, W. (1985) Evaluation of a short form of POMS-Depression Scale. *J. Clin. Pyschol.*, **41**, 389–391.

Massie, M.J. and Holland, J.E. (1988) Consultation and liaison issues in cancer care. *Psych. Med.*, **5**, 343–359.

Mayou, R., Hawton, K. and Feldman, E. (1988) What happens to medical patients with psychiatric disorder? *J. Psychosom. Res.*, **32**(415), 541–549.

McNair, D.M., Lorr, M. and Droppleman, L.F. (1971) *Profile of Mood States*. Educational and Industrial Testing Service, San Diego.

Meares, A. (1982/1983) A form of intensive meditation associated with the regression of cancer. *Am. J. Clin. Hypn.*, **25**(2–3), 114–121.

Moorey, S. and Greer, S. (1989) Adjuvant psychological therapy: A cognitive behavioral treatment for patients with cancer. *Behav. Psychother.*, **17**, 177–190.

Morrow, G.R. and Morrell, L. (1982) Behavior treatment for the anticipatory nausea and vomiting induced by cancer chemotherapy. *New Engl. J. Med.*, **307**, 1476–1480.

Nelson, D., Friedman, L., Baer, P., Lane, M. and Smith, F. (1989) Attitudes to cancer: Psychometric properties of fighting spirit and denial. *J. Behav. Med.*, **12**(4), 341–355.

Nerenz, D., Leventhal, H. and Love, R. (1982) Factors contributing to emotional distress during cancer chemotherapy. *Cancer*, **50**(5), 1020–1027.

Petersen, H.E., Smith, D.F. and Enig, B. (1988) The severity of depression in cancer patients. *Scand. J. Psychol.*, **29**, 126–128.

Phillips, L. and Osborne, J. (1989) Cancer patients' experiences of forgiveness therapy. *Can. J. Counselling*, **23**(3), 236–257.

Pullin, W.M. and Stam, H.J. (1986) *Psychosocial predictors of lagtime to diagnosis in cancer*. Paper presented at the 47th annual convention of the Canadian Psychological Association, Toronto.

Radloff, L.S. (1977) The CES-D Scale: A self-report depression scale for research in the general population. *App. Psycholog. Meas.*, **1**, 385–401.

Rait, D. and Lederberg, M. (1989) *The Family of the Cancer Patient*. In Holland, J. and Rowland, J. (eds). *Handbook of Psychooncology*. Oxford University Press, New York, pp. 585–597.

Razavi, D., Delvaux, N., Farvacques, C. and Robaye, E. (1990) Screening for adjustment disorders and major depressive disorders in cancer in-patients. *Br. J. Psych.*, **156**, 79–83.

Redd, W.H., Andresen, G.V. and Minagawa, R.Y. (1982) Hypnotic control of anticipatory emesis in patients receiving cancer chemotherapy. *J. Consult. Clin. Psychol.*, **50**, 14–19.

Ringler, K., Whitman, H., Gustafson, J. and Coleman, F. (1981) Technical advances in leading a cancer patient group. *Int. J. Group Psychother.*, **31**(3), 329–343.

Robinson, J., Boshier, M., Dansak, D. and Peterson, K. (1985) Depression and anxiety in cancer patients: Evidence for different causes. *J. Psychosom. Res.*, **29**(2), 133–139.

Rodin, G. and Voshart, K. (1986) Depression in the medically ill. *Am. J. Psych.*, **143**(6), 696–697.

Roud, P.C. (1986/1987) Psychosocial variables associated with the exceptional survival of patients with advanced malignant disease. *Int. J. Psych. Med.*, **16**(2), 113–122.

Sampson, W.I. and Whitfield, C.L. (1977) On dying at home. *Emergency Medicine*, **9**, 137–141.

Schag, C.C. and Heinrich, R.L. (1989) Anxiety in medical situations: Adult cancer patients. *J. Clin. Psychol.*, **45**(1), 20–27.

Schipper, H., Clinch, J., McMurray, A. and Levitt, M. (1984) Measuring the quality of life of cancer patients: The Functional Living Index – Cancer: Development and validation. *J. Clin. Oncol.*, **2**, 472–483.

Schwartz, M.D. (1977) An information and discussion program for women after a mastectomy. *Arc. Surg.*, **112**, 277–281.

Shacham, S. (1983) A shortened form of the Profile of Mood States. *J. Person. Ass.*, **47**, 305–306.

Siegel, B.S. (1986) *Love, Medicine, and Miracles*. Harper & Row, New York.

Simonton, D.C., Matthews-Simonton, S. and Creighton, J.L. (1978) *Getting Well Again*. Tarcher-St. Martins, Los Angeles.

Spiegel, D. and Glafkides, M. (1983) Effects of group confrontation with death and dying. *Int. J. Psychother.*, **33**(4), 433–447.

Spiegel, D. and Yalom, I.D. (1978) A group support for dying patients. *Int. J. Group Psychother.*, **28**, 233–245.

Spiegel, D., Bloom, J.R. and Yalom, I. (1981) Group support for patients with metastatic cancer – a randomized prospective outcome study. *Arch. Gen. Psych.*, **38**, 478–486.

Spiegel, D., Bloom, J.R., Kraemer, H.C. and Gottheil, E. (1989) The effect of psychosocial treatment on survival of patients with metastatic breast cancer. *Lancet*, **ii**(8668), 888–891.

Spielberger, C.D., Gorsuch, R.L. and Lushene, R. (1970) *The State-Trait Anxiety Inventory Manual*. Consulting Psychological Press, Palo Alto, California.

Stam, H.J. (1989a) From symptom relief to cure: Hypnotic interventions in cancer. In Spanos, N.P. and Chaves, J.F. (eds). *The Cognitive–Behavioral Perspective*. Prometheus Books, Buffalo, pp. 313–339.

Stam, H.J. (1989b) *Depression in cancer patients*. Paper presented at Psychologists Association of Alberta Annual Meeting, Calgary, Alberta.

Stam, H.J. and Bultz, B.D. (1986) The treatment of severe insomnia in a cancer patient. *J. Behav. Ther. Exp. Psych.*, **17**, 33–37.

Stam, H.J. and Steggles, S. (1987) Predicting the onset or progression of cancer from psychological characteristics: Psychometric and theoretical issues. *J. Psychosoc. Oncol.*, **5**(2), 35–46.

Stam, H.J., Bultz, B. and Pittman, C. (1986) Psychosocial problems and interventions in a referred sample of cancer patients. *Psychosom. Med.*, **48**(8), 539–548.

Stam, H.J., Goss, C., Rosenal, L., Ewens, S. and Urton B. (1985) Aspects of psychological distress and pain in cancer patients undergoing radiotherapy. In Fields, H.L., Dubner, R. and Cervero, F. (eds). *Advances in Pain Research and Therapy*, Vol. 9. Raven Press, New York, pp. 569–573.

Stam, H.J., Koopmans, J.P. and Mathieson, C.M. (1991) The psychosocial impact of a laryngectomy: A comprehensive assessment. *J. Psychosoc. Oncol.* (in press).

Stewart, M. and Roter, D. (eds) (1989) *Communicating with Medical Patients*. Sage Publications, Newbury Park.

Strauss, A., Fagerhaugh, S., Suczek, B. and Wiener, C. (1985) *Social Organization of Medical Work*. University of Chicago Press, Chicago.

Tarrier, N. and Maguire, G.P. (1984) Treatment of psychological distress following mastectomy: An initial report. *Behav. Res. Ther.*, **22**, 81–84.

Tarrier, N., Maguire, G.P. and Kincey, J. (1983) Locus of control and cognitive behavior therapy with mastectomy patients: A pilot study. *Br. J. Med. Psychol.*, **56**, 265–270.

Taylor, S.E., Falke, R., Shoptaw, S. and Lichtman, R.R (1986) Social support, support groups, and the cancer patient. *J. Consult. Clin. Psychol.*, **54**(5), 608–615.

Telch, C.F. and Telch, M.J. (1985) Psychological approaches for enhancing coping among cancer patients: A review. *Clin. Psychol. Rev.*, **5**, 325–344.

Telch, C. and Telch, M. (1986) Group coping skills instruction and supportive group therapy for cancer patients: A comparison of strategies. *J. Consult. Clin. Psychol.*, **54**(6), 802–808.

Vachon, M.L.S., Lyall, W.A.L., Rogers, J., Crochane, J. and Freeman, S.J.J. (1982) The effectiveness of psychosocial support during post surgical treatment of breast cancer. *Int. J. Psych. Med.*, **11**, 365–372.

van den Borne, H.W., Pruyn, J.F.A. and van Dam-de Mey, K. (1986) Self-help in cancer patients: A review of studies on the effects of contacts between fellow-patients. *Patient Education and Counseling*, **8**, 367–385.

Vinokur, A., Threatt, B., Vinokur-Kaplan, D. and Satariano, W. (1990) The process of recovery from breast cancer for younger and older patients. *Cancer*, **65**, 1242–1254.

Ware, J.E. (1984) Conceptualizing disease impact and treatment outcomes. *Cancer*, **53**(10), 2316–2326.

Weisman, A., Worden, W. and Sobel, H. (1980) *Project Omega: Psychosocial Screening and Intervention with Cancer Patients*. Department of Psychiatry, Harvard Medical School, Boston.

Welch-McCaffrey, D.W., Hoffman, B., Leigh, S., Loescher, L.J. and Meyskens, F. (1989) Surviving adult illness (part II): Psychosocial implications. *Ann. Intern. Med.*, **111**(6), 517–524.

Wellisch, D.K., Mosher, M.G. and Van Scay, C. (1978) Management of family emotion-stress: Family group therapy in a private oncology practice. *Int. J. Group Pyschother.*, **28**(2), 225–231.

Wellisch, D., Landsverk, J., Guidera, K., Pasnau, R. and Fawzy, F. (1983) Evaluation of psychosocial problems of the homebound cancer patient: 1: Methodology and problem frequencies. *Psychosom. Med.*, **45**(1), 11–21.

Wolpe, J. (1958) Psychotherapy and Reciprocal Inhibition. Stanford University Press, Stanford.

Zimpfer, D.G. (1989) Working with groups: Groups for persons who have cancer. *Spec. Group Work*, **14**(2), 98–104.

9

Coping and Adaptation in Cancer

EDGAR HEIM

Department of Psychiatry, University of Bern, Bern, Switzerland

The boom in publications on coping and cancer is well known to all those active in the field. Most studies are concerned with coping style or strategies as intervening factors in somatic outcome, mostly expressed as relapse or survival time (Heim, 1988; Levy and Schain, 1988; Levy and Wise, 1988; Watson, 1988). True, in-depth studies are needed to test the potential influence of the more recent psychoneuroimmunological models (e.g. Schultz and Raedler, 1986; Sabbioni and Hürny, 1990; see also Chapter 1). There remains the risk, however, that coping research in cancer will become more or less one-sided by neglecting the effect of psychosocial responses to cancer on adaptation in a broader sense.

THEORETICAL ASSUMPTIONS

Most researchers nowadays would agree that coping is best described as a transactional process (Beutel, 1988; Ell, 1986; Heim *et al.*, 1983, 1986; Folkman and Lazarus, 1985). Thus coping is always related to the specific demands (or stressors) of a given situation in cancer, e.g. the initial psychological impact of diagnostic procedures, the side-effects of aggressive chemotherapy and/or radiotherapy or the long-lasting challenges of rehabilitation. Depending on how the demands can be met the process will result in more or less successful adaptation, a term which must be described more accurately. The coping process depends not only on situational factors such as the stressors but also on the intrinsic and

Cancer and Stress: Psychological, Biological and Coping Studies
Edited by C. L. Cooper and M. Watson. © 1991 John Wiley & Sons Ltd

extrinsic resources of the person, mostly his or her personality assets and support systems. Within the transactional process with many mutually dependent feedback and feedforward loops, coping acts as a mediator with a preventing or buffering effect against the negative impact of the stressors. This leads to the following definition of coping:

Coping refers to the attempt to ward off, to reduce or to assimilate an existing or expected demand (or stressor) either by intrapsychic effort (cognition- or emotion-related) or by action (field-related).

The human potential to cope with demands is much greater than is usually assumed. Rarely will one coping mode, such as repression or sensitization, be the answer, mostly it is a pattern which expresses what has been called a "person–situation fit" (French *et al.*, 1974). A number of studies show that the repertoire is rather broad, e.g. in one study on cancer an average of 10 different coping modes per illness situation were found (Heim *et al.*, 1987). Within an individual's repertoire there are some constant and some variable coping patterns.

The moderating or mediating effort in coping may be successful, but this is not necessarily so. There is always a chance of "bad" or otherwise unfavourable coping with a negative outcome. What determines a good or bad outcome is a question of viewpoint, with those involved in the illness process (patient, family or health professionals) taking different perspectives. This becomes more obvious when looking at a list of the different adaptive goals of these groups: see Table 1.

As described in Table 1 the patient's subjective priority is to keep up an acceptable intrapsychic and interpersonal psychosocial equilibrium; the family wants to see the patient as a functioning member of the social network at large, whereas doctors and other healthcare providers expect optimal compliance, in view of difficult and sometimes even harmful medical procedures. So adaptation to illness is a wide-ranging and demanding process, sometimes including conflicting goals. Moreover, it includes goals on an individual, an interpersonal and, as social roles change, even on an institutional level (Beutel, 1988). It is all the more surprising that the interest of many psychosocial researchers is predominately in pathophysiological changes. Only more recently have adaptive needs been rediscovered under the heading of quality of life research (Joyce, 1988). The concepts are related but not identical. Quality of life research in cancer developed because many medical interventions were not only unhelpful to psychosocial adjustment, but harmful. This is especially true for chemotherapy where ever more aggressive treatments exact a high cost in relation to psychological morbidity.

In the context of coping a preferable term is adjustment or adaptation. It refers in a very broad and comprehensive sense to the psychological and

Table 1. Adaptive goals of coping process as expressed by patient, family and healthcare providers

---

Patient's expectations
  Regaining wellbeing (after pain, discomfort, etc.)
  Restoring or preserving emotional balance (e.g. after distress)
  Adjusting or restoring body integrity after mutilation or loss of body functions
  Overcoming insecurity and loss of control in view of self-image and orientation
    toward the future
  Adapting to uncommon (medical) situations, such as hospitalization with new
    interpersonal relationships
  Mastering existential threat, e.g. in view of terminal illness
  Preserving a meaningful quality of life under whatever circumstances

Family's and social network's expectations
  Getting well
  Regaining or re-establishing roles in family and social network
  Preserving or regaining an acceptable relationship with spouse
  Reassuring job position or adapting to change in occupation
  Securing family's financial and social resources
  Sustaining social relationship with friends and acquaintances

Health professional's expectations
  Complying optimally to all diagnostic and/or therapeutic procedures
  Enduring painful and/or discomforting interventions
  Adjusting to the new role demands of medical setting (including hospitalization)
  Active cooperation in rehabilitation
  Preserving emotional stability in spite of long-term illness or progressive impair-
    ment, including terminal outcome

---

behavioural goals of the healing process. It includes the adjustment reaction to the illness, the integration of changing demands on the patient, adjustment responses in interpersonal relationships and adaptation to social roles. Factors mediating this process may be intrapsychic (cognitive/emotional) or behavioural. We have to recognize that these goals are part of different value systems, as listed in Table 1. What is good and desirable and what is harmful and to be eschewed are judgments acquired through socialization. Their impact on adjustment is considerable as Pearlin (1989) states: "Values ... regulate the effects of experience by regulating the meaning and the importance of the experience". This is particularly relevant when ethnic–social–demographic differences are taken into consideration. Sarell *et al.* (1983), for example, pointed out that coping and adjustment differences in Israeli cancer patients depended on their ethnic and religious background.

These differences in value systems are also noticeable in research strategies relating to coping and cancer. As mentioned before, many investigators give preference to medical and biological markers in studies on outcome of coping with cancer. This, of course, is not only desirable but also necessary in our understanding of the mediating effect of coping on the underlying biological processes such as psychoneuroimmunological changes. But this might be at the expense of a better understanding of the multiple psychosocial changes going on at the same time. Whereas the former strategies see psychosocial processes mostly as independent or mediating factors and the biological changes as dependent factors, it is important to acknowledge the impact of the disease "cancer" as an independent influence on psychological equilibrium. This is especially meaningful in view of the high incidence of cancer. Cancer will strike almost every third individual and three out of four families are involved. With increasing survival time it is all the more important to study the adjustment process. Although not all cancer patients are failing or struggling to adapt all have to cope with the many demands already mentioned. It is therefore important to understand accurately in what way the quality of life of cancer patients is affected by coping strategies and how these can be improved. The preferred strategy is to contextualize the study of coping in cancer as a biopsychosocial process. Researchers in the behavioural sciences can, in cross-disciplinary collaboration, contribute a great deal to a comprehensive understanding of the illness process. Their expertise lies in knowing the appropriate methods or instruments to use to monitor changes in psychosocial adjustment to cancer. These instruments must fit the goals mentioned above, such as assessing wellbeing or distress, psychopathology, self-image, body-image, attribution, locus of control, role strain, adaptation in family and job, social activities and relationships, compliance and illness behaviour.

Now that the coping process and the adaptive goals have been outlined it should be possible to clarify in what way the coping process might affect psychosocial adjustment. Analogous to what is known in social support (Wortman, 1984; Cohen, 1988), coping can also be seen as having a preventive, buffering or restoring effect on psychosocial adjustment. The *preventive* aspect particularly concerns the emotional impact experienced, i.e. the amount of distress suffered. Initial denial of an unfavourable or fearful diagnostic assessment often provides a certain limited peace of mind. In the immediate present, at least, a repressing patient will not have to deal with unpleasant emotions. Other patients will seek support and attention and thus, early in the process, gain adequate information which allows for appraisal of the risks involved. Probably the major mediating effect of coping is through *buffering*. Although the impact of the demands or stressors is present initially, its lasting influence is reduced or compensated for. Again, most importantly, seeking attention and care (e.g. from the spouse) will reduce the threat of an uncertain prospect; the ability to divert attention from the side-effects of chemotherapy may bring considerable relief; to go reasonably about one's problems may be helpful in order to regain control. Finally, coping is extremely important in long-term adjustment, that is in securing rehabilitation and overcoming potential losses. Here the task is to *regain an appropriate equilibrium*, whether intraphysically or in relationships or social obligations. To find meaning in the experience of a serious illness may make up for loss of social interactions; to join a self-help group may provide self-esteem through solidarity; to tackle training in a new occupation may secure one's role as a provider for the family.

These, of course represent examples of the positive effect of coping on adaptation. The effect need not be positive, however, as many studies on psychosocial outcome show. A patient might respond to the threatening bodily change, such as a lump in the breast or blood in faeces with denial and repression. Ruminating or self-blame will not only worry the patient, it might also discourage adherence to treatment programmes. Although, to some extent, social withdrawal may facilitate the patient regaining intrapsychic balance, it can easily give way to a fatalistic–regressive attitude with no effort whatsoever in rehabilitation.

These few examples suggest that the adjustment process is strongly dependent on the mediating effect of coping. We should expand our assessment in both areas to clarify the efficacy of both, the intervening and the depending variable. Only exceptionally do investigations allow for this; shortcomings mostly concern both the range and relevance of coping modes assessed and the narrow definition of psychosocial adjustment. The obvious example of denial has to be quoted again: whatever the initial buffering effect of denying or repressing painful emotions may be, it could, in the long-term, interfere with compliance to treatment.

The demands and tasks of the illness process change enormously. Schain (1976), in an account of the course of breast cancer, lists about a dozen different stages, starting from threatening expectations over initial changes to diagnostic confrontation of cancer; from major surgery and/or chemotherapy and radiotherapy to convalescence, to social reintegration, potential relapse and death. In studying adaptation, the illness stages and their specific tasks should be considered when the outcome of coping is the issue. Pearlin (1989) pointed out that primary stressors must be distinguished from secondary stressors. *Primary stressors* refer to undesired and disruptive events, such as a sudden loss or confronting life-threatening illness. *Secondary stressors* are the consequences of the former, insofar as overall adjustment is endangered. They are secondary only in respect to the sequence in which they occur and not to the meaning. "On the contrary once established social stressors independently may become capable of producing even more intensive stress than those we consider to be primary" (Pearlin, 1989). Cancer disease with succeeding stages includes many secondary stressors or demands which in themselves are highly challenging. We know that for many women the loss of a breast through mastectomy has a stronger impact than the progressing disease. Comparably a male patient treated for cancer of the prostate may suffer most from impaired sexual function after prostatectomy; a colorectal cancer patient may be handicapped particularly by the stoma, which he or she often considers an inhibiting social stigma. We have elsewhere demonstrated that the coping process can only be meaningfully understood by studying changes over time and situations (Heim *et al.*, in preparation). The same is true for adaptation. Only in prospective long-term studies can we analyse the mediating influence of coping on adaptation. The criteria used must be sensitive to repeated measure and changes over time and situations. A cross-sectional approach is too limiting and might even result in confounding independent and dependent variables.

SURVEY OF INVESTIGATIONS

This chapter assumes that theoretical conceptualization allows for appropriate research strategies. There is a gamut of questions to be asked in respect to psychosocial adaptation (PSA) in cancer. Here the term is used in a very broad sense including all psychosocial factors relevant for adjustment in cancer. Potential questions are as follows:

(1) What differences are noticeable in respect to the different areas of adjustment, e.g. wellbeing, psychopathology, family harmony, work adjustment, social activities?
(2) What PSA can be observed in distinct stages of the illness? Does PSA differ over time and situations? Is there progressive impairment in some areas compared with others?
(3) How is PSA related to coping? Are certain coping strategies related to good or bad PSA? Do certain coping strategies affect distinct areas of PSA differently? What is the meaning of a broad compared with a narrow repertoire of coping? What of stable versus changing coping?

I will attempt to answer these questions as well as the present body of research allows.

Procedure

A critical survey of controlled prospective studies of coping with cancer (Heim, 1988) indicated that only two (out of 15) used psychosocial factors as dependent variables whereas all other studies preferred survival or relapse time as the dependent variable.

A more recent search included all data from the US National Library of

Medicine from the time period 1983–1990 (February). The keywords used were: cancer, coping and good/bad; adaptive/maladaptive, outcome, distress, discomfort, emotion, adjustment, survival. The number of relevant publications listed was about 1500 (with considerable overlap in publication output depending on the different keywords). It is noticeable that the replication of the 1988 search in 1990 showed almost a tripling of output, i.e. the number of publications in the last quarter of the search period was almost three times that of the 1983–88 period. This in itself documents a quantitative productivity in the field. The qualitative aspects, however, are less encouraging. Only around two dozen publications out of hundreds met the following selection criteria:

● Empirical design
● Intelligible statements on independent and dependent factors observed, relating in a very general way to coping and PSA

Therefore, no studies with strictly biological outcome criteria (e.g relapse or survival time) were included. All cancer subjects were considered, independent of localization, staging and biological markers. Although this implies the doubtful assumption of comparable disease it was assumed that PSA includes many common features in spite of different biological criteria. To allow for comparisons between studies, an effort was made to "translate" the respective authors' definition or description of the coping process to a common terminology. To do so an interviewer-rating instrument developed by our group for long-term research in cancer was applied: the Bernese Coping Modes (BECOMO)* (Heim *et al.*, 1987). This instrument allows an observer to rank or rate on a five-point-scale 26 different coping modes which can be classified as behavioral, cognitive or emotion-oriented coping. A detailed, 70-page manual operationalizes defined coping modes. The observer's rating sheet is given in Appendix 1. Selection and operation of the coping modes are partly based on theoretical assumptions, partly on empirical observation. The instrument has adequate construct properties which are detailed in the manual. Inter-raterreliability of different research groups and interraterstability satisfied psychometric requirements. The different coping modes proved to be independent; less than 11% of all intercorrelations were significant ($P < 0.01$).

Such a procedure has its own pitfalls. Some authors extensively defined their coping modes, but only a few included operationalizations. The question also remains of whether the authors would agree with our "translation" of their term. To control for some of the methodological weaknesses we took two steps: (1) rating the degree of "subjective

---

* All coping modes in quotation marks refer to defined BECOMO (Appendix 1).

confidence" in attributing our rating concept to the author's terms (on a five-point-scale) (from "not secure" to "very secure"); (2) two independent raters (the author and his co-worker, Dr Liliane Schaffner) assessed the respective authors' terminology and translated it into the appropriate coping modes as BECOMO. The interrater agreement of the two judges was good overall: full agreement in seven (out of 15) publications; in four one or two modes more rated, in three one or two different modes rated. Based on the selection criteria cited above the following publications shown in Table 2 were rated.

Overall it is surprising that so few studies, out of some hundreds, provided answers to the questions asked. It is also noticeable that six out of 15 studies are published in German and therefore risk going unnoticed by most of the scientific community. Even those meeting our selection criteria did so to varying degrees; it is therefore questionable if they are comparable at all. It is only in view of the unchallenged need to gain a better integrated understanding of the research going on in the field that we decided to go ahead with the presented meta-analysis.

When looking at the differences or weaknesses in some of these studies, one is struck by the fact that only a few include specific hypotheses addressing PSA. Furthermore, most authors used a cross-sectional approach (nine out of 15 studies), which of course limits any interpretation of process.

Within the instruments used we have separated those addressing the dependent and those the independent or rather intervening variable, namely coping. Here, none of the instruments were identical, very few are well known in the field. It is not surprising that those giving a clear definition or even an operationalization of the coping modes studied could easily be translated in our own "language", i.e. BECOMO. It seemed as if the 26 coping modes defined by us amply covered the modes defined by other authors. One difficulty persisted in those studies dealing with the control process (e.g. locus of control) – although quite a few of the BECOMO include control aspects they were not defined for that purpose. Studies of those few authors who limited the coping process to cognitive control could not be included, in spite of interesting designs and meaningful results. Others were included, but the score of "subjective confidence" in transforming the control rating in BECOMO was very low (e.g. Jenkins and Pargament, 1988). Although some of the authors applied aggregated measures the transformation to a common terminology could not do justice to these efforts. This may eschew some of the study findings. Coping mostly functions in patterns, even including contradictory modes, so that reducing its expression does not do justice to the process. The same is true for the individual repertoire, which on average includes about a dozen different coping modes per illness situation.

Furthermore, the populations studied seemed to differ substantially. Not all investigations clearly define their subjects on demographic and biological parameters. The range of the age, sites and staging makes the samples even less comparable. Nevertheless, *in toto*, a patient population of over 2000 subjects is included in this survey. Whatever the criteria such a number is in itself representative as far as the distribution of general PSA is concerned. In addition the questions asked are more on a descriptive level and do not include inference statistics.

In spite of the numerous methodological limitations it is quite surprising that this summary of the contributing coping modes (Table 3) shows good agreement between the different findings. To a large extent this corroborates clinical experience. Furthermore, it is impressive to note that the most important coping modes named, in either a favourable or unfavourable context, are identical with those found to be contributing to the biological course of cancer (Table 4). These data, dealing with all controlled studies known to us at present (Heim, 1988) were analysed using a comparable procedure. The surprising agreement on what has to be considered as "good" or "bad" coping in dealing with cancer, whether in the biological or in the psychosocial process, warrants the conclusion that they express more general coping patterns.

In *good* or *favourable coping* an active, tackling behaviour by the patient, combined with a supportive and responsive environment is central. Reasonably assessing the options open to the individual patient further enhances their chances of survival or of psychosocial adjustment. In a limited, probably stage-dependent sense, denying some of the illness demands also favours this process.

There are additional coping modes found in this meta-analysis which have different weights in relation to psychosocial or biological adjustment: in PSA we note a set of instrumental coping modes, such as distracting oneself by different activities, by being optimistic, by comparing oneself to others, building up self-esteem or sheer acceptance of the illness process.

In contrast, those predictive studies investigating biological course parameters, such as survival time, include an expressive emotional pattern such as rebelling against the disease, releasing emotions or focusing on an optimistic outlook.

For *bad* or *unfavourable coping* there is some agreement: here resignation/fatalism (i.e. a "giving up attitude") dominates, a finding barely any clinician would challenge. It is interesting that the second most frequently used coping response includes a repressive, denying attitude, a cognitive response such as repression, dissimulation or preserving composure, or an emotion response such as isolation or suppression of feelings. Social withdrawal reflects the same attitude and at the same time is the opposite to what we call "attention and care", i.e. seeking social support,

Table 2. Overview on publications (1983–1990) addressing coping and psychosocial adaptation

Author	Patients	Observation time	Demands	Outcome criteria	Coping criteria	Coping effect (BECOMO) Positive/negative
Baider *et al.*, 1988	Breast cancer (62)	Cross-sectional, 1 × 1.5 year postops S5	Global adjustment	BDI, STAS, PAIS	SSCT (Shanan) Active vs passive SC 1-2	*Positive* Attention and care tackling
Buddeberg (personal communication)	Breast cancer (107)	Longitudinal, 36-month S 1-5	Subject coping success	Subject score	ZKV/FKV SC 4-5	*Negative* Resignation Problem analysis Dissimulation Isolation Preserv. comp Withdrawal
Burgess *et al.*, 1988	Breast cancer (107); Hodgkin/ non-Hodgkin lymphoma (61)	Longitudinal, 3 + 12 months after diagnosis All stages S 1-6	Global adjustment	STAI, Wakefield Depression Locus of control	Hopeless/ helpless Denial/ avoidance Fighting Fatalistic SC 3	*Negative* Resignation Self-accusation *Positive* Tackling Dissimulation Acceptance/ stoicism
Ell *et al.*, 1989	Diff. cancer (253) female + male	Diagnosis, 1 + 2 year post-diagnosis S 2-7	Global adjustment	Mental Health Index (MHI) wellbeing and distress	Perceived support Social integration Personal sense of control SC 3	*Positive* Attention and care Valorization Problem analysis

Feifel et al., 1987	Diff. cancer (74)	Cross-sectional, 1×	Life-threatening illness	Adjustment Effectiveness of coping (patient, doctor, family)	MCMQ Confrontation Avoidance Acceptance/resignation SC 4	*Negative* Dissimulation Diversion Resignation
		S 4				
Filipp et al., 1988	Diff. cancer (333) female + male	Longitudinal, first observation average 11 months	Emotional adjustment	Wellbeing Self-validation Rosenberg life orientation Scheier and Carver	Rumination Social involvement Fighting Threat Religion Seeking information	*Positive* Attention and care Diversion as ACT Dissimulation Optimism Tackling Problem analysis Religion *Negative* Rumination Withdrawal
		S 2–6			SC 4	
Herschbach et al., 1985	Breast cancer (385); Genital cancer (95 female)	Cross-sectional, 1× Rehabilitation	Psychological and social adjustment	Subjective score of being stressed	Reduced dissonance Fighting Seeking information Resignation Catharsis Divert/avoid SC 5	*Positive* Tackling Relativizing *Negative* Resignation Diversion/ dissimulation
		S 3–5				

(continued)

Table 2. (continued)

Author	Patients	Observation time	Demands	Outcome criteria	Coping criteria	Coping effect (BECOMO) Positive/negative
Herschbach and Henrich, 1987	Diff. cancer (308 female + male)	Cross sectional, 1× Rehabilitation S 3–5	Psychological and social adjustment	Subjective score what helps?	15 Coping strategies SC 5	*Positive* Relativizing Diversion as ACT Optimism Tackling Attention and care
Jenkins and Pargament, 1988	Diff. cancer (62 female + male)	Cross-sectional >3 month diagnosis S 3–6	Perceived life threat	Rosenberg Self esteem MBHI BUMP GAIS	Global coping PIER MMPI Lie scale SC 2	*Positive* Religion Relativizing Accept/stoicism Valorization
Lakomy, 1988	Diff. cancer (84 female)	Cross-sectional, pre- and post-diagnosis S 1 and 2	Threat of illness	STAI Depression	Different coping strategies SC 2–3	*Positive* Problem analysis Dissimulation *Negative* Resignation
Manual *et al.*, 1987	Head and neck cancer (5 male + female)	Longitudinal, 3 days, 4–6 weeks, 2–3 months after diagnosis	Threat of illness Effect of chemo- and radiotherapy	SCL-90 R Sympt. Distr. PAIS	IES: avoidance vs. approach	*Positive* Problem analysis Tackling Attention and care

Reference	Sample	Design	Stage (S)	Focus (S1)	Distress measures	Coping (authors' terms, SC)	Translation into BECOMO
Thomas *et al.*, 1988	Diff. cancer (91 male and female)	Longitudinal, postoperative and 3 and 12 months	S 2–4	Threat of illness	Distress as depression, Anxiety	SC 3–4	Dissimulation, Diversion, Passive cooperation, Optimism; *Negative* Resignation
Watson *et al.*, 1984	Breast cancer (24)	Cross-sectional, postoperative	S 2–7	Threat of diagnosis	STAI, POMS	Denial, Stoicism/acceptance, Fighting spirit, Helpless/hopeless, SC 5	*Positive* Tackling, Acceptance/stoicism; *Negative* Dissimulation, Resignation
Ziegler *et al.*, 1984	Diff. cancer (31 male and female)	Cross-sectional, 1 × 1 month to 15 year illness	S 2	Threat of illness	STAI, Depression	Denial, Different mode, Acceptance, SC 5	*Positive* Dissimulation, Problem analysis, Diversion
			S 2–7			Coping competence, SC 2–3	*Positive* Problem analysis, Valorization, Dissimulation, Attention and care

S1, Detection of change, preliminary diagnosis; S2, hospitalization; S3, postdischarge and convalescence; S4 postdischarge and adjunctive chemotherapy and/or radiotherapy; S5, rehabilitation and adaptation, latency; S6, metastatic disease, recurrence; S7, terminal illness; SC, subjective confidence score: 1, "not secure" to 5, "very secure" in "translating" authors' terms of coping in Bernese Coping Modes (BECOMO). For definition of BECOMO see Appendix 1.

Coping and Psychosocial Interventions

Table 3. Summary of good/bad coping in psychosocial adaptation.
(Survey of 15 publications 1983–1990)

Good coping		Bad coping	
Naming	Mode	Naming	Mode
7	Attention and care	7	Resignation/fatalism
7	Tackling	4	Dissimulation
6	Problem analysis	2	Diversion
5	Dissimulation	2	Social withdrawal
3	Acceptance/stoicism	1	Isolation/suppression
3	Diversion as action	1	Preserving composure
3	Optimism	1	Problem analysis
3	Relativizing	1	Rumination
3	Valorization	1	Self-accusation
2	Religion		
1	Passive cooperation		

"Naming" means in how many studies is coping (positively/negatively) related to PSA. For definition of coping modes see Appendix 1.

predominant in favourable coping. Again, the clinical notion of what is considered unfavourable coping is confirmed experimentally.

It certainly would do more justice to the richness of the studies mentioned if they could be analysed separately. But at the same time the reader will agree that this probably is beyond the scope of this contribution. A few comments will have to suffice.

Table 4. Summary of good/bad coping in biological disease process.
(Survey of 15 prospective studies 1975–1985)

Good coping		Bad coping	
Naming	Mode	Naming	Mode
7	Tackling	8	Resignation/fatalism
5	Attention and care	6	Isolation/suppression
4	Rebelling	3	Dissimulation
3	Dissimulation	3	Social withdrawal
3	Emotional release	2	Rebelling
3	Problem analysis	1	Religion
2	Optimism	1	Release of anger
1	Constructive activity	1	Rumination
1	Preserving composure		
1	Social withdrawal		

"Naming" means in how many studies is coping (positively/negatively) related to biological criteria (e.g. survival or relapse time). For definition of coping modes see Appendix 1.

What I mentioned above as a critical statement, namely how non-comparable the designs and samples are, has at the same time a positive connotation: in spite of this disparity there is a high agreement in evaluating the coping process. Some researchers based their observations on the patient's self ratings (e.g. Buddeberg, 1990; Filipp *et al.*, 1988; Herschbach *et al.*, 1987) as dependent variables. Other authors, predominantly of the English speaking community, preferred standardized instruments, such as the PAIS, STAI, MHI, MBHI, SCL-90 etc. Some authors report on the family's or doctor's observations as well (e.g. Baider *et al.*, 1988; Feifel *et al.*, 1987). These not only confirm the patient's self-rating but enhance the findings. In other studies (e.g. Burgess *et al.*, 1988) the authors had developed very elaborate instruments which somehow got lost either in the aggregation (as in this study by focusing on four factors) or by transforming them in our rating system (BECOMO). Another limiting factor is that not all coping modes defined by the different investigators (as a matter of fact only a limited number of them) showed significant relations to the dependent variables (e.g. Lakomy, 1988; Ziegler *et al.*, 1984). These non-contributing modes are not included, in order to avoid an even more complicated listing in Table 3. Finally, a few authors decided to express their outcome variables in a positive *and* negative context (e.g. Burgess *et al.*, 1988; Filipp *et al.*, 1988; Herschbach, 1987; Manuel *et al.*, 1987) whereas most only addressed one or the other dimension.

Some of the studies with a longitudinal prospective design (such as Ell *et al.*, 1989) showed how the PSA varies over time and with it also the interdependency of coping. Furthermore, the demands to be coped with, which are of major importance in any illness process, were often not mentioned at all or only implicitly, or very generally stated. In only a few studies were they specified and the coping related to the different tasks stemming from the illness situations. It is regrettable again, that a meta-approach cannot do justice to these refined findings.

THE BERNESE BREAST CANCER STUDY

This prospective longitudinal study of coping with cancer was started in 1983.* The study was originally planned to answer a number of questions:

(1) Do cancer patients cope differently from non-cancer patients in comparable situations?

(2) What is the range or repertoire of coping modes used both by groups and individuals over time?

---

* Besides this writer the following participated in this project: K.F. Augustiny, P. Ballinari, A. Blaser, C. Bürki, D. Kühne, M. Rothenbühler, L. Schaffner and L. Valach.

(3) How effective is adjustment to the demands of different illness stages as expressed in social adaptation and emotional distress?
(4) Is there any way to differentiate good from bad copers and do they remain stable over time?

In this chapter only those questions concerning psychosocial adaptation (PSA) are addressed, as expressed by questions 3 and 4.

Subjects

The subjects consisted of 151 female patients with breast disease: 72 with breast cancer, 55 with fibrocystic disease and 24 with mastodynia (pain and tension in the breast). Results are presented only for the cancer patients. Their mean age at the beginning of the study was 57.7 years (range 37 to 83).

Procedure

This has been described elsewhere in more detail (Heim *et al.*, 1987; Heim, 1990). The subjects have been followed continuously for five years. For the first two years observations were made every three months, after this every six months unless there were somatic complications, then our field worker would see them at the time the complications arose. Results for the first two years are reported. A semistructured interview addressed the immediate past and actual illness situation with their demands, life circumstances in general, social and emotional adjustment and coping behaviour. The interview lasted 2–3 h. Initially patients were seen in the hospital, then mostly in their homes at follow-up.

Measures

Coping: (1) The Bernese Coping modes (BECOMO) further, not reported in this chapter; (2) Coping questionnaire SVF by Janke *et al.* (1985); (3) Sense of coherence questionnaire SOC by Antonovsky (1987) (only at end of the study).

Adjustment: (4) Social adjustment scale (SAS) Heim *et al.* (1982); (5) Emotional State Scale Bf-s by von Zerssen (1976) further, not reported in this chapter; (6) Compliance questionnaire by Wengele (unpublished); (7) Freiburger Anpassungsinventar by Koch *et al.* (1986) (only at end of the study).

Medical details were obtained via the GYN and oncology university clinics in Bern (including TNM-staging). This design shares some of the shortcomings mentioned above. Probably the most important one is that the breast cancer patients could not be matched for TNM-stages and other biological markers. Therefore no prediction of the biological course (especially survival or relapse time) based on psychosocial factors was attempted. Furthermore, due to the clinical complications (eight patients died during the first two years; two dropped out and some were too sick to complete questionnaires at times) some missing values could not be avoided.

Results

Coping

The following is a summary of specific results on coping reported extensively elsewhere (Heim *et al.*, in preparation).

Frequencies: All modes of the rating instrument developed by us, the Bernese Coping Modes (BECOMO) (see above) were more or less regularly apparent, i.e. the coping spectrum was very broad. As shown by the rank order on 10 different observation points (Table 5) the distribution is quite uneven: some modes were frequently employed and others more rarely. Of the top 10 ranks listed only two coping modes are always within the first ranks: "attention and care" and "acceptance–stoicism". Others, such as "problem analysis", "tackling" around operation time or "thought or action as diversion" are also outstanding.

Table 6 lists the different dimensions (or "factors") over the 10 observations made during the first two years. Here again, some coping modes are very important at all stages observed: in dimension I again "attention and care" and "acceptance–stoicism", in dimension II "dissimulation" and in dimension III "diversion". Complementary to the robustness of these three modes a whole gamut of different modes is associated with them over time.

Some of these observations are in favour of overall stable coping, others vary and are in favour of situation-dependent patterns. It should be kept in mind, however, that these are all group values which do not do justice to the richness of individual patterns. We have reported elsewhere that patients differ considerably in respect to specifically determined repertoire and stability coefficients (Heim, in preparation).

Coping and Psychosocial Interventions

Table 5. Frequencies of the Bernese Coping Modes (BECOMO) (expressed as mean ranks out of 26 possible ranks)

Hospitalization			12 Months		
R	$n = 72$	MR	R	$n = 54$	MR
1	Attention and care	4.9	1	Acceptance–stoicism	7.4
2	Acceptance–stoicism	8.6	1	Attention and care	8.4
3	Problem analysis	9.2	3	Thought as diversion	8.7
4	Valorization	10.4	4	Problem analysis	9.5
5	Passive cooperation	10.5	5	Activity as diversion	9.8
5	Tackling	10.5	6	Relativizing	10.6
3 Months			*18 Months*		
R	$n = 66$	MR	R	$n = 50$	MR
1	Attention and care	6.1	1	Acceptance–stoicism	6.7
2	Acceptance–stoicism	9.5	1	Attention and care	6.8
3	Activity as diversion	9.3	3	Problem analysis	9.1
4	Thought as diversion	9.5	4	Relativizing	9.7
5	Preserving composure	9.7	5	Thought as diversion	9.9
6	Valorization	9.7	6	Tackling	9.9
6 Months			*24 Months*		
R	$n = 60$	MR	R	$n = 47$	MR
1	Attention and care	7.5	1	Acceptance–stoicism	5.4
1	Acceptance–stoicism	7.5	2	Attention and care	8.4
3	Thought as diversion	8.8	3	Relativizing	8.5
4	Activity as diversion	9.0	4	Problem analysis	9.9
5	Problem analysis	9.4	5	Optimism	10.5
6	Tackling	9.5	6	Altruism	10.7

R, rank; MR, mean rank.

Social adaptation

The instrument used in the longitudinal part of the study is the Social Adaptation Scale (SAS) originally developed by Barrabee *et al.* (1955) and later on modified by us (Heim *et al.*, 1982). It has proven useful in a number of studies since the early seventies, a time when very few adaptation scales for patients were available. It covers most areas of adaptation, compared to more recent scales on quality of life. A clinical interview allows for a five-point rating-type Likert scale. The results presented here are based on 495 protocols rated over the first two years. Since no normative values for a nonmedical population are available the distributions rather than the raw scores will be presented in a descriptive way (i.e. as "box plots"; Tukey, 1977). We consider the median with the first and third quartile to be especially helpful, since here 50% of all values are included.

Table 6. Multidimensional scaling (MDS) of the Bernese Coping Modes (BECOMO) (solutions in three dimensions)

Observation period	I	SC	II	SC	III	SC
Hospitalization (n=72)	Attention and care	4.0	Dissimulation	2.7	Thought as diversion	1.8
	Acceptance–stoicism	2.3				
	Problem analysis	1.8				
3 Months (n=66)	Attention and care	3.2	Dissimulation	2.0	Altruism	1.8
	Acceptance–stoicism	2.7	Isolation–suppression	1.7	Thought as diversion	1.7
	versus					
	Resignation–fatalism	−1.8				
	Release of anger	−1.8				
6 Months (n=60)	Acceptance–stoicism	2.8	Dissimulation	1.8	Activity as diversion	1.6
	Attention and care	2.3	Problem analysis	1.9	versus	
	Thought as diversion	1.9			Problem analysis	−1.7
	versus					
	Activity as diversion	1.7				
12 Months (n=53)	Acceptance–stoicism	3.3	Dissimulation	−1.8	Thought as diversion	−2.2
	Attention and care	1.7	versus		versus	
	versus		Attention and care	2.2	Problem analysis	1.6
	Resignation–fatalism	−1.7				
18 Months (n=50)	Acceptance–stoicism	3.6	Relativizing	2.1	Valorization	2.0
	Attention and care	2.4	Activity as diversion	1.6	versus	
	Problem analysis	1.7	versus		Thought as diversion	−1.8
	Tackling	1.5	Tackling	−1.6		
			Problem analysis	−1.5		
24 Months (n=47)	Acceptance–stoicism	−4.2	Thought as diversion	1.7	Problem analysis	−2.1
	Attention and care	−2.7				
	Relativizing	−2.5				

Dimensions

Figure 1 gives the distribution of the total psychosocial adaptation (PSA) over the first two years. Most values are between scale score 4 and 5, i.e. between good and excellent adaptation. Figure 2 shows the different categories. Most values of PSA in the core family and occupation are 4 and higher; those in the other three categories are significantly lower, with scores on social life often lowest. Before going into any details, we can already see how the course of the illness affects psychosocial adaptation: at time of "hospitalization" psychosocial life during the preceding weeks is reflected. Here, as a rule the values are highest, i.e. adaptation is best. In contrast, three months later (i.e. at post-discharge convalescence or for some patients at time of adjunctive chemotherapy and/or radiotherapy), PSA value is lowest. It takes 18 months for the median to return to the prehospitalization adaptation level.

The distribution of the occupation scores in Figure 3 shows a comparable variation. Here it becomes obvious that we are not dealing with a uniform sample, but with a group of patients where some had very low initial occupational adjustment. As an addendum it should be mentioned that household chores in this sample of middle-aged Swiss women were considered comparable with being employed and therefore rated identically. Even so, responses in the subcategory of "level of work" varied most

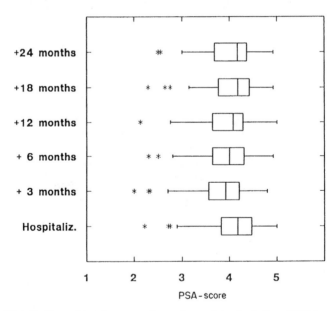

Figure 1. Distribution of total scores of psychosocial adaptation (PSA) over the first two years of observation ("box plot"). Boxes describe median with the first and third quartile (including 50% of all values). $n = 48-67$

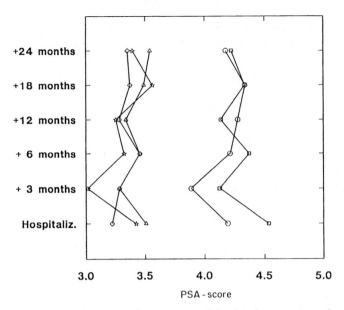

Figure 2. Distribution of means (five-point scale) of subcategories of total PSA (blow-up of scale from 3.0–5.0). Adjustment to: ☆ social life; ◇ family of origin; □ core family; △ financial situation; ○ occupation

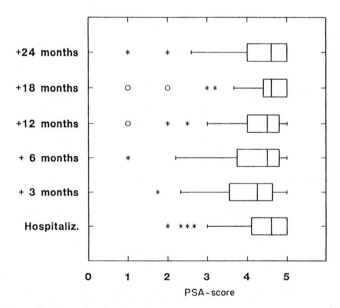

Figure 3. Distribution of adjustment to occupation over two-year observation period in "box plot". The broad range is marked by stars and open circles. $n = 46$–64

between subjects. This means that, depending on the state of their health, certain patients were, at given times, absent from work. The best scores are those of "working hours" and of "attitude to work". This might reflect the willingness of these patients to get back to work as soon as possible.

Score values of 3 in "financial situation" (see Figure 2) mean that the patients were able to maintain their usual standard of living, provided insurance cover was sufficient. This socioeconomic level corresponds to lower middle-class and does not change considerably over time. Most subjects, in spite of obvious limits in income, seem satisfied with their financial situation (scores around 4).

The scores of "core-family" adjustment are high overall, between 4 and 5 on a five-point scale. Lowest points are at three and 12 months. This is best explained by the inability to cover the usual responsibilities for the family at a time when the impact of the illness is worst. This can also be seen in Figure 4 which shows the subcategories and a significant drop in the ability to care for the family (family responsibility) at three months. But married life and relationships with children also seem to suffer before they regain more or less the usual level after six months. Adaptation to partnership is not very satisfactory, with values around 3 points, meaning that there is some agreement on the meaning of the relationship; but the partnership is seen as not very rewarding and in addition there are some disruptions in sexual relations. Improvement over time is limited.

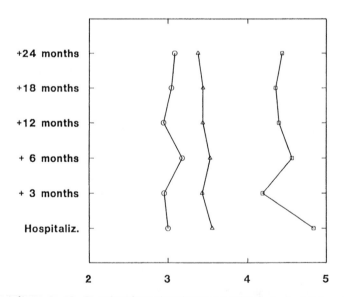

Figure 4. Adjustment in core family to family responsibility (□), children (▵) and marriage/partner (○)

Adaptation to "family of origin", i.e. to parents and siblings, is satisfactory in view of the high mean age of our sample. In this age group the relationship to the family of origin may not be close. It might event be that the roles are reversed in the sense that the younger generation scares for the elderly parents. This could explain the low values at time of hospitalization and the peak score after six months.

"Social life" is strongly influenced by the course of the illness (Figure 5). On average the mean values of "social contacts" are half a point higher than those of "social activities". This corresponds to satisfying contacts with friends and relatives, although the ties might not be that strong. A score of 3 in activities means that the person participates in cultural events or club activities in only a limited way, regardless of whether this is due to illness or lack of interest. Again, we found lowest scores after three months, with a more or less steady increase in the old interests and activities over following months.

A caveat is justified here: we only report on the first two years out of the five years observed so far. Few of the subjects relapsed or died during this period; that is months 12 to 24 are a period of convalescence or latency with no new signs or symptoms. At this point it is therefore hard to tell if this surprisingly good adjustment will continue in the years to follow. Furthermore, although on inspection we can detect some trends it is difficult to show statistical proof of significant changes in time series.

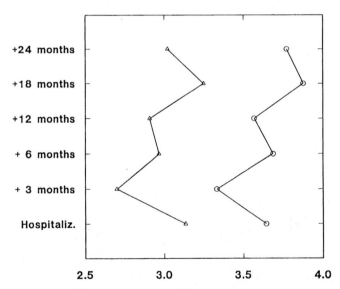

Figure 5. Adjustment to social life. ▵ activities; ○ contacts

When we compare these findings to what is known from the literature there is some agreement and some disagreement. In general these subjects show a good PSA which improves over time. The only observation period with significantly impaired adjustment in respect to all criteria is the posthospitalization time at month three. We cannot differentiate as yet if this is a general drop or if it is due to subjects undergoing chemotherapy or radiotherapy. A further analysis in respect to distinct illness stages will clarify this issue. On average it took the subject 18 months after diagnosis to reach the same level of PSA as shown at prehospitalization. Most studies on PSA report that 12–18 months are needed to regain a psychosocial balance (Andersen, 1989; Cohen et al., 1988a; Sullivan et al., 1988; Wolberg et al., 1989).

The Californian–Swedish Comparative Study on cancer survivors (Cohen et al., 1988a,b; Sullivan et al., 1988) points out that the period of diagnosis is the most stressful (for about one-quarter of all patients), but later stages may still be quite stressful for a substantial number of patients. Their 2–3-year follow-up also showed overall good adjustment, with varying adaptation in different areas. Within this large sample, breast cancer patients were only moderately affected, compared with patients with oral, prostate or lung cancer. One other long-term follow-up study, however, described a decline of PSA over the first two years (Ell et al., 1989). This surprising difference may be due to their different assessment method, as the Mental Health Index focuses more on psychopathology than psychosocial criteria.

The Californian–Swedish study also confirmed that at times two-fifths of the patients felt that their present physical condition limited their ability to work. Another Californian study (Heinrich et al., 1984) found two-thirds complained about occupation problems. That the financial situation is primarily culturally determined is convincingly demonstrated by the comparison with Swedish patients who suffered fewer financial difficulties than those in California due to the Swedish social welfare system. The Swiss conditions in this respect might be closer to Sweden than California. The same study also showed, however, that the Californians had a stronger informal, family-oriented, support system than the Swedes. Ell et al. (1989) found as we did that "the emotional support from close social relationships" (i.e. family) decreases over time but "distant social ties" become stronger.

Distress or emotional adjustment

The "emotional state scale Bf-s" by von Zerssen (1976) is widely used in German speaking countries. It assesses distress: the higher the score the worse the patients feel. It is a standardized instrument with scores

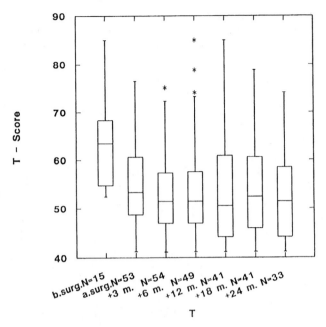

Figure 6. Distribution of distress score in "box-plot"

expressed as T-values. Figure 6 gives the distribution over time and subjects. For all observation points the T-scores are widely distributed. The mean at prehospitalization (a small subsample of 15 patients was assessed) is highest (65), later levelling out to around 55. These scores are astonishingly low when compared with a student sample showing T-scores of 51.1 one month before a major examination, 58.1 at time of exam and 45.5 one month later (Sabbioni *et al.*, in preparation).

The correlation of the total social adaptation score with the distress score Bf-s was highly significant ($r = -0.48$ ($P < 0.01$)): those patients feeling strongly distressed did worse in social adaptation and vice versa. This interdependence was true for all observation points over the two years reported here.

Regaining an emotional balance by one year postsurgery is what most studies report (Andersen, 1989; Bloom, 1987; de Haes *et al.*, 1986). There seems to be considerable consistency of this finding in most studies carried out in the 1980s compared with the earlier English studies. Maguire *et al.* (1978) and Morris *et al.* (1977) still found increased psychopathology (especially depression) in breast cancer patients in about 20% of their sample. A more recent study (Cohen *et al.*, 1988b) confirmed that the greatest distress for patients, in both Sweden and California, was immediately after diagnosis. More than one-third felt overwhelmed and showed different signs of distress. After 2–3 years, however, only about 6% still suffered from depression and anxiety.

Interdependence of coping and psychosocial adaptation

In the theoretical model presented earlier coping is conceived as the mediating force serving either to avoid or to buffer the negative impact of illness demands. The characteristics of psychosocial adaptation as dependent variables express to what extent the mediating effect was successful or not. In this respect we can approach the differentiation of favourable and unfavourable, or "good" and "bad" coping.

Only our preliminary findings are reported here. Our approach is exploratory. The following description of the findings is based on the Mann–Whitney U test which allows a first approximation in order to examine if those patients using a given coping mode differ in PSA from those not using it. Only strong trends in this computation are reported.

To start with emotional wellbeing or alternatively "distress"; we found astonishingly consistent interrelationships. High distress scores related to "resignation", "social withdrawal", "rumination" and "emotional release". In contrast low distress is reported when patients prefer "dissimulation" or "isolation/suppression" as coping modes. One-quarter of all computations proved to be significant (at conventional probability levels).

Total social adaptation shows some, but not many, significant interrelationships with coping (24/156 computations): it is especially in the later stages of illness (after 12 months) that some of the emotion-related BECOMO was associated with low social adaptation such as "resignation", "rumination", "release of anger" and "emotional release".

The interrelationship of coping and adaptation varies in the different categories. In occupation and financial status significant values are rare and each is limited to different observation times.

When we look at what coping response contributes positively to high adjustment in the core family we find that for the second year "optimism" and "acceptance/stoicism" are important. Much clearer than the positive is the negative interrelationship between coping and family adjustment. Coping that hinders good adjustment includes "resignation" and "self accusation", and to a lesser degree "rumination" and "social withdrawal".

Social life *in toto* is supported by "acceptance/stoicism" and "attention and care". In the subcategory "social contacts" we further find "optimism", "giving meaning" and "constructive activities". Negative influences are more scattered, with "social withdrawal" and, to a lesser degree, "resignation" as outstanding coping modes. Figure 7 shows how those patients who named "attention and care" in adjustment to social life

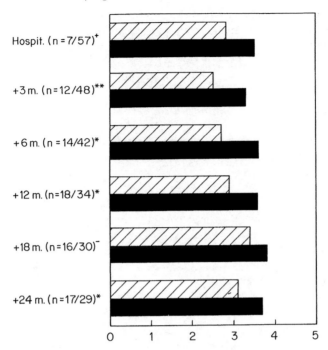

Figure 7. Interdependence of "attention and care" as coping with adjustment in social life. *n* refers to "not named"/"named", e.g at time of hospitalization the raters had seven patients without "attention and care" observed. The bar charts give the differences of mean scores. Significance (Mann-Whitney U-test, 2-tailed). + $P < 0.10$; * $P < 0.05$; ** $P < 0.01$; –, no sign. ▨ not named; ■ named

differed from those not naming it. Those patients seeking "attention and care" had a more active social life over the total observation period.

Discussion and conclusion

In this study psychosocial adaptation (PSA) is operationalized as a sum score of different categories, including wellbeing or lack of distress.

The results indicate a clear-cut relationship between distress and certain coping modes; "dissimulation" and "isolation–suppression" going with lower distress and "resignation–fatalism", "social withdrawal", "rumination" and "emotional release" with higher distress. The results confirm everyday experience that ignoring negative emotions may contribute to a (superficial?) wellbeing. It is even more evident that certain unfavourable coping patterns, as mentioned above, lack not only a buffering effect but increase negative emotional experiences.

The connection of the total social adjustment score with coping is less conclusive, less also than in some categories studied, i.e. "core family" and "social life". It appears that summing scores for distinct areas of adaptation disguises rather than clarifies true relationships. Furthermore, the impact of coping seems to vary over time, with late observations indicating a stronger relationship of coping to PSA than earlier ones. One explanation could be that only when a certain level of social adaptation is reached can one detect interdependency of coping and adaptation. Methodologically one must conclude that to determine mutual effects of coping and adjustment different areas of adjustment and distinct illness stages must be observed. This is similar to a long term study by Ell *et al.* (1989) who found a change over time among all study variables and the significance of the changes for psychological adaptation. It is also important to remember that in chronic illnesses as a rule demands in many different areas have to be met, in respect to occupation, financial consequences, family affairs and social life. To test adaptation by selecting only a few of the many different psychosocial demands, will not do justice to the adaptive efforts of the patients.

Our results also indicate that changes over time are important. Although conclusions are limited by this exploratory descriptive approach we find certain time-dependent tendencies. There is a trend that overall adjustment in the early stages of illness was positively related to diverting activities and finding a meaning in the illness. In the middle stage seeking support, mostly through the family, was additionally helpful. In the last third of this two-year observation period, patients who accepted their disease with a stoical attitude and who were still socially supported seemed to do best. One certainly should be prudent not to overstretch interpretation of these findings, but they clearly indicate a time effect. Probably the most convincing effects of different observation times can be found by looking at a single constellation, for example the interdependency of coping – here dissimulation – and distress over time. By looking at dissimulation (Figure 8) as a global category for all forms of denial, one finds a differential effect on distress over time. When comparing those patients who used "dissimulation" with those not using it the strong initial relationship at hospitalization time disappears over the following observation periods, so that there is no significant relationship by 18 and 24 months. This means that "dissimulation" originally had a strong buffering effect on distress, i.e. patients with high "dissimulation" suffered less from distress and vice versa. It has often been reported that denial refers to a complex concept including reduced perception in respect to threat, to meaning of illness, to emotional impact etc. (Breznitz, 1983). It seems that not only the meaning of denial is changing over the illness course, but also its buffering effect as coping. Watson *et al.* (1984), in a

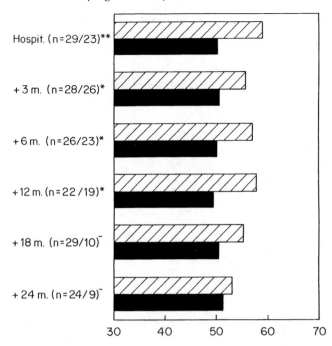

Figure 8. Interdependence of "dissimulation" ("not named"/"named") and distress (T-score). For details see Figure 7

cross-sectional study at time of initial hospitalization of breast cancer patients, found comparable results: "deniers" had fewer mood disturbances than "acceptors", a differentiation which was not confirmed for trait anxiety.

Finally, the question remains to be answered whether these results contribute to the understanding of "good" versus "bad" or favourable versus unfavourable coping. The theoretical issues involved were addressed at the beginning of this chapter. What is known from the literature was analysed here in a special survey. The bearing of this study on this question has already been alluded to. First a negative outcome must be mentioned: some modes contribute surprisingly little, such as "religion", "tackling" and "passive cooperation". Most astonishing is the almost absent impact of "tackling" on adjustment, a coping mode otherwise found to be very influential. This finding is all the more surprising since in the rank order of all BECOMO it was always named within the 10 most important modes. A possible explanation could be that in this rural sample of middle-aged women where accepting of the illness is so dominant a more aggressive approach to the illness just does not fit the cultural pattern to resolve illness problems.

As in the survey outlined above "attention and care" again has the strongest impact on good psychosocial adjustment. It reflects seeking and perceiving support, as mentioned earlier. The concept of social support has many facets, as is well known. It includes informational and emotional attention, it assumes involvement and profit from close and more distant networks. Its protective function against very different stressors, whether they are illness-related or more general life events, is well documented (e.g. Wortman, 1984; Kessler *et al.*, 1985). The second most important coping mode in our study is "acceptance/stoicism", probably a specific cultural finding for this Swiss sample. In the survey mentioned earlier, however, it was also among modes that contributed the most to PSA. A particular feature of this coping mode is that it is based on an attitude of self-confidence, of trust and perhaps also of internal control. It reminds one of Antonovsky's (1987) salutogenetic principle where an attitude of "coherence" turned out to be particularly protective. In his concept stimuli derived from one's internal or external environment are predictable and explicable and allow for stoical acceptance. A second point concerns resources that are available to meet the demands of the illness. This is related to "attention and care". Finally Antonovsky postulates that these demands are seen as challenges and this refers to the optimistic outlook. "Optimism" in this context and "diversion as action" are most likely action and future oriented. In our study they were among those modes that related most to PSA.

Pearlin (1989) has postulated that the primary stressor may be followed by different secondary stressors, conceivably the opposite also holds true: demands met and goals reached allow the person to achieve new tasks or goals. So the "primary success" may stimulate people to go to many different "secondary successes". Once a minimal adjustment is reached, e.g. in household chores, this primary goal stimulates the subject to attain other goals, i.e. to meet other demands of the illness process. The consequence could be that activities in the broader network of social contacts become possible and that they contribute to the overall adjustment. For these successfully coping subjects it is probably not important in which area they make progress but rather that they are successful. This is a well known therapeutic principle where nothing is more successful than success. It also suits one other positive attitude – hope. In this respect people keep motivating themselves by holding on to positive signs of the illness process or by encouragement from their support system.

Opposed to this are the hopeless patients. In our findings the single most frequent contributing factor is probably the significant intercorrelation of "resignation/fatalism" to poor psychosocial adjustment. Again, this is in agreement with the findings described in the survey, but also with many theoretical concepts, such as Engel's (1962) "giving up–given up complex" or Seligman's (1975) helplessness. Resignation is not only a strong predictor of negative outcome to PSA but also to the biological course of the disease. Its deleterious effect on cancer was also documented in animal experiments (Levy and Wise, 1988; Levy and Schain, 1988); for further discussion see Chapter 2. The other modes related to poor PSA have a common denominator, i.e. denying and avoiding reality, by avoiding treatment adherence, by avoiding social contacts and thus support and by avoiding thoughts of the illness process; they all refer to an attitude of not tackling the disease and of not solving the problems involved. This implies not only a lack of compliance in the therapeutic process, but also is an attitude prone to the above-mentioned resignation and helplessness. Clinicians are aware of these "bad copers", who cannot be reached and helped.

One final conclusion: research on appropriate versus inappropriate coping is goal oriented. The better our understanding becomes the easier it will be to modify the coping process. The next consequence is to develop intervention strategies fitting the needs of the patient in his or her illness situation, the possibilities of a therapeutic framework (intervention by whom?) and the goals to be achieved. The individual patient might be helped considerably by learning to avoid the unfavourable coping modes described above. He or she might even profit by more learning to apply new and more appropriate coping modes. Elsewhere we have screened for the coping intervention strategies in cancer and have suggested an intervention model (based on crisis and cognition theory) suiting the conditions just mentioned (Heim, 1991).

Summary

Psychosocial adjustment (PSA) in this sample of originally 72 women with breast cancer is satisfactory overall. In some areas (core family, occupation) adjustment reaches higher levels than in others (finances, family of origin, social life). Differences within categories (e.g. regarding occupation, working hours versus working relations; regarding core family, marital relationship against responsibility to total family; regarding social life, contacts vs activities) call for differential assessments of PSA since the sum score may turn out to be a crude measure. Distress as measured by a standardized instrument (Bf's v.Zerssen) is acceptable on most observation times.

There are *differences over time* when PSA is assessed at three-month intervals. PSA of the prehospitalization time in most areas is reached again after 18 months. It is poorest three months after surgery, i.e. initial hospitalization. This is true for adjustment in all categories rated. Distress, however, was worst during hospitalization, following diagnosis, with scores levelling out after 3–6 months. A caveat is justified: results presented here only concern the three-month observation interval during the first two years, with few patients relapsing or dying during this period. In a further, stage-oriented evaluation, including the total observation time of five years, more pronounced differences may become detectable. Already it has become clear, however, that PSA is a process over time, corresponding to the changing demands and challenges of the illness.

Coping as rated with an observer-rating instrument, the Bernese Coping Modes (BECOMO) is variable and stable over the first two years. Rank order of frequencies and aggregation patterns in Multi-Dimensional Scaling (MDS) indicates some constant modes, such as "attention and care", "acceptance–stoicism" and "diversion" (cognitive and behavioural) – besides some other frequently observed modes as "problem analysis" or "relativizing". The other 26 modes rated vary over the 10 different observation times and stages.

There are certain significant *interrelationships between PSA and coping*. They vary over time and areas of PSA, with some observation periods and psychosocial criteria indicating more meaningful relationships than others. In an attempt to test effectiveness of coping, with PSA as the dependent criterion, certain trends regarding "good" or "poor" coping, or appropriate versus inappropriate coping can be tentatively described. "Good" coping includes seeking and perceiving social and emotional support and an attitude of stoical acceptance of the cancer illness. Poor PSA goes with a coping pattern of resignation–fatalism, combined with a passive-avoiding attitude. High distress as a dependent variable is related to resignation, withdrawal, ruminating and emotional release. Distress is low, or wellbeing high, when emotions are denied, isolated and suppressed.

Overall these findings are in agreement with those of other authors. A survey on 15 studies answering comparable questions gave good concordance in a meta-analysis. Different clinical implications have to be considered, the most important one being to develop *intervention strategies* to support poor copers by modifying their coping pattern.

ACKNOWLEDGEMENTS

The author wants to thank K. Augustiny, P. Ballinari, A. Blaser, M. Haour and L. Valach for valuable suggestions. He is especially indebted to M. Watson, the co-editor of this book, for her assistance in the preparation of the manuscript.

REFERENCES

Andersen, B.L. (1989) Health psychology's contribution to addressing the cancer problem: update on accomplishments. *Health Psychol*, **8**(6), 683–703.

Andersen, B.L., Anderson, B. and deProsse, C. (1989) Controlled prospective longitudinal study of women with cancer: II. Psychological outcomes. *J. Consult. Clin. Psychol.*, **57**, 692–697.

Antonovsky, A. (1979) *Health, Stress, and Coping*. Jossey-Bass, San Francisco.

Antonovsky, A. (1987) *Unraveling the Mystery of Health. How People Manage Stress and Stay Well*. Jossey-Bass, San Francisco.

Baider, L.A. and Kaplan De-Nour, A. (1988) Breast cancer – a family affair. In. Cooper, C.L. (ed.) *Stress and Breast Cancer*. John Wiley, Chichester.

Barrabee, P. *et al.* (1955) A normative social adjustment scale. *Am. J. Psych.*, **112**(4), 252–259.

Beutel, M. (1988) *Bewältigungsprozesse bei chronischen Erkrankungen*, edition medizin VCH, Weinheim.

Bloom, J.R. (1987) Psychological response to mastectomy. A prospective comparison study. *Cancer*, **59**, 189–196.

Breznitz, S. (1983) The seven kinds of denial. In Breznitz, S. (ed.) *The Denial of Stress*. IUP, New York, pp. 257–280.

Burgess, C., Morris, T. and Pettingale, K.W. (1988) Psychological response to cancer diagnosis – II. Evidence for coping styles (coping styles and cancer diagnosis). *J. Psychosom. Res.*, **32**, 263–272.

Cohen, S. (1988) Psychosocial models of the role of social support in the etiology of physical disease. *Health Psychol.*, **7**(3), 269–297.

Cohen, J., Sullivan, M. and Branehög, I. (1988a) *A Psychosocial Study of Cancer Survivors in California, USA and the Western Region of Sweden. (Part 1: Crosscultural Comparisons)*. University of California at Los Angeles, Gothenburg University.

Cohen, J., Sullivan, M. and Branehög, I. (1988b) Psychosocial responses to cancer in California and Western Sweden: A comparative study. *J. Psychosoc. Oncol.*, **6**(3/4), 29–40.

de Haes, J.C.J.M., van Oostrom, M.A. and Welvaart, K. (1986) The effect of radical and conserving surgery on quality of life of early breast cancer patients. *Eur. J. Surg. Oncol.*, **12**, 337–342.

Ell, K.O. (1986) Coping with serious illness: On integrating constructs to enhance clinical research, assessment and intervention. *Int. J. Psych. Med.*, **15**(4), 335–356.

Ell, K., Nishimoto, R., Morvay, T., Mantell, J. and Hamovitch, M. (1989) A longitudinal analysis of psychological adaptation among survivors of cancer. *Cancer*, **63**, 406–413.

Engel, G.L. (1962) *Psychological Development in Health and Disease*. Saunders, Philadelphia.

Feigel, H., Strack, S. and Tong Nagy, V. (1987) Degree of life-threat and differential use of coping modes. *J. Psychosom. Res.*, **31**(1), 91–99.

Filipp, S.H., Ferring, D., Freudenberg, E. and Klauser, Th. (1988) Affektivmotivationale Korrelate von Formen der Krankheitsbewältigung. Erste Ergebnisse einer Längsschnittstudie mit Krebspatienten. *Psychother. Med. Psychol.*, **38**, 37–42.

Folkman, S. and Lazarus, R.S. (1985) If it changes it must be a process. *J. Person. Soc. Psychol.*, **48**, 140–170.

French, J.R.P., Rodgers, W. and Cobb, S. (1974) Adjustment as personal–environment fit. In Coelho, G.V., Hamburg, D.A. and Adams J. (eds) *Coping and Adaptation*. Basic, New York, pp. 316–333.

Heim, E. (1988) Coping und Adaptivität: Gibt es geeignetes oder ungeeignetes Coping? *Psychother. Med. Psychol.*, **38**, 8–18.

Heim, E. (1991) Coping als Interventionsstrategie bei psychosozialer Belastung durch somatische Krankheiten. In Brähler, E., Geyer, M. and Kabanov, M. (eds). Westdeutscher Verlag, Opladen.

Heim, E. and Willi, J. (1986) *Psychosoziale Medizin, Klinik und Praxis*. Springer-Verlag, Berlin.

Heim, E., Adler, R. and Moser, A. (1982) Beeinträchtigung der psychosozialen Anpassung durch terminale Krankheit. *Zschr. Psychosom. Med.*, **28**, 347–362.

Heim, E., Augustiny, K.F., Blaser, A., Bürki, C., Kühne, D., Rothenbühler, M., Schaffner, L. and Valach, L. (1987) Coping with breast cancer – a longitudinal prospective study. *Psychother. Psychosom.*, **48**, 44–59.

Heim, E., Augustiny, K.F., Ballinari, P., Blaser, A., Kühne, D., Rothenbühler, M., Schaffner, L. and Valach, L. (in preparation) A prospective longitudinal study of coping with breast cancer: the issues of stability and variability.

Heinrich, R.L., Schag, C.C. and Ganz, P.A. (1984) Living with cancer: The cancer inventory of problem situations. *J. Clin. Psychol.*, **40**(4), 972–980.

Herschbach, P. and Henrich, G. (1987) Probleme und Problembewältigung von Tumorpatienten in der stationären Nachsorge. *Psychother. Med. Psychol.*, **37**, 185–192.

Herschbach, P., Rosbund, A.M. and Brengelmann, J.C. (1985) Probleme von Krebspatientinnen und Formen ihrer Bewältigung. *Onkologie*, **8**, 219–231.

Janke, W., Erdmann, G. and Kallus, W. (1985) *Stressverarbeitungsfragebogen (SVF)*. Göttingen, Hogrefe.

Jenkins, R.A. and Pargament, K.I. (1988) Cognitive appraisals in cancer patients. *Soc. Sci. Med.*, **26**, 625–633.

Joyce, C.R.B. (1988) Quality of life: The state of the art in clinical assessment. In Walker, S.R. and Rosser, R.M. (eds). *Quality of Life. Assessment and Application*. MTP Press, Lancaster.

Kessler, R.C., Price, R.H. and Wortman, C.B. (1985) Social factors in psychopathology: Stress, social support and coping processes. *Ann. Rev. Psychol.*, **36**, 531–572.

Koch, U., Haag, G. and Muthny, F.A. (1986) Erleben und Verarbeitung der Brustkrebs-Erkrankung. Fragebogen für Patientinnen in der Heilbehandlung. Abtlg. Rehabilitationspsychologie der Universität Freiburg, Belfortstrasse 16, DW-7800 Freiburg.

Lakomy, D.K. (1988) Art und Effizienz des Copingverhaltens der Frau under der Erstbedrohung eines Mamma- oder Zervixkarzinoms. *Psychother. Med. Psychol.*, **38**, 43–47.

Levy, S.M. and Schain, W.S. (1988) Psychologic response to breast cancer: Direct and indirect contributors to treatment outcome. In Lippman, M.E., Lichter, A.S. and Danforth, D.N. (eds) *Diagnosis and Management of Breast Cancer*. W.B. Saunders, London.

Levy, S.M. and Wise, B.D. (1988) Psychosocial risk factors and cancer progression. In Cooper, C.L. (ed.) *Stress and Breast Cancer*, John Wiley, Chichester.

Maguire, G.P., Lee, E.G., Bevington, D.J., Kucherman, C.S., Crabtree, R.J. and Cornell, C.E. (1978) Psychiatric problems in the first year after mastectomy. *Br. Med. J.*, **61**(18), 963–965.

Manuel, G.M., Roth, S., Keefe, F.J. and Brantley, B.A. (1987) Coping with cancer. *J. Human Stress*, **13**(4), 149–158.

Morris, T., Greer, H. and White P. (1977) Psychological and social adjustment to mastectomy. *Cancer*, **40**, 2381–2387.

Pearlin, L.I. (1989) The sociological study of stress. *J. Health Soc. Behav.*, **30**, 241–256.

Sabbioni, M. and Hürny, C. (1990) Psychoneuroimmunological studies. In Holland, J.C. and Zittoun, R. (eds) *Psychosocial Aspects of Oncology*. Springer Monographs, Berlin, Heidelberg.

Sabbioni, M., Valach, L., Heim, E., de Weck, L. and Pichler, W. (in preparation) Changes in distress and immune functions during an examination period.

Sarell, M., Baider, L. and Edelstein, E. (1983) A judgmental measure of coping with cancer and its social, psychological and medical correlates: An exploratory study of Israeli patients. *Isr. J. Psych. Relat. Sci.*, **20**(3), 242–253.

Seligman, M.E.P. (1975) *Helplessness: On Depression, Development and Death*. Freeman, San Francisco.

Sullivan, M., Cohen, J. and Branehög, I. (1988) *A Psychosocial Study of Cancer Survivors in California, USA and the Western Region of Sweden. Part II. Response patterns and determinants of adjustment to cancer in Sweden*. Gothenburg University, University of California at Los Angeles.

Schain, W. (1976) Psychological impact of the diagnosis of breast cancer on the patient. *Front. Rad. Ther. Oncol.*, **11**, 68–89.

Schulz, K.H. and Raedler, A. (1986) Tumorimmunologie und Psychoimmunologie als Grundlagen für die Psychoonkologie. *Z. Psychother. Med. Psychol.*, **36**, 114–129.

Thomas, C., Turner, P. and Madden, F. (1988) Coping and the outcome of stoma surgery. *J. Psychosom. Res.*, **32**(4/5), 457–467.

Tukey, J.W. (1977) *Exploratory Data Analysis*. Addison-Wesley, Reading.

von Zerssen, D. (1976) *Die Paranoid-Depressivitätsskala*. Beltz, Weinheim.

Watson, M. (1988) Breast cancer: Psychological factors influencing progression. In Cooper, C.L. (ed.) *Stress and Breast Cancer*. John Wiley, Chichester.

Watson, M., Greer, S., Blake, S. and Shrapnell, K. (1984) Reaction to a diagnosis of breast cancer. Relationship between denial, delay and rates of psychological morbidity. *Cancer*, **53**, 2008–2012.

Wolberg, W.H., Rosaas, E.P., Tanner, M.A. and Malec, J.F. (1989) Psychosexual adaptation to breast cancer surgery. *Cancer*, **63**, 1645–1655.

Wortman, C.B. (1984) Social support and the cancer patient. Conceptual and methodologic issues. *Cancer*, **53**, 2339–2362.

Ziegler, G., Pulwer, R. and Koloczek, D. (1984) Psychische Reaktionen und Krankheitsverarbeitung bei Tumorpatienten – erste Ergebnisse einer empirischen Untersuchung. *Psychother. Med. Psychol.*, **34**, 44–49.

Appendix 1. Rating sheet and short version of Bernese Coping Modes (BECOMO)

1. ACTION-RELATED

A1 ACTIVITY AS DIVERSION

0	1	2	3	4
Not present	Mild	Moderate	Severe	Very Severe

A familiar activity is engaged in the sense of a diversion: "I'm throwing myself into my work in order to forget my illness".

A2 ALTRUISM

0	1	2	3	4
Not Present	Mild	Moderate	Severe	Very Severe

One's own needs are placed after those of others; one does things for others: "I want to be here for my family as long as I can".

A3 ACTIVE AVOIDANCE

0	1	2	3	4
Not Present	Mild	Moderate	Severe	Very Severe

Necessary medical action is not undertaken or discounted; e.g. consulting a doctor, mediation, rehabilitation etc.

A4 COMPENSATION

0	1	2	3	4
Not Present	Mild	Moderate	Severe	Very Severe

Wish fulfillment as diversion: shopping, eating, tranquillizer, alcohol, doing anything pleasurable: "When I am not feeling well, I buy myself something nice, even if I don't really need it".

A5 CONSTRUCTIVE ACTIVITY

0	1	2	3	4
Not Present	Mild	Moderate	Severe	Very Severe

Something constructive is done, something seen as needed (perhaps for a long time). For example: developing one's creativity, travelling etc.: "I'm finally taking some time for myself".

A5 WITHDRAWAL (social)

0	1	2	3	4
Not Present	Mild	Moderate	Severe	Very Severe

The need to be alone in order to recharge one's energies; to reflect on matters, to stand aside: "I need peace and quiet. I want to be able to find myself".

Seizing the opportunity; taking the initiative oneself in relation to clarification and therapy; an illness-related search for information; resorting to help; cooperation in clarification and therapy: "A lot now depends on what I do and how I take part".

A7 TACKLING

0 Not Present	1 Mild	2 Moderate	3 Severe	4 Very Severe

The need to feel fulfilled, to speak out and to be heard, to have support: "Up to now there has always been someone who has listened/understood".

A8 ATTENTION AND CARE

0 Not Present	1 Mild	2 Moderate	3 Severe	4 Very Severe

2. COGNITION-RELATED

Attention to the illness is directed towards something else: "This is more important to me than the illness at the moment".

C1 THOUGHT AS DIVERSION

0 Not Present	1 Mild	2 Moderate	3 Severe	4 Very Severe

The illness is accepted as a matter of fate and as being unalterable and is endured with composure: "This is simply the way it is. I'm trying to resign myself to it".

C2 ACCEPTANCE–STOICISM

0 Not Present	1 Mild	2 Moderate	3 Severe	4 Very Severe

The illness is played down, denied, minimized and ignored: "It's really not so bad – actually I'm feeling quite well".

C3 DISSIMULATION

0 Not Present	1 Mild	2 Moderate	3 Severe	4 Very Severe

An attempt is made to keep one's poise and (emotional) self-control in front of others and in relation to oneself: "I have to pull myself together. No one must notice anything".

C4 PRESERVING COMPOSURE

0 Not Present	1 Mild	2 Moderate	3 Severe	4 Very Severe

Cognitive analysis of the illness and its consequences: recognition, careful consideration, making a decision: "I'm trying to explain to myself what is actually happening".

C5 PROBLEM ANALYSIS

0 Not Present	1 Mild	2 Moderate	3 Severe	4 Very Severe

(continued)

Appendix 1. (*continued*)

One's own burden is placed in relation to the (hard) lot of others. Comparing oneself with others, playing down one's fate: "I'm in relatively good shape compared with others who have lost a leg".

C6 RELATIVIZING

0 Not Present	1 Mild	2 Moderate	3 Severe	4 Very Severe

Religious faith as a support: illness as God-given, indicted upon mankind: "Everyone's time comes, but God is with me".

C7 RELIGIOUSNESS

0 Not Present	1 Mild	2 Moderate	3 Severe	4 Very Severe

The illness is clung to mentally brooding, aimless reflection and reconsideration: "Is it really so, or isn't it ...? I can't get it off my mind".

C8 RUMINATION

0 Not Present	1 Mild	2 Moderate	3 Severe	4 Very Severe

The illness is given meaning. It is seen as a responsibility, as a chance to alter one's view of life, one's set of values: "Through my illness, I've discovered my true self".

C9 GIVING MEANING

0 Not Present	1 Mild	2 Moderate	3 Severe	4 Very Severe

Being conscious of one's own worth, remembering successful experiences, a positive evaluation of one's own attitude (including toward the illness): "I've succeeded in doing other important things up to now. Actually, I've been quite brave about it all".

C10 VALORIZATION

0 Not Present	1 Mild	2 Moderate	3 Severe	4 Very Severe

3. EMOTION-RELATED

Resistance is shown towards the illness and its consequences; protest, quarrelling with one's lot: "Why me?"

E1 REBELLING

0 Not Present	1 Mild	2 Moderate	3 Severe	4 Very Severe

E2 EMOTIONAL RELEASE

Emotional release is brought about through the expression of feelings engendered by the illness: affliction, fear, anger, despair, despondency ... possibly even courage, love, hope are expressed: "I feel so miserable, at least crying seems to help a bit".

0 Not Present	1 Mild	2 Moderate	3 Severe	4 Very Severe

E3 ISOLATION–SUPPRESSION

Feelings adequate to the situation are not admitted: "I'm not in the least worried by the whole thing".

0 Not Present	1 Mild	2 Moderate	3 Severe	4 Very Severe

E4 OPTIMISM

Confidence that the (momentary) crisis can be overcome: "If I only have faith, then everything will surely be better".

0 Not Present	1 Mild	2 Moderate	3 Severe	4 Very Severe

E5 PASSIVE COOPERATION

One commits oneself to another's care. In the knowledge that help is available, that responsibility can be entrusted to qualified persons, one feels oneself to be in good hands: "They know what they're doing".

0 Not Present	1 Mild	2 Moderate	3 Severe	4 Very Severe

E6 RESIGNATION–FATALISM

One gives up, resigns oneself, loses all hope: "I don't believe there's any point in continuing any more".

0 Not Present	1 Mild	2 Moderate	3 Severe	4 Very Severe

E7 SELF-ACCUSATION

One blames oneself for the illness. One looks for mistakes in oneself, guilt is expiated: "I don't deserve any better".

0 Not Present	1 Mild	2 Moderate	3 Severe	4 Very Severe

E8 RELEASE OF ANGER

Stowed-up anger is given expression. One is indignant, annoyed, irritable: "I am so angry that this illness has got me".

0 Not Present	1 Mild	2 Moderate	3 Severe	4 Very Severe

10

Counselling and Stress in HIV Infection and AIDS

JOHN GREEN and BARBARA HEDGE

Psychology Department, St Mary's Hospital, London, UK

AIDS-related tumours are the most frequent tumours in young men under the age of 40 years in North America, much of western Europe and sub-Saharan Africa. The arrival of AIDS has made Kaposi's Sarcoma, previously one of the rarest of tumours in the west, a common clinical finding. The tumours seen in AIDS are present because the individual has an underlying immune deficiency. AIDS therefore appears, superficially at least, to be a potentially rich source of information about the interactions between mind, the immune system and cancers.

AIDS, the acquired immune deficiency syndrome, has a history which spans less than a decade, although unrecognised cases undoubtedly occurred before that time. It is an area of intense research and more has probably been discovered in a short period about AIDS than about any other disease. Nevertheless there is a great deal which remains unknown.

The disease is caused by one of two viruses, the Human Immuno-deficiency Viruses (HIV) Types 1 and 2. HIV-2 is mainly confined to parts of West Africa although cases have occurred elsewhere and there are signs that the virus is spreading. In this chapter "HIV" is used to refer to HIV-1, although the similarity in mode of action of the viruses suggests that what applies to HIV-1 is likely to apply to HIV-2.

HIV is a retrovirus, part of a family of viruses found widely amongst mammals and birds (Shaw et al., 1988). It is an enveloped virus containing a single strand of RNA. HIV particularly infects the CD4+ subset of T-cells, the so-called "T-helper" or T4 cells. These play a key role in switching on the immune system in response to infection and affect the

Cancer and Stress: Psychological, Biological and Coping Studies
Edited by C. L. Cooper and M. Watson. © 1991 John Wiley & Sons Ltd

activity of cytotoxic T-cells, B-cells production of antibodies and Natural Killer (NK) Cells. Directly or indirectly they play a central role in immune system functioning.

The HIV virus infects T-cells by binding to the CD4 receptor on the cell surface (Koenig and Fauci, 1988). It is then absorbed into the cell and the coat stripped off. The virus then makes a double-stranded DNA copy of the RNA genome which is usually incorporated into the host cell genome. Activation of the T-cell by external factors and internal action of the viral genes is thought to cause production by the cell of new virus particles. Infection with the virus is lifelong and productive, with the infected person being potentially infectious to a greater or lesser degree throughout the infection.

The virus also infects other cells of the immune system, including the monocyte-macrophage population of the brain, leading in some cases to a dementia.

The virus impairs the activity of the immune system in a variety of different ways, most imperfectly understood (Koenig and Fauci, 1988). Infected T-cells are killed by HIV and, probably, by the immune system. However, there is evidence that uninfected T-cells and other immune system cells may be impaired, although the mechanism is unclear.The overall result is that as the disease progresses the number of T-cells falls. This sharp fall also suggests that the mechanisms for replacing T-cells are also impaired, probably through damage to progenitor cells.

HIV is transmissible in a limited number of ways, involving trans-mission of infected material or cells. Transmission is bidirectional in vaginal and anal intercourse, occurs through transfer of infected blood or blood products and tissues and, probably in rare cases, breast milk. Materno–fetal transmission also occurs either *in utero* or at birth; the reported rate of materno–fetal transmisson varies widely from study to study and it is possible that the health of the mother may affect the probability of transmission (Peckham and Newell, 1990).

Transmission through sex is the most common route worldwide. As with other sexually transmitted diseases transmission from infected to uninfected partner is by no means universal (Turner, 1989). It is possible to be infected through a single exposure but there are many couples recorded in which hundreds of episodes of sex have not led to the infection of the partner of an infected person. However, even where infection has not occurred on, say, the first hundred episodes of sex it seems possible for it to occur on the hundred-and-first. It is not clear whether failure of transmission is a result of variations in the infectivity of the infected individual, resistance of some sort in the uninfected partner, or both. Transmission is aided by lesions in the genitalia, for instance caused by other sexually transmitted diseases, but can occur readily in the absence of such lesions.

The ready transmissibility of the virus has led to it becoming one of the major causes of death in young adults worldwide. Estimates of the numbers of people in the world infected vary but a figure in the 5–10 million range by the end of the 1980s seems reasonable. The virus is still spreading very rapidly on a global level. No effective vaccine is available and there is as yet no drug which can reverse or halt the symptoms in the long term.

Infection with HIV causes the production of antibodies against various viral antigens; however, while these may be protective in the short to medium term they do not provide long-term protection in a large proportion of subjects, if any (Bolognesi, 1989). The presence of antibodies allows testing of subjects for infection.

THE COURSE OF THE DISEASE

Initial infection may be asymptomatic, although some patients report a brief glandular fever-like illness at the time of seroconversion (the appearance of antibodies). An asymptomatic period usually follows. Some patients show a persistent generalised lymphadenopathy (PGL) but the prognosis in PGL does not seem to be any worse than in asymptomatics. After year one of infection there is a steady 4–6% rate of developing AIDS at least up to year 10, data beyond that time not being available (Moss and Bacchetti, 1989). Some patients are diagnosed as having AIDS from being asymptomatic, however, other patients pass through a period of lesser symptoms with weight loss, night sweats, malaise and minor signs of immunodeficiency. This syndrome is usually referred to as AIDS-related complex (ARC).

AIDS itself is a clinical diagnosis rather than an assessment of immunodeficiency as such. The diagnosis is made on the basis of an opportunist infection, an opportunist tumour or HIV-related dementia, which can occasionally occur in the absence of other symptoms. There is a range of opportunist infections in AIDS, with *Pneumocystis carinii* pneumonia, cryptococcal infections, cytomegalovirus infections and atypical tuberculosis being common. The most common opportunist tumours are Kaposi's sarcoma, which is most common in homosexual men and African populations but rare in other groups, non-Hodgkin's lymphoma and anorectal carcinoma.

The underlying immunodeficiency is related in a complex way to the expression of disease. Many asymptomatic patients show signs of underlying immune problems but no single indicator of immune functioning correlates at more than a rather gross level with clinical disease. CD4+ T-cell levels in patients with AIDS are sometimes higher than in some patients with ARC or even asymptomatics although there is a strong trend towards lower T-cell levels being associated with more and more severe symptoms (Fernandez-Cruz *et al.*, 1990, Schecther *et al.*, 1989).

The mean survival time after diagnosis of AIDS is 18–20 months. Putting an absolute value on survival time is difficult, in part because it is the opportunist infections and tumours which kill the patient, not HIV itself. Consequently the steady improvement in treatment of opportunist infections and tumours during the 1980s has led to a shifting picture. Populations are also not always comparable because a diagnosis of AIDS encompasses a spectrum of disease and some patients, particularly those with Kaposi's sarcoma only, have a rather better mean survival time, probably because Kaposi's sarcoma can appear at rather lower levels of immunodeficiency.

DIRECT EFFECTS OF STRESS ON PROGNOSIS IN HIV INFECTION

In view of the evidence that stress can affect the functioning of the immune system it appears that AIDS is an obvious disease in which to look for evidence of an impact of stress. It would appear reasonable to hypothesise that stress might have an additive or synergistic effect on progression of the disease or might even be involved in mediating susceptibility to infection. Many researchers have embarked on this path, but few have reported. It is important to understand the problems involved in researching the area to see why the results have been rather inconclusive.

Some of the problems are outlined below.

Finding an outcome

The most obvious outcome to use in a study on the effects of stress on the course of HIV infection is the development of symptoms. In theory it is possible to take a cohort of infected individuals, measure their levels of stress in some way and then analyse the relationship between stress and the probability of developing, say, AIDS over a given time period.

The first difficulty with this approach is the size of the cohort required and/or the time period necessary to follow the cohort. Only 4–6% of individuals in the cohort will go on to develop AIDS in any one year. Suppose that a measurable level of stress made a further 10% of individuals develop AIDS in that year. One might then expect a further 0.4–0.6% increase in morbidity in that cohort. In order to obtain a statistically significant difference it would be necessary either to follow the cohort over a long period of time or to have an extremely large cohort.

Rather than looking directly at the incidence of disease it might, then, be possible to look at some surrogate marker of immune functioning – the obvious marker to look at in this case would be CD4+ T-cell levels. However, this is an approach not without its own problems. As indicated above, T-cell levels fluctuate considerably in a single individual and, while there is a marked general trend towards lower T-cell levels in those worse affected by the virus this does not hold up quite so well at the individual level. Moreover, even if more stress leads to a greater drop in T-cell levels that, in itself, does not prove that the observation is of any clinical significance: it only tells you what you first set out to measure, i.e. that stress affects T-cell levels. In other words, observations based on T-cells have to be backed up by clinical observations if they are to have any significance.

Exactly the same considerations apply to other measures of immune system functioning. The situation is worsened by the fact that not only are other measures of immune functioning no more strongly related to disease stage or progression than levels of T-cells, but they are frequently only weakly related to each other. At the gross level T-cell levels and other measures of immune functioning are likely to be worse in someone with AIDS than in an asymptomatic patient, but a finer level of discrimination is likely to be needed if they are to prove a better measure of the effects of stress than simple clinical outcome.

Using a sample of patients with ARC might improve the probability of finding an effect of stress on disease progression; our own observations suggest that probably 50% of people with ARC will progress to AIDS in a year if untreated. However, there is a very large area of overlap between AIDS and ARC, with many patients diagnosed as having ARC probably being as immunosuppressed as some patients with AIDS. Under these circumstances whether an individual develops an infection or tumour indicative of AIDS may have a strong chance element.

Another possible approach is to look at time of death in people with AIDS and, perhaps, ARC. Here the measure is straightforward and our own research is along these lines. This approach is also not without major problems. For AIDS sufferers much of the stress in their lives is likely to be directly or indirectly associated with the disease and, particularly, with episodes of illness. A man with repeated bouts of opportunist infections is likely to lose work time and eventually give up work, to reduce social contact markedly and to experience greatly increased difficulties in personal relationships. For instance, many couples where one partner has AIDS find that the well partner has to spend a great deal of time looking after the other and the whole balance of the relationship often changes, particularly if the ill partner had been the more dominant.

Opportunist infections and tumours, then, are likely both to be a source of stress and to lead directly to death. In general terms the more illnesses a person has the worse their health and the more likely they are to die soon, and the greater the degree of stress in their lives. Separating the two influences on time to death is not easy.

As with studies on the progression of asymptomatics considerable numbers of patients need to be followed up in detail to obtain a measurable effect. The disease shows a very variable course and a long study with large numbers is necessary to measure any reasonably-sized effect over and above background variance.

Direct or indirect effects of stress

One of the major areas of interest in AIDS has been the possible role of cofactors in progression to disease. There are several possible physical cofactors, which can be divided into two main groups: infectious diseases and other physical agents.

Infection with various pathogens causes T-cell activation and proliferation (Roitt *et al.*, 1985). The activation of T-cells should, theoretically, increase viral production because of increased activity in host cell, and hence incorporated viral, DNA.

Additionally activation of T-cells may make them more susceptible to infection with HIV. Some viruses may have a direct influence on HIV replication in that their genes (aimed at promoting their own replication) may also promote replication of HIV; human retroviruses are a case in point but other DNA viruses may have the same effect. Many pathogens may in themselves be immunosuppressive (Nelson *et al.*, 1990).

It follows that catching other infectious diseases after infection with HIV may lead to a worsened prognosis: one obvious group of pathogens in this case is other sexually transmitted diseases. These are especially important because if stress were to cause people to change their behaviour sexually, to have more or less sexual partners, then progression might be affected. The same applies potentially to other physical agents. While there is no clear evidence that opiates or other recreational drugs directly affect immune functioning the possibility cannot be ruled out. A range of other drugs (including nicotine and alcohol) might also affect immune functioning in a complex way. Smoking, for instance, raises CD4 + T-cell levels in uninfected individuals but increases them to a lesser extent in HIV-positive individuals and is then associated with a more rapid reduction in T-cell levels (Royce and Winkelstein, 1990). Smoking and heavy drinking might be expected also to directly affect susceptibility to certain opportunist infections. Nutritional status has been widely suspected, although not proven, to influence prognosis in HIV infection.

It follows from the above that any study of the effects of stress on prognosis or time to death needs to take into account other confounding factors such as changes in sexual behaviour, eating and drug usage. These effects might produce an apparent direct effect of stress on prognosis but might also mask any such effect, depending on their direction.

Therefore a good study of the effects of stress on prognosis needs to pay particular attention to possible behavioural changes.

Effects of medication

A further complicating factor in longitudinal studies of HIV is the rapid changes in treatment which have occurred and which continue to occur. The major drug for the treatment of HIV disease of the 1980s was zidovudine (AZT), an antiretroviral drug. Most individuals with AIDS, many patients with ARC and increasing numbers who are asymptomatic, are now enrolled on a course of AZT. Many patients are also involved in experimental trials of other drugs. In addition to antivirals there are many treatments for opportunistic infections and tumours, and there has been a notable shift towards prophylactic treatment for opportunist infections, particularly *Pneomocystis carinii* pneumonia. This shifting treatment background makes analysis of other influences on progression difficult to assess. It is further complicated by the fact that our own preliminary data, and other data (Jacobsen *et al.*, 1987) suggest that there may be psychological differences between those who enrol on drug trials for experimental drugs and those who choose not to. Being enrolled in a drug trial may itself affect stress levels (Melroe *et al.*, 1990).

In view of the difficulties of carrying out research it is hardly surprising that most published work is theoretical and the available data on the effects of stress on prognosis are preliminary and, often, poor. Antoni *et al.* (1990) reviewed the effects of aerobic exercise on seronegatives and asymptomatics. Temoshok and colleagues have reported on the applications of psychoimmunology to HIV disease (Solomon *et al.*, 1987; Temoshok, 1988). They looked at a group of 43–55 AIDS/ARC patients and found a positive relationship between a range of standardised measures of psychological distress and total white blood cell count, numbers of polymorphonuclear leukocytes and lymphocytes. Given that the effect is in the opposite direction to what might be expected the author remarks that "the relative lymphocytosis in more distressed individuals is difficult to interpret" (Temoshok, 1988). The possible effects of early bacterial infection were suggested as a reason for this finding. However, Barnes *et al.* (1989) have also reported a positive relationship between better immune functioning and emotional distress.

In a small study of 15 men with AIDS, Temoshok *et al.* (1990) found that positive affect, coping and heart rate reactivity were related to survival time. When the results were adjusted for CD4 levels the effect was weakened, though not eliminated.

Kemeny *et al.* (1990) reported on a study of 35 chronically depressed seropositives matched against non-depressed seropositive controls. The depressed individuals showed a sharper drop in CD4+ T-cells over five years than did the controls. Kemeny suggested, cautiously, that chronic depression might be a possible cofactor in progression of HIV disease; however, no data were presented on disease progression *per se*. On the other hand, Perry *et al.* (1990b) reported that, while anxiety and death of a partner within the past two years was related to CD4+ T-cell levels at entry to their study, there was no relationship between 22 psychological variables including anxiety or bereavement three months later, once entry levels of T-cells were controlled for.

Robertson *et al.* (1990) reported that titres of herpes simplex virus, a virus which causes particularly unpleasant symptoms in people with AIDS and a possible (though unproven) cofactor for progression, were related to psychological distress in seropositives. Cortisol levels were elevated and there was transient immunosuppression in men entering a research study testing their serostatus (Fletcher *et al.*, 1990).

Overall, then, the available data do not allow any conclusions to be drawn about the role of stress in prognosis of HIV disease. Only Temoshok *et al.* (1990) address the problem head-on. However, the area is an important and intriguing one and it is to be hoped that further data will be forthcoming in the future, in spite of the formidable methodological problems involved.

COUNSELLING IN HIV AND AIDS

AIDS is an unusual disease in that the central role of counselling was recognised right at the beginning of the epidemic (Green, 1989). This is in part a response to the infectious nature of HIV, in part it reflects existing practice with respect to other conditions in sexually transmitted diseases and in part reflects the fact that HIV is a disease of the 1980s and 1990s and the response to it incorporates up-to-date thinking about the comprehensive care of the patient. It is likely that the model developed in HIV, particularly around testing for HIV, will be applied to other "new" conditions, for instance to carrier screening for genetic disease such as cystic fibrosis and for the screening for genetic susceptibility to various conditions which appears to be just over the horizon.

There are two main aims of counselling in HIV/AIDS: first to help the individual to make changes to his or her lifestyle which will reduce their risk of transmitting HIV, or if they are uninfected of acquiring the infection, and secondly to maximise quality of life for the infected person.

All individuals coming for HIV testing in the UK are offered pre- and post-test counselling (McCreaner, 1988). Testing is confidential and that confidentiality is protected by law. Persons coming for the test may, if they wish, use an alias. Confidentiality is central to the provision of testing

(Fehrs *et al.*, 1988; Kegeles *et al.*, 1990). In practice most testing is carried out in clinics for sexually transmitted diseases.

Pretest counselling aims to ensure that anyone coming for a test is fully informed about the nature of the test and its consequences and is able to give informed consent to testing. The psychological consequences of being tested and the legal implications in terms of access to, say, life and health insurance, employment and travel are considerable and it is important that the individual is aware of these before being tested. It is also clear from clinical practice that an individual who has thought through the implications of the test before being tested is likely to suffer less distress if they have a positive test result. Those few individuals we have seen where pretest counselling has not occurred for some reason have particular problems in adjusting to the result (Green, 1988).

Post-test counselling is also regarded as crucial for the seropositive to help them deal with telling others and to take steps to protect his or her health. Seropositives are also likely to need help in adjusting to the diagnosis. However, seronegatives also need help to reduce any risk that they might be at.

Counselling in HIV is not limited to the time around the test. Infected individuals are offered counselling throughout the course of the infection. This is not usually continuous; individuals come for counselling when they have particular problems. Most individuals will return for counselling when they become symptomatic. Counselling often extends beyond the individual to their lovers, partners and informal carers. Green and McCreaner (1988) have provided an outline of current practice in HIV counselling in the UK.

From a strictly research point of view, the stress on counselling has its problems. Ethically and practically it is considered unacceptable not to offer counselling to an individual who is either coming for testing or who has had a positive or negative test result. To withhold counselling from an individual who might infect others or who might catch another sexually transmitted disease and worsen their own prognosis, is clearly not acceptable. A placebo-controlled or a no-treatment controlled trial of pre- and post-test counselling would not be considered acceptable and we are not aware of any such trial having been carried out.

Similar problems apply to the counselling of individuals with AIDS. Levels of distress are high in such patients and their life expectancy is short. To withhold support and counselling or to put such patients on a waiting list has not been regarded by most workers as acceptable if such services are available. It might be argued that research into counselling is going on without these constraints in other terminal or potentially terminal diseases; however, it is one prospect to add counselling to a service which doesn't already have it and a very different prospect to remove it from a service where it is widely seen as essential.

AIDS is also unusual in the amount of voluntary support available to the patient. In London alone there are at least a dozen major HIV support organisations offering counselling and help, and many smaller support groups. Many organisations with wider briefs than AIDS also offer support and help. Patients themselves, particularly homosexual men, are extremely well-informed about HIV and the services they should be receiving. They will, rightly, demand these of hospitals and social work departments and if they fail to get them will seek elsewhere. People with HIV infection are also, typically, part of informal networks; they know other people with HIV and receive support and help from them (Hart *et al.*, 1990). The person with HIV infection or AIDS who wants help but is receiving none at all is likely to be unusual.

Support services for gay men and haemophiliacs tend to be more common than those for injecting drug users, the latter being less "club-bable" and sometimes having difficulty in organising a structure and finding someone to take a lead. However, there are examples of successful self-help groups for drug users and ex-users. Self-help is also important with a disease where most individuals infected are very cautious about whom they tell, and where. Even given this caution at least one-quarter report rejection by those people they do tell (King, 1989).

Given the considerable difficulty of carrying out no-treatment, placebo-controlled or waiting-list based studies of counselling in HIV infection and AIDS most workers have chosen to compare different approaches to counselling, to report on uncontrolled trials or to seek for an analogue approach to studying counselling.

STUDIES ON THE PSYCHOLOGICAL DISTRESS IN INDIVIDUALS WITH HIV INFECTION AND THE EFFECTS OF INTERVENTIONS

It is generally assumed that finding out that one is infected with HIV will in itself lead to behavioural change, but there seems little evidence that this is, in fact, the case. Most of the data come from cohort studies. These are cohorts of men recruited (usually in the early 1980s) to study the natural history of HIV, or sometimes hepatitis B. Sera were collected over a period of time from these individuals and around 1985 it became possible to test for the presence of antibodies to HIV. Many studies then offered the opportunity to individuals in the cohorts to find out their antibody status.

These studies have generally failed to find a marked effect on behaviour of knowing one's HIV status, or have found only a relatively slight effect (Centres for Disease Control, 1988; Fox *et al.*, 1987; Ostrow *et al.*, 1989). Two studies are of particular interest.

In one study (Fox *et al.*, 1987) 1001 individuals in a cohort were offered the opportunity to learn their status, of whom 670 elected to do so. Over the period of the study there was a marked shift in risk behaviours in all subjects, with those individuals aware of being seropositive changing more than those who chose not to discover their status. However, those who became aware that they were not infected changed significantly less than either of the other two groups. The differences between the groups were small in comparison to the overall change in all three groups. Those who became aware of being seropositive showed a small increased tendency to depression, and some showed increased stress and anxiety.

Ostrow *et al.* (1989) found no effect of finding out serostatus in individuals with high levels of risk behaviours but an increase in risk behaviour regardless of status in individuals with low initial risk levels. They reported that those who found out that they were seropositive showed reduced wellbeing and increased depression, anxiety, obsessive–compulsive problems and distress. This contrasted with relatively stable mental health prior to disclosure.

Neither of these groups of researchers were able to separate satisfactorily counselling from disclosure. The study populations were enrolled in cohort studies (which might be expected to affect behaviour in itself), were highly educated and motivated and had access to counselling both within the studies and, presumably, from outside it. In both studies seropositives, seronegatives, and those who chose not to know their results were subsets of the same single population. It is very likely that there were differences between those who elected to know their status and those who did not. Nevertheless, the available data suggest that simply knowing whether one is seropositive or not in itself does not change risk behaviour, or does not change it very much, and the pattern of change may be very complex. On the other hand, even with a cohort of well-informed individuals offered counselling, finding out serostatus has psychological costs for the individual in terms of increased stress.

These studies are matched by a variety of other studies showing adverse psychological effects of finding out that one is infected with HIV. Perry *et al.* (1990a) reported that both seropositive and seronegative subjects showed high levels of anxiety, depression and psychiatric symptomatology. After receiving their test results the seronegatives showed a drop in levels of distress which was, not surprisingly, sustained at 10 weeks. The seropositives showed a slight drop in most measures of distress on receiving their results, which was increased at 10 weeks, but their distress still remained elevated relative to seronegatives. It might be expected that the period when individuals are attending for testing might be a time of maximal stress and that even a positive test result might fail to elevate distress any further. Also the results for seronegatives are relative to the time they were contemplating being tested, not their general levels of distress. Thus the authors' view that the study shows the benefits of a negative test result need to be viewed with some caution, although the results do suggest that for some individuals taking a test may be reassuring, particularly if it is negative.

Jadresic *et al.* (1989) reported that, in a cohort of individuals attending for testing levels of anxiety and depression at the time of testing fell within the borderline pathological range but six months later had fallen to normal levels, suggesting that over a longer period individuals may adjust to being seropositive. However, the numbers involved in the trial were small and the sample may not have been representative.

Overall the available data suggest that knowing one's HIV status may help some individuals, but the evidence that testing individuals *in itself* leads to public health benefits is not strong, although a case can be made in terms of the value of partner notification at least where an individual's partner could have had no idea that they might have been at risk. In Sweden a strong pro-testing approach has been taken; however, while many individuals not at risk have been tested there is little evidence that the approach is of value in public health terms, and some evidence that those at risk have become less keen to be tested (Mansson, 1990). This paralleled the experience in our own hospital where government health education campaigns have markedly increased the numbers of individuals not at risk coming forward for testing but have not affected the rates of individuals who *are* at risk requesting tests.

One obvious way to look at stress in people with HIV disease is to look cross-sectionally at samples and to try to establish the extent to which they show psychiatric and psychological distress. The results are not always what might be expected.

Chuang *et al.* (1989) looked at 65 gay or bisexual men with HIV disease, using standardised psychiatric and psychological measures of distress and symptomatology. They found that patients with ARC and asymptomatics showed significantly higher levels of anxiety, depression and mood disturbance than people with AIDS but did not differ from each other. All three groups showed significant levels of distress. However, at the same time subjects reported reasonable levels of subjective wellbeing. This latter finding is of considerable interest. Most workers have assumed that psychological distress is the inverse of quality of life, or life satisfaction; there is no reason whatsoever to suppose that this is true.

King (1989) reported on the psychosocial status of 192 individuals with HIV and AIDS at a London hospital. He reported that 31% showed significant psychiatric symptoms. There were no differences with respect to stage of HIV disease although there was a trend towards ARC patients reporting higher levels of distress. Past history of psychiatric problems strongly predicted current problems. Three out of eight men tested without consent reported psychiatric symptoms which they blamed on the manner of their testing. King did not use a seronegative control group. However, he did compare his results to published studies of other outpatient and inpatient samples and concluded that "in this unselected group of patients with HIV infection, psychiatric disorder was no more common than among patients in other medical settings".

Tross *et al.* (1987) reported higher levels of psychological distress in patients with ARC (63%) than in those with AIDS (52%) or seronegative controls (31%). The overall level of psychiatric morbidity in patients with HIV disease may have been caused by an atypical patient population. However, the high levels of distress in ARC patients matches the findings of King and Perry and our own clinical observations.

Most studies have reported on homosexual men, however, Catalan (1990) reported higher levels of mood disturbance in HIV infected haemophiliacs than in seronegatives.

Most studies reporting high levels of distress in HIV-infected individuals have reported on mood disturbances. While there are anecdotal reports of major psychotic episodes in individuals infected with HIV it is not known whether the rates are higher than in seronegatives (Miller and Riccio, 1990).

One of the key weaknesses in all the available studies is the lack of appropriate control groups. Catalan *et al.* (1981) showed high levels of psychiatric disturbance in attenders at sexually transmitted disease clinics. Similarly, in a study of infected and uninfected homosexual men higher levels of psychiatric disturbance were found relative to heterosexual controls both currently and, in the case of seropositives, prior to knowledge of infection (Atkinson, *et al.*, 1988). It might be expected that any group of individuals subjected to systematic prejudice would show elevated levels of psychological distress, and most individuals at high risk of HIV infection are subject to such prejudice.

Assuming that levels of psychological distress are, in fact, higher in those infected with HIV than in controls the question arises as to whether these are the effects of knowing that one is infected with the disease, a reaction to being physically ill, or some direct effect of HIV on the brain. HIV, as noted above, directly infects the brain and can cause a dementia in severely affected individuals (Brew *et al.*, 1988). There is considerable debate as to whether some asymptomatics may show mild signs of cognitive impairment (Kocsis, 1990). HIV might, then, cause mood disturbance or frank psychiatric symptomatology either directly or indirectly, for instance through the release of endogenous interferons. However, there is little evidence for such an effect (Maj, 1990). Kessler *et al.* (1988) showed that psychological distress is not related to serostatus in individuals unaware of whether they are infected; however, it is related to subjectively perceived symptoms of HIV infection. Similar results were reported from a study by Ostrow *et al.* (1989) of 4954 men enrolled in a cohort study. Levels of depression were related more strongly to perceived physical symptoms and reported level of social support than to serostatus.

Given the reports of high levels of psychological distress and psychiatric symptomatology in people with HIV infection one might expect to find a large literature on interventions in HIV. However, for reasons given above the field is a particularly difficult one in which to carry out research.

The difficulties of changing behaviour should not be underestimated. For instance Silvestre *et al.* (1989) found that in men who seroconverted, most engaged in unsafe sexual practices after an educational programme because of strong emotional responses to partners or because of alcohol or drug-related problems. Additionally there is evidence which links the way in which individuals cope with being infected with HIV to their psychological distress levels (Catalan, 1990; Namir *et al.*, 1987) with individuals who adopt active behavioural coping strategies and actively seek the help of others doing better (Zich and Temoshok, 1987).

It has generally been found that the best predictor of future risk behaviours is past risk behaviours (McCusker *et al.*, 1989). Particularly among homosexual men, change towards safer sexual behaviour has already occurred on a large scale through awareness of HIV; individuals at continuing high risk have already made most of the adjustments which they can easily make or have already resisted behavioural change for some reason.

As part of their study Perry *et al.* (1990a) carried out three different interventions; a one-hour pretest and one-hour post-test counselling session, six weekly sessions of a stress prevention training programme or three weekly psychoeducational interactive video sessions. There were no differences between treatments on any of the visual analogue scale measures. The overall effects of intervention could not, of course, be assessed since all subjects had an intervention post-test and all subjects had undergone pretest counselling. The authors themselves were clear that they felt that appropriate counselling was essential.

Valdiseri *et al.* (1989) reported that in a randomised trial of two approaches to helping homosexual and bisexual men to change their risk behaviours the one which emphasised training in negotiating and practical skills led to a greater adoption of condom usage. Fawzi *et al.* (1989) reported that a group intervention reduced distress and improved coping skills in a group of seropositive homosexual men. Moulton *et al.* (1990) reported that an eight-week psychoeducational group was more effective than a waiting list control in reducing psychological distress and increasing coping. Hedge and Glover (1990) showed that an educational group provided support and relieved distress in group participants as well as providing information.

Garcia-Huete (1990) reported a study of behavioural treatment of individuals with HIV and AIDS using a control intervention and pre- and post-intervention measures. He reported that the behavioural treatment approach led to significantly reduced distress which was maintained at six months follow-up.

Hedge *et al.* (1990) reported on 32 people with HIV and AIDS provided with individual cognitive–behavioural counselling. They reported significant reductions in anxiety and depression and increases in self-esteem in patients, but no change in subjective feelings of ability to cope. George (1988) reported on a 6–12 month follow-up of HIV/AIDS patients involved in cognitive–behavioural counselling. Patients reported sustained improvements in anxiety, depression and distress levels which they attributed to the counselling.

OVERVIEW

It is a truism in all reviews to say that further research is needed. However, in the field of the interaction of stress and HIV the available data are only a starting point. There is need for much more research on the effects of learning that one is infected with HIV on stress levels, and a need for a much better understanding of how individuals can better be helped to adjust to the infection.

The next few years will be particularly difficult ones. HIV continues to spread rapidly. As new treatments become available the emphasis on early identification of individuals who have been infected so that they can be treated earlier will inevitably increase. Both of these factors will increase the need for effective counselling and the numbers seeking it.

The existing research is mainly on homosexual men and there is a need to extend research to other risk groups, not just injecting drug users but also heterosexuals in general. In global terms most people affected by HIV are heterosexual and there are a number of promising research projects under way in developing countries which should report soon. Counselling alone is not always going to be enough to achieve behavioural change; programmes such as syringe exchange (Stimson, 1989), condom programmes and health education programmes need to be rigorously evaluated and the lessions learnt applied to practice.

Despite the difficulties there is a real need to try to find out the extent to which stress itself influences disease progression in HIV.

AIDS presents a particular opportunity to study the links between stress, immune functioning and cancer discussed elsewhere in this book (Chapter 1), as long as researchers understand the major methodological problems to be overcome. We still do not know whether the severe effects of HIV on the immune system may simply "drown out" any other influences.

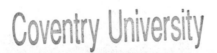

It is to be hoped that the next few years will provide answers to some of the pressing questions which remain unanswered today.

REFERENCES

Antoni, M.H., Schneiderman, N., Fletcher, M.A., Goldstein, D.A., Ironson, G. and Laperriere, A. (1990) Psychoneuroimmunology and HIV-1. *J. Consult. Clin. Psychol.*, **58**, 38–49.

Atkinson, J.H., Grant, I., Kennedy, C.J., Richman, D.D., Spector, S.A. and McCutchan, J.A. (1988) Prevalence of psychiatric disorders among men infected with human immunodeficiency syndrome. *Arch. Gen. Psych.*, **45**, 859–864.

Barnes, R., Calzavara, L., Coates, E.S., Read, S., McFadden, F., Johnson, K., Fanning, M. and Shepherd, S. (1989) *Emotional states in relation to immune function in a cohort of male sexual contacts of men with HIV disease.* Results presented at the Vth International Conference on AIDS, Montreal, June 1989, Abstract TDP63.

Bolognesi, D.P. (1989) HIV antibodies and vaccine design. *AIDS*, **3** (suppl 1), S111–S118.

Brew, B., Rosenblum, M. and Price R.W. (1988) Central and peripheral nervous system complications of HIV infection and AIDS. In DeVita, V.T., Hellman, S. and Rosenberg, S.A. (eds) *AIDS: Etiology, Diagnosis, Treatment and Prevention.* Lippincott, Philadelphia, pp. 185–198.

Catalan, J. (1990) *Psychological and psychiatric disturbance in haemophiliacs.* Presented at the Satellite Conference on Neurological and Neuropsychiatric Aspects of AIDS, Monterey, Ca., June 1990.

Catalan, J., Bradley, M. and Gallwey, J. (1981) Sexual dysfunction and psychiatric morbidity in patients attending a clinic for sexually transmitted diseases. *Br. J. Psych.*, **138**, 292–296.

Center for Disease Control (1988). *Report on consultation on disclosure of antibody status in Human Immunodeficiency Virus infection.* Atlanta, Georgia.

Chuang, H.T., Devins, G.M., Hunsley, J. and Gill, M.J. (1989) Psychosocial distress and well-being among gay and bisexual men with Human Immunodeficiency Syndrome. *Am. J. Psych.*, **146**, 876–880.

Fawzy, F.I., Namir, S. and Wolcott, D.L. (1989) Structured group intervention model for AIDS patients. *Psychiat. Med.*, **7**, 35–45.

Fehrs, L.J., Fleming, D., Foster, L.R., McAlister, R.O., Fox, V., Modesitt, S. and Conrad, R. (1988) Public Health: trial of anonymous versus confidential human immunodeficiency virus testing. *Lancet*, **ii**, 379–382.

Ferenandez-Cruz, E., Desco, M., Montes, M.G., Longo, N., Gonzalez, B. and Zabay, J.M. (1990) Immunological and serological markers predictive of progression to AIDS in a cohort of HIV-infected drug users. *AIDS*, **4**, 943–951.

Fletcher, M.A., Antoni, M., Klimas, N., LaPerriere, A., Ironson, G. and Schneiderman, N. (1990) *Psychoneuroimmunologic aspects of HIV-1 serostatus.* Results presented at the VI International Conference on AIDS, San Francisco, June 1990, Abstract SB367.

Fox, R., Odaka, N.J., Brookmeyer, R. and Polk, F.B. (1987) Effect of HIV antibody disclosure on subsequent sexual activity in homosexual men. *AIDS*, **1**, 247–255.

Garcia-Huete, E. (1990) *Treatment of the psychological disturbance in HIV infected people.* Results presented at the VI International Conference on AIDS, San Francisco June 1990, Abstract SB396.

George, H. (1988) *AIDS: Factors identified as helpful by patients*. Presented at the IVth International Conference on AIDS, Stockholm, June 1988.

Green, J. (1988) Post-test counselling. In Green, J. and McCreaner, A. (eds) *Counselling in HIV Infection and AIDS*. Blackwell Scientific, Oxford, pp. 28–68.

Green, J. (1989) Counselling for HIV infection and AIDS: the past and the future. *AIDS Care*, 1, 5–10.

Green, J. and McCreaner, A. (eds) (1988) *Counselling in HIV Infection and AIDS*. Blackwell Scientific, Oxford.

Hart, G., Fitzpatrick, R., McLean, J., Dawson, J. and Boulton, M. (1990) Gay men, social support and HIV disease, a study of social integration in the gay community. *AIDS Care*, 2, 163–170.

Hedge, B. and Glover, L. (1990) Group intervention with HIV seropositive patients and their partners. *AIDS Care*, 2, 147–154.

Hedge, B., James, S. and Green, J. (1990) *Evaluation of focussed cognitive-behavioural intervention with HIV seropositive individuals*. Results presented at the VI International Conference on AIDS, San Francisco, June 1990, Abstract SC689.

Jacobsen, P., Perry, S. and Roberts, R. (1987) *Psychological reactions of individuals at risk of AIDS entering an experimental treatment trial*. Presented at the IIIrd International Conference on AIDS, Washington DC, June 1987, abstract MP195.

Jadresic, D., Riccio, M., Hawkins, D., Wilson, B. and Thompson, C. (1989) *Impact of HIV diagnosis on mood, the St. Stephen's cohort*. Presented at the Vth International Conference on AIDS, Montreal, June 1989, Abstract WBP201.

Kegeles, S.M., Catania, S.J., Coates, T.J. and Pollack, L.M. (1990) Many people who seek anonymous HIV antibody testing would avoid it under other circumstances. *AIDS*, 4, 585–588.

Kemeny, M.E., Duran, R., Taylor, S.E., Weiner, H., Visscher, B. and Fahey, J.L. (1990) *Chronic depression predicts CD4 decline over a five year period*. Results presented at the VI International Conference on AIDS, San Francisco, June 1990, Abstract Th.C.676.

Kessler, R.C., O'Brien, K., Joseph, J.G., Ostrow, D.G., Phair, J.P., Chmiel, J.S. and Wortman, C.B. (1988) Effects of HIV infection, perceived health and clinical status on a cohort at risk for AIDS. *Soc. Sci. Med.*, 27, 569–578.

King, M.B. (1989) Prejudice and AIDS; the views and experiences of people with HIV infection. *AIDS Care*, 1, 137–152.

Kocsis, A.E. (1990) *Neuropsychological impairment in asymptomatic individuals and those with AIDS*. Presented at the German Conference on neurological and neurophysical aspects of AIDS, Gottingen, November 1990.

Koenig, S. and Fauci, A. (1988) AIDS: Immunopathogenesis and immune responses to the Human Immunodeficiency Virus. In DeVita, V.T., Hellman, S. and Rosenberg, S.A. (eds) *AIDS: Etiology, Diagnosis, Treatment and Prevention*. Lippincott, Philadelphia, pp. 61–78.

McCreaner, A. (1988) Pre-test counselling. In Green, J. and McCreaner, A. (eds) *Counselling in HIV Infection and AIDS*. Blackwell Scientific, Oxford, pp. 21–27.

McCusker, J., Stoddard, A.M., Zapka, J.G., Zorn, M. and Mayer, K.H. (1989) Predictors of AIDS-preventive behaviour among homosexually active men: A longitudinal study. *AIDS*, 3, 333–339.

Maj. M. (1990) Organic mental disorders in HIV-1 infection. *AIDS*, 4, 831–840.

Mansson, S.A. (1990) Psychosocial aspects of HIV testing – the Swedish case. *AIDS Care*, 2, 5–12.

Melroe, N.H., Robiner, W.N., Campbell, S. and Rahe, S. (1990) *Psychological response to participation and non-participation in a placebo controlled drug trial*. Results presented at the VI International Conference on AIDS, San Francisco, June 1990, Abstract SB407.

Miller, J.D. and Riccio, M. (1990) Non-organic psychiatric and psychosocial syndromes associated with HIV-1 infection and disease. *AIDS*, **4**, 381–389.

Moss, A.R. and Bacchetti, P. (1989) Natural history of HIV infection. *AIDS*, **3**, 55–61.

Moulton, J., Gorbuz, G., Sweet, D., Martin, R. and Dilley, J. (1990) *Outcome evaluation of eight-week educational support groups, validating the model using control group comparisons.* Results presented at the VI International Conference on AIDS, San Francisco, June 1990, Abstract SB400.

Namir, S., Wolcott, D.L., Fawzy, F.I. and Alumbaugh, M.J. (1987) Coping with AIDS: psychological and health implications. *J. App. Soc. Psychol.*, **17**, 309–328.

Nelson, J.A., Ghazal, P. and Wiley, C.A. (1990) Role of opportunistic viral infections in AIDS. *AIDS*, **4**, 1–10.

Ostrow, D.G., Joseph, J.G., Kessler, R., Soucy, J., Tal, M., Eller, M., Chmiel, J. and Phair, J.P. (1989) Disclosure of antibody status: Behavioural and mental health correlates. *AIDS Education and Prevention*, **1**, 1–12.

Peckham, C.S. and Newell, M-L. (1990) HIV-1 infection in mothers and babies. *AIDS Care*, **2**, 205–213.

Perry, S., Jacobsberg, L.B., Fishman, B., Weiler, P.H., Gold, J.W.M. and Frances, A.J. (1990a) Psychological responses to serological testing for HIV. *AIDS*, **4**, 145–152.

Perry, S., Jacobsberg, L. and Fishman, B. (1990b) *Relationship between CD4 lymphocytes and psychosocial variables amongst HIV seropositive adults.* Results presented at the VI International Conference on AIDS, San Francisco, June 1990, Abstract ThB27.

Robertson, K.R., Bowdre, W.J., van der Horst, C., Snyder, C., Fryer, J. and Hall, C. (1990) *Psychological influences on herpes simplex virus titers in HIV+ subjects.* Results presented at the VI International Conference on AIDS, San Francisco, June 1990, Abstract FB417.

Roitt, I., Brostoff, J. and Male, D. (1985) *Immunology.* Churchill Livingstone, Edinburgh.

Royce, R.A. and Winkelstein, W. (1990) HIV infection, cigarette smoking and CD4+ T-lymphocyte counts: preliminary results from the San Francisco men's health study. *AIDS*, **4**, 327–333.

Schechter, M.T., Craib, K.J.P. and Le, T.N. (1989) Progression to AIDS and predictors of AIDS in seroprevalent and seroincident cohorts of homosexual men. *AIDS*, **3**, 347–353.

Shaw, G.M., Wong-Staal, F. and Gallo, R.C. (1988) Etiology of AIDS: Virology, molecular biology and natural history of human immunodeficiency viruses. In DeVita, V.T., Hellman, S. and Rosenberg, S.A. (eds) *AIDS: Etiology, Diagnosis, Treatment and Prevention.* Lippincott, Philadelphia, pp. 11–32.

Silvestre, A.J., Lyter, D.W., Valdisseri, R.O., Huggins, J. and Rinaldo, C.R. (1989) Factors related to seroconversion in homosexual and bisexual men after attending a risk-reduction session. *AIDS*, **3**, 647–650.

Solomon, G.F., Temoshok, L., O'Leary, A. and Zich, J. (1987) An intensive psychoimmunologic study of long-surviving persons with AIDS. Pilot work, background studies, hypotheses and methods. *Ann. NY Acad. Sci.*, **496**, 647–655.

Stimson, G.V. (1989) Syringe exchange programmes for injecting drug users. *AIDS*, **3**, 253–260.

Temoshok, L. (1988) Psychoimmunology and AIDS. In Bridge, T.P. (ed.) *Psycho-*

logical, Neuropsychiatric and Substance Abuse Aspects of AIDS. Raven Press, New York, pp. 86–94.

Temoshok, L., O'Leary, A. and Jenkins, S.R. (1990) *Survival time in men with AIDS.* Results presented at the VI International Conference on AIDS, San Francisco, June 1990, Abstract 3133.

Tross, S., Holland, J., Hirsch, D., Schiffman, M., Gold, J. and Safai, B. (1986) *Psychological and social impact of AIDS spectrum disorders.* IInd International Conference on AIDS, Paris, June 1986, Abstract 63,S6C.

Tross, S., Holland, J., Hirsch, D., Schiffman, M., Gold, J. and Safai, B. (1987) *Determinants of current psychiatric disorder in AIDS spectrum patients.* Presented at the III International Conference on AIDS, Washington DC, June 1987, Abstract T10.5.

Turner, C.F. (1989) Research on sexual behaviours that transmit HIV: progress and problems. *AIDS,* **3** (suppl 1), S63–S69.

Valdiseri, R.O., Lyter, D.W, Leviton, C., Callahan, C.M., Kingsley, L.A. and Rinaldo, C.R. (1989) AIDS prevention in homosexual and bisexual men, results of a randomized trial evaluating two risk reduction interventions. *AIDS,* **3,** 21–26.

Zich, J. and Temoshok, L. (1987) Perceptions of social support in patients with ARC and AIDS. *J. App. Soc. Psychol.,* **17,** 309–328.

Index

Index compiled by Liza Weinkove